Experiential Therapies for Treating Trauma

Experiential Therapies for Treating Trauma offers 17 chapters, with 15 of them focusing on a different experiential psychotherapy for treating trauma, written by clinicians with expertise in that modality. No other book contains descriptions of such a wide array of experiential therapies under one cover. Readers will obtain both a comprehensive overview of the many experiential therapies that are currently utilized and specific knowledge regarding how to utilize each of them in psychotherapy practice. The authors of each chapter emphasize that in working with clients impacted by trauma, there is a need for the use of therapeutic modalities that go beyond the cognitive processes central to talk therapy and incorporate more holistic, sensory approaches that emphasize the building of a strong relationship between the client and therapist. Both experienced clinicians and students will find this book to be an invaluable resource to enhance their knowledge of how to use experiential therapies and to motivate them to obtain advanced training in modalities that spark their interest.

Evan Senreich, PhD, LCSW, is a professor of social work at Lehman College, City University of New York, and a graduate of Gestalt Associates for Psychotherapy in New York.

Shulamith Lala Ashenberg Straussner, PhD, LCSW, is professor emerita of New York University and was honored by NASW as a Social Work Pioneer for contributions in the areas of trauma and addictions.

Jordan Dann, LP, is the author of *Somatic Therapy for Healing Trauma* and a faculty member at Gestalt Associates for Psychotherapy in New York.

A must read! There is a slow but sure consensus growing among mental health professionals and researchers that experiential work is a missing key ingredient to achieving profound clinical change. Many already suspect this but wonder how to actually implement it with their clients. This important volume answers this question, providing clear rationales, guidelines, and examples on how to unlock the powerful benefits of experiential treatments.

Alexandre Vaz, *PhD, director of training, Sentio Marriage and Family Therapy Program and Sentio Counseling Center*

Every psychotherapist must learn about trauma and its treatment, and the field of contemporary psychotherapy includes more methods and forms of treatment than ever. This timely and tremendously valuable book provides a clear, balanced, and conveniently structured resource for understanding the similarities, differences, strengths, and limitations of therapies from an essential domain of trauma treatment.

David S. Elliott, *PhD, co-author of Attachment Disturbances in Adults*

Experiential Therapies for Treating Trauma is a well-written book about an area of importance to all counselors and psychotherapists. The format offers the reader an opportunity to sample 15 different evidence-based approaches described by experts. I appreciated its breath and depth. It is a must read for anyone who works with trauma, whether a beginner or expert. I highly recommend it.

Joseph Melnick, *PhD, founding editor of Gestalt Review and co-author of The Evolution of the Cape Cod Model: Gestalt Conversation, Theory and Practice*

Highlighting the critical role of the body in trauma recovery, Experiential Therapies for Treating Trauma is a vital resource for practitioners looking to deepen their understanding of integrative approaches to healing.

Scott Lyons, *founder of the Embody Lab*

Experiential Therapies for Treating Trauma

EDITED BY
EVAN SENREICH, SHULAMITH LALA
ASHENBERG STRAUSSNER AND
JORDAN DANN

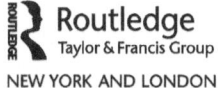

Routledge
Taylor & Francis Group

NEW YORK AND LONDON

Designed cover image: stellalevi @ Getty Images

First published 2025
by Routledge
605 Third Avenue, New York, NY 10158

and by Routledge
4 Park Square, Milton Park, Abingdon, Oxon, OX14 4RN

Routledge is an imprint of the Taylor & Francis Group, an informa business

Library of Congress Cataloging-in-Publication Data
Names: Senreich, Evan, editor. | Straussner, Shulamith Lala Ashenberg, editor. | Dann, Jordan, editor.
Title: Experiential therapies for treating trauma / edited by Evan
Senreich, Shulamith Lala Ashenberg Straussner and Jordan Dann.
Description: New York, NY : Routledge, 2025. | Includes bibliographical references and index. |
Identifiers: LCCN 2024032734 (print) | LCCN 2024032735 (ebook) | ISBN 9781032595528
(hardback) | ISBN 9781032595085 (paperback) | ISBN 9781003455851 (ebook)
Subjects: MESH: Stress Disorders, Traumatic--therapy | Psychotherapy--methods
Classification: LCC RC552.P67 (print) | LCC RC552.P67 (ebook) |
NLM WM 172.5 | DDC 616.85/21--dc23/eng/20240930
LC record available at https://lccn.loc.gov/2024032734
LC ebook record available at https://lccn.loc.gov/2024032735

ISBN: 978-1-032-59552-8 (hbk)
ISBN: 978-1-032-59508-5 (pbk)
ISBN: 978-1-003-45585-1 (ebk)

DOI: 10.4324/9781003455851

Typeset in Bembo
by SPi Technologies Private Limited, India (Straive)

CONTENTS

ACKNOWLEDGMENTS

The editors would like to thank the 22 contributing authors of this book for the creative energy that they put into this endeavor. We appreciate their love of experiential methods and their keen knowledge and sensitivity regarding working with clients impacted by trauma. We are also grateful for their timeliness in completing their chapters and their openness to discussions of revisions. The editors also wish to thank Anna Moore, publisher at Routledge, Taylor & Francis Group, for her immediate recognition of the unique contribution that this book could make in the field of psychotherapy and her steadfast guidance throughout the publishing process. Last, we would like to wholeheartedly acknowledge the founders and developers of the 15 experiential therapies explicated in this book for their invaluable contributions to clinical psychotherapeutic work. Their treatment modalities foster deep respect for the struggles of human beings navigating the vicissitudes of life and the profound healing impact of a meaningful, authentic relationship between the therapist and client.

ABOUT THE CONTRIBUTORS

Lia Avellino, LCSW
Psychotherapist, columnist, and CEO of Spoke Circles, LLC
MSW from Columbia University School of Social Work, 2016

Sara K. Bridges, Ph.D.
Associate Professor of Counseling Psychology, The University of Memphis
Ph.D. from the University of Memphis, 1999
Co-director, Coherence Psychology Institute

Haydn Briggs LCSW, CGP, CET III
Founder and director, Healing Self Psychotherapy
MSS from Bryn Mawr College, 2020

Jennifer Byxbee ART-BC, LCAT, CGT
Founder of Creative Arts Psychotherapy NYC
Masters in Professional Studies from the School of Visual Arts, Art Therapy, 2007

Alan Cohen, LCSW, LP
Senior faculty, Gestalt Associates for Psychotherapy
MSW Washington University, St Louis, 1974
Visiting faculty, GATLA International Training Conferences

Jordan Dann, LP
Author of *Somatic Therapy for Healing Trauma*
Creator of the "Relationship Transformation School"
Faculty, Gestalt Associates for Psychotherapy

Bruce Ecker, MA, LMFT
Co-director, Coherence Psychology Institute, LLC
M.A. from John F. Kennedy University, 1984
Independent psychotherapy practice

Anna Gartshore, MSW, RSW
Registered social work psychotherapist in private practice, Ontario, Canada
MSW from Laurier University, Lyle S. Hallman Faculty of Social Work, 2009
IFS Institute Approved Clinical Consultant and Trainer

Scott Giacomucci, DSW, LCSW, BCD, CGP, FAAETS, TEP
Director, founder, and owner, Phoenix Center for Experiential Trauma Therapy, Media, Pennsylvania
Adjunct professor and research associate, Bryn Mawr College Graduate School of Social Work and Social Research
Author of *Social Work, Sociometry, & Psychodrama* (2021) and *Trauma-Informed Principles in Group Therapy, Psychodrama, & Organizations* (2023)

Amanda Garcia Torres, LMHC
Co-Director, Chairwork Psychotherapy Initiative
Master of Arts in Counseling for Mental Health and Wellness, New York University, 2014
Certified chairwork psychotherapist

Amy Gladstone, PhD, LCSW
Professor of Social Work, Seton Hall University
Faculty, Sensorimotor Psychotherapy Institute
Faculty, Integrative Trauma Program, National Institute for the Psychotherapies

Benjamin Kagedan, PsyD, CHT, PATP
Practitioner and supervisor in somatic and psychedelic therapies
Psy.D. from Rutgers University Graduate School of Applied and Professional
    Psychology, 2017
Faculty, Hakomi Institute

Scott Kellogg, PhD
Director, Chairwork Psychotherapy Initiative
Ph.D. in Clinical Psychology, Graduate Center of the City University of New York, 1994
ISST–Certified Advanced Schema Therapist

Ben Medley, LCSW
Senior faculty, AEDP Institute
M.S.W. from NYU Silver School of Social Work, 2006

Patricia O'Keefe Monteleone, LCSW
Psychotherapist; trauma specialist
ISTDP Core Training
Parnell Institute Faculty, Consultant and Facilitator
EMDRIA Consultant

Jeffrey L. Morrison, MA, LMHC
Certifying coordinator and focusing trainer
Executive director of the Seattle Focusing Institute
MA in Existential Phenomenological Psychology, Seattle University, 1986

Noora Niskanen, LCSW, MFA
EMDR trauma therapist in private practice, New York, NY
MSW from Lehman College, City University of New York, 2012
MFA from NYU, 2006

Riley Paterson, MA, LMHC
Psychotherapist in Seattle, Washington
Master of Arts in Psychology from Seattle University, 2019

Benjamin Seaman, BFA, LCSW
Certificate in Psychoanalytic Psychotherapy, Psychoanalytic Psychotherapy Study Center
Psychotherapist in private practice
Former adjunct lecturer, NYU Silver Graduate School of Social Work

Evan Senreich, PhD, LCSW
Professor of social work, Lehman College, City University of New York
Ph.D. New York University Silver School of Social Work, 2007
Graduate of Gestalt Associates for Psychotherapy, 1994
Author of over 40 published research and conceptual journal articles

Rebecca Stone, LCSW
Founder and clinical director, Brooklyn Somatic Therapy
Certified teacher, The Hakomi Institute
Certified EFT therapist and supervisor candidate
MSW from Silberman School of Social Work, Hunter College, 2014

Shulamith Lala Ashenberg Straussner, PhD, LCSW
Professor Emerita, New York University Silver School of Social Work;
Founding editor, *Journal of Social Work Practice in the Addictions*
NASW Social Work Pioneer;
Fulbright Scholar; board member, *Fulbright Israel Interest Group*

Dennis Tirch, PhD
Founding director, The Center for Compassion Focused Therapy
Chairperson, The Compassionate Mind Foundation, USA
Past president and Fellow, Association for Contextual Behavioral Science

Talya Vogel, PsyD
Director of Trauma, Transformation, and Resilience (TTR) Program, The Center for
    Compassion Focused Therapy
Senior psychologist, The Center for Compassion Focused Therapy
Psy.D. from PGSP-Stanford PsyD Consortium, 2020

1

CHAPTER 1
INTRODUCTION

Overview of Experiential Psychotherapies for the Treatment of Trauma

Shulamith Lala Ashenberg Straussner,
Evan Senreich and Jordan Dann

Addressing traumatic experiences is a frequent occurrence in current psychotherapy practice. Many contemporary authors and clinicians who focus on the treatment of trauma point out the need for the use of therapeutic modalities that go beyond the cognitive processes central to talk therapy and incorporate more integrative, experiential sensory or somatic approaches (Dann, 2022). The number of experiential psychotherapies has grown substantially over the past four decades, and there is a great need for practicing clinicians and students to become familiar with the variety of these newer treatment approaches. This book provides an overview of 15 different types of contemporary experiential psychotherapies and how each one can be utilized in the treatment of trauma. The chapters include a brief history of a specific experiential psychotherapy approach, its main clinical concepts, how it is practiced, an assessment of its evidence base and how it can be utilized in the treatment of trauma utilizing fictional case examples.

This introductory chapter has four sections. In the first, the definition and characteristics of experiential psychotherapy are briefly delineated. The second section presents an overview of trauma and clinical issues pertaining to it. This is followed by a section on the neurophysiology of trauma and how this knowledge can be applied when using experiential therapies. The final section provides a historical overview of experiential psychotherapy and includes a brief description of the 15 treatment modalities presented in this book.

EXPERIENTIAL PSYCHOTHERAPY: DEFINITION AND DESCRIPTION

The term *experiential therapy* applies to an increasing number of psychotherapeutic modalities developed since the mid-20th century (with the exception of psychodrama) that share a number of common features. In defining the key element of experiential therapy, the American Psychological Association's (APA) *Dictionary of Psychology* states:

DOI: 10.4324/9781003455851-1

A core belief of the approach is that true client change occurs through direct, active experiencing of what the client is undergoing and feeling at any given point in therapy, both on the surface and at a deeper level.

(VandenBos & American Psychological Association, 2015, p. 396)

In other words, in experiential psychotherapies there is less emphasis on clients talking about current and former life events in a narrative form and much greater focus on what the client is fully experiencing in the room in the presence of the therapist. In addition, many of the early experiential therapies were developed in tandem with humanistic approaches, such as the person-centered psychotherapy of Carl Rogers and the existential psychotherapy of Rollo May, Irvin Yalom, and others. Therefore, there is usually a strong emphasis in experiential therapies on the importance of an authentic relationship between the therapist and client, in which the latter feels that their worldview is confirmed and validated (Watson et al., 1998). Geoghegan (2019), a contemporary practitioner of coherence therapy, has clearly delineated five key characteristics that specifically apply to the vast majority of experiential psychotherapies described in this book. First, the therapist utilizes prompts during sessions to tap directly into the client's experiences in the moment rather than just talking about the client's life experiences. Second, the therapist encourages the client to attend closely to sensations and feelings that occur during the session in a mindful way. Third, experiential therapists do not take on the role of expert, but instead foster a collaborative relationship with clients, assisting them to discover and integrate the disparate parts of their selves. Fourth, in order to alleviate the client's symptoms, the therapist does not try to counter or override them, but instead focuses on their meaning. Last, Geoghegan emphasizes that by demonstrating a genuine curiosity about the client's perceptions without challenging them, a warm relational field is developed in which clients feel respected, valued, and safe.

It is important to clarify that the attention paid to clients' experiences during the therapy session does not in any way de-emphasize the importance of processing life events outside of the therapy room. However, whereas most psychotherapy modalities focus on the client's discussion of these events, experiential therapies stress that the client explore their *current* thoughts, feelings, and body sensations regarding these events while in the presence of the therapist. This is particularly important when assisting clients working through past traumas while at the same time focusing on their lived experiences in the room within the context of a warm, reparative client-therapist relationship.

Although most experiential therapies include the five key elements identified here by Geoghegan (2019), there is considerable diversity among them regarding theoretical orientation, terminology, and practice. However, the development of a number of these experiential therapies were profoundly influenced by each other. Therefore, it is quite common for contemporary experiential clinicians to be trained in more than one such approach and to utilize elements of more than one experiential modality in their psychotherapy practice.

OVERVIEW OF TRAUMA AND TRAUMATIC EXPERIENCES

The term "trauma" comes from the Greek language meaning a "wound" or "hurt" (Oxford Dictionaries, 2013). Psychologically, "trauma" refers to an experience that is emotionally painful, distressful, or shocking; one that often has long-term negative mental, physical, and neurological consequences. An event is thought to produce a traumatic response when the stress resulting from that event overwhelms the individual's psychological ability to cope.

Although we often think of trauma as being synonymous with the identified *objective* cause of the trauma, such as a woman being raped or someone who has experienced war-related violence, the effect of the trauma is always *subjective* and refers to the impact – the perceived "wound" or "hurt" as identified by the early Greeks – that it has on the individual (Straussner & Calnan, 2014). Thus, what might be a traumatizing, life-shattering event for one individual might have minimal effects on another. Such differential reaction is based on many factors, including the individual's age, sex and gender, pre-morbid ego strength, genetics, epigenetics, previous traumatic experiences, the chronicity of the trauma, family history of trauma, current life stressors, social supports, and one's cultural, religious, or spiritual attitude toward adversity (Amir & Lev-Wiesel, 2003; Straussner & Phillips, 2004).

HISTORICAL AWARENESS OF TRAUMA

Awareness of the destructive physical and mental impact of trauma was first identified centuries ago by the ancient Egyptians and Greeks in relation to historic wars, as reflected by the writings of the Greek historian Herodotus in the 5th Century BCE. In the 17th Century, Swiss and German military physicians identified illnesses that caused combat soldiers to experience such symptoms as melancholy, physical weakness, anxiety, insomnia, heart palpitations, and homesickness (Osei-Boamah et al., 2013). In the United States, the growing recognition of trauma-related symptoms can be traced to the US Civil War, where they were known as "irritable" or "soldiers' heart" conditions (Pizarro et al., 2006). The terms "combat fatigue" and "shell shock" were introduced during World War I, while Freud suggested that these mental symptoms represented "combat neurosis" that resulted from the conflict between a soldier's "war ego" and "peace ego" (Jones, 1918). During and following World War II the cluster of trauma symptoms that manifested in soldiers were referred to collectively as "war neurosis" (van der Kolk et al., 2005), and studies of survivors of the Nazi-caused Holocaust (Krystal & Niederland, 1968) and of the atomic bombing of Hiroshima and Nagasaki, Japan by the United States introduced the concept of "survivors' guilt" (Lifton, 1968).

The mental sequelae of traumatic events were early recognized in civilian life as well.

Traumatic reactions to events such as sexual assault or exposure to domestic violence or to deadly accidents has made what was eventually termed post-traumatic stress disorder (PTSD), a widely recognized condition throughout the world. A famous description of an early civilian accident-related trauma and its impact was that experienced by the writer Charles Dickens who, in 1865, was a passenger on a boat-train to London that derailed, killing and injuring many passengers. Dickens was not hurt and tried to aid the victims, some of whom died while he was trying to help them. The experience affected him greatly, as he lost his voice for two weeks and afterwards tried to avoid travelling by train. Dickens died at age 58, five years to the day after the accident. According to his son, he had never fully recovered from this incident (Lewis, 2012).

NATURE OF TRAUMA: ACUTE, COMPLEX, AND DEVELOPMENTAL TRAUMA

There are many different kinds of traumas and many ways of conceptualizing them. In the contemporary literature, they are often categorized as "acute," "complex," and "developmental" trauma. Acute trauma refers to one-time events that can impact individuals, families, groups, and communities and include physical and sexual assaults; natural disasters such as hurricanes, floods, and wildfires; car or airplane accidents; mass violence; and other traumatizing events. Complex trauma (Herman, 1992) includes ongoing traumatic situations such as physical and/or sexual abuse spanning several years, child abuse, wars, and repeated acts of terrorism. They may also involve being bullied in school or in the workplace (Idsoe et al., 2012), being stalked by someone (Purcell et al., 2005), living in severe poverty (Kiser, 2007), or being the recipient of ongoing individual discrimination because of one's race, religion, gender, or sexual orientation. These traumas often go unrecognized and unacknowledged while still causing much psychic pain and damage to one's mental health and may lead to the development of complex post-traumatic stress disorder (C-PTSD) (van der Kolk, et al., 2005).

The concept of developmental trauma overlaps with complex trauma but relates specifically to issues of attachment. Attachment refers to a psychobiological principle rooted in evolutionary development and agreed upon to be the most significant factor in human development (Bowlby, 1969). It is an inborn primary motivational system that guides interactions between the caregiver and infant and is the governing factor in mediating affective attunement as well as emotional and physiological regulation. The attachment pattern established in early development forms an enduring intersubjective context for the ongoing cognitive, affective, and interpersonal development of the child. Attachment formation also plays a key role in psychosocial functions such as empathy, mentalization, and metacognition, which are key to forming secure and stable social relationships. Early adversity and traumatic experience, such as caregivers' physical and emotional neglect, various forms of abuse, or any environmental factors that lead to a feeling of disorganization or insecurity can result in ongoing developmental trauma throughout early development and into adulthood (Lahousen et al., 2019). According to psychiatrist and trauma expert Judith Herman:

> … repeated trauma in childhood forms and deforms the personality. The child trapped in an abusive environment is faced with formidable tasks of adaptation. She must find a way to preserve a sense of trust in people who are untrustworthy, safety in a situation that is unsafe, control in a situation that is terrifyingly unpredictable, power in a

situation of helplessness. Unable to care for or protect herself, she must compensate for the failures of adult care and protection with the only means at her disposal, an immature system of psychological defenses.

(Herman, 1992, p. 96)

The recognition and growing literature focusing on adverse childhood experiences, known as ACEs, encompasses a variety of different types of childhood trauma, including but not limited to sexual abuse, family violence, neglect, and poverty (Felitti, et al., 1998). The number of ACEs have been showed to be highly correlated with a person experiencing mental health disorders, substance misuse issues, and even physical health problems later in life.

DIAGNOSING TRAUMA AND POST-TRAUMATIC STRESS DISORDER

The idea that trauma could result in specific clusters of symptoms first became formalized by the inclusion of the diagnosis of post-traumatic stress disorder (PTSD) in the third edition of the *Diagnostic and Statistical Manual of Mental Disorders* (DSM III; American Psychiatric Association [APA], 1980) under the category of *Anxiety Disorders*. This new diagnosis was precipitated by awareness of the psychological problems experienced by returning Vietnam War veterans in the 1970s and the growing literature by European writers such as Gunter Grass, Primo Levy, and Eli Wiesel among others who survived their own traumatic experiences during World War II and who vividly described the profound impact of mass violence on individuals, families, and communities (Straussner & Phillips, 2004).

In the *DSM-5* (APA, 2013), PTSD was removed from the category of *Anxiety Disorders* and placed under the new category of *Trauma- and Stressor-Related Disorders* along with adjustment disorder, reactive attachment disorder, disinhibited social engagement disorder, and acute stress disorder. Prolonged grief disorder was added to this category in the *DSM-5-TR* (2022). The diagnoses in the *Trauma- and Stressor-Related Disorders* category are distinct among psychiatric disorders in the DSM in that they require exposure to a stressful event as a precondition. Over the years, there has been an increase in the symptom groups required for an individual to receive a PTSD diagnosis. They now include intrusion symptoms, avoidance of stimuli associated with the traumatic event, negative alterations in cognition and mood, and marked alterations in arousal and reactivity.

Although widely debated, what was not included in the DSM-5 was the diagnosis of complex post-traumatic stress disorder (C-PTSD), even though it has been included in the 2019 World Health Organization (WHO) 11th revision of the International Classification of Diseases (ICD-11) (World Health Assembly, 72, 2019). The main differences between diagnosing PTSD and C-PTSD are the length of trauma and the symptoms. Both PTSD and C-PTSD involve symptoms of psychological and behavioral stress responses such as flashbacks, hypervigilance, and efforts to avoid distressing reminders of the traumatic event(s). However, people with C-PTSD typically have additional symptoms, including chronic and extensive issues with emotion regulation, issues with identity and sense of self, and problematic interpersonal relationships often related to such traumatic situations as prolonged domestic violence, childhood sexual or physical abuse, torture, genocide, or slavery (U.S. Department of Veterans Affairs, 2022). Clinicians with expertise in trauma have noted that most individuals diagnosed with borderline personality disorder (BPD) have been exposed to developmental and/or complex trauma in their early lives, resulting in the emotional pain and interpersonal volatility characteristic of this disorder (Herman, 1992). van der Kolk (2014) reported on a study that indicated that 81% of patients diagnosed with BPD at Cambridge Hospital in Massachusetts were subject to histories of severe child abuse and/or neglect. Earlier, Herman (1992) noted how mental health professionals stigmatize individuals with the diagnostic label of BPD by viewing them as difficult patients, in effect re-traumatizing those who are in desperate need of help due to their early adverse experiences.

More recently, it has been suggested that trauma disorders may be best viewed as a spectrum condition across different DSM diagnoses that share common neurobiological brain features such as smaller hippocampal volume (Bremner & Wittbrodt, 2020). According to this theory, trauma spectrum disorders include PTSD, BPD, dissociative disorders, and a certain subgroup of major depressive disorder. Awareness of the interplay between environmental stressors, especially in early childhood, and their effects on brain and neurobiology across the life span is important in understanding these disorders and in the development of therapeutic interventions (Bremner & Wittbrodt, 2020).

EPIGENETICS AND TRAUMA

While still in its infancy, there is a growing body of research in the study of epigenetics that continues to examine the intersection of nature and nurture, or gene and environment. Epigenetics is defined as the study of changes in organisms caused by modification of gene expression rather than alteration of the genetic code itself. Epigenetics has more recently come to refer to direct alteration of DNA regulation that are "on top of" or "in addition to" the traditional genetic code (Howie et al., 2019). The converging evidence of the field of epigenetics and trauma indicates that exposure to extremely adverse environmental circumstances and events impacts individuals so severely that future generations continue to grapple with the inheritance of that trauma (Yehuda & Lehrner, 2018).

The dynamics of *intergenerational transmission of trauma* were first identified in studies of children of Holocaust survivors (Danieli, 1998; Yehuda et al., 2001). Earlier, in a vivid description of three patients presented for psychiatric treatment, Rakoff (1966) noted,

> The parents are not broken conspicuously, yet their children, all of whom were born after the Holocaust, display severe psychiatric symptomatology. It would almost be easier to believe that they, rather than their parents, had suffered the corrupting, searing hell.
>
> (p. 20)

The growing attention in the United States on what is being termed *historical trauma* related to Native American populations (Brave Heart, 1999), and *Post Traumatic Slave Syndrome* (DeGruy, 2017), which focuses on the long-term consequences of slavery on African Americans, points to the increasing recognition and need to address the psychological, social, political, and cultural impact of widespread trauma *over time*. The emerging body of research on epigenetics and trauma is still very young, but what is evident is that some populations and individuals are more biologically susceptible to PTSD, highlighting the importance of clinicians' socio-cultural competency and the incorporation of understanding how catastrophic historical events and familial history may play a highly significant role in the treatment of trauma and PTSD (Ford et al., 2015).

EPIDEMIOLOGY OF TRAUMA AND POST-TRAUMATIC STRESS DISORDER

The experience of trauma is fairly common. A 2016 general population survey conducted in 24 countries showed that more than 70 percent of respondents experienced a traumatic event, and over 30 percent had experienced four or more events (Benjet et al., 2015). Although there is a lack of recent national epidemiological findings in the United States focusing on trauma, studies during the 1990s found that over 60 percent of men and 51 percent of women reported having experienced at least one traumatic event during their lifetime (Kessler et al., 1995).

Nonetheless, while the experience of trauma is common, PTSD diagnosis is much less prevalent. The estimated lifetime prevalence rate of PTSD in the United States has been found to range between 6.1 to 8.3% percent (APA, 2022), although the initial prevalence rates among active-duty military exposed to war conditions and survivors of mass trauma, such as the 2001 destruction of the World Trade Centers in New York, can be as high as 30 percent (Galea, et al., 2005). According to the DSM-5-TR, the "[h]ighest rates (ranging from one-third to more than one-half of those exposed) are found among survivors of rape, military combat and captivity, and ethnically or politically motivated internment and genocide" (APA, 2022, p. 308). While a study published in 2015 found that 6% of a sample of US adults had a lifetime PTSD prevalence, such disorder was twice as high among women (8%) as among men (4%) despite the fact that men are more likely to be exposed to traumatic events (Atwoli et al., 2015). A study based on findings from the 2004–2005 wave of the National Epidemiologic Survey on Alcohol and Related Conditions (NESARC; Roberts et al., 2011) found that the lifetime prevalence of PTSD in the United States was highest among Black individuals (8.7%), intermediate among Hispanics and Whites (7.0% and 7.4%), and lowest among Asians (4.0%). All minority groups were less likely to seek treatment for PTSD than Whites, with fewer than half of minorities with PTSD seeking treatment (range: 32.7–42.0%). Incidence of both trauma and PTSD are higher among lesbian, gay, bisexual, and transgender individuals than among sexual majority individuals. Studies of self-identified gay, lesbian, and bisexual (LGB) individuals found that 83% reported going through adverse childhood experiences (ACE) such as sexual and emotional abuse and having a greater risk for mental health conditions as adults when compared to their heterosexual peers. More than half, 52%, of LGB adults reported three or more ACEs compared to 26% of their heterosexual counterparts (Tran et al., 2022). Reliable prevalence studies on trauma and/or PTSD among transgender individuals are lacking although they are very likely to be much higher than among other populations.

PTSD can affect all aspects of a person's functioning and well-being. It is frequently comorbid with anxiety disorders, major depressive disorder, and substance use disorders, with all of the co-occurring disorders requiring attention during treatment (Qassem et al.,

2021). Overall, PTSD is associated with poorer physical health and greater health care utilization. Findings on mortality are mixed, but generally show that PTSD is associated with increased rates of death due to accidental causes (Goldstein et al., 2016).

THE NEUROPHYSIOLOGY OF TRAUMA AND ITS RELATIONSHIP TO EXPERIENTIAL APPROACHES

Traumatic stress can change the brain's chemistry and structure. Studies suggest that trauma is associated with permanent changes in key areas of the brain, including the *amygdala* – the part of the brain that processes fear and other emotions; the *hippocampus* – the part that is largely responsible for learning and memory; and the *prefrontal cortex* – the part of the brain that is involved in executive functions, such as planning, decision-making, personality expression, and social behavior. The coordination of these three key areas is essential for stress management, affect regulation, and effective functioning of the autonomic nervous system and is associated with increased cortisol and norepinephrine responses to subsequent stressors (Carrion & Wong, 2012). Some neuroimaging studies show that brain changes are more severe in people with C-PTSD compared to people with PTSD.

It is clear that acute trauma, developmental trauma, and C-PTSD all impact both the emotional and physical state of a person. When an individual experiences a traumatic event, the amygdala (emotional and survival center) goes into overdrive and the autonomic nervous system (ANS) goes into survival mode, sending signals to the muscles to prepare for mobilization (fight or flight). If the threat cannot be fought against or escaped from, the autonomic nervous system utilizes its third threat response: Freeze. The freeze response initiates an emotional and psychological shutdown, a safety mechanism to prevent the psyche from becoming too overwhelmed. Meanwhile, trauma also leads to reduced activity in the hippocampus, one of whose functions is to distinguish between the past and present. In other words, the brain cannot tell the difference between the actual current traumatic event and a memory of it. It perceives things that trigger memories of traumatic events as threats themselves. Consequently, during a future time, the nervous system can misinterpret safe environments or situations as life-threatening, leading to the use of maladaptive responses (Ehlers, 2015).

Terpou et al. (2019) differentiated PTSD symptoms into two categories with opposing physiological defense reactions: 1. Hypervigilance and exaggerated sensitivity to stress with increased sympathetic nervous system activation, usually as a result of a single traumatic event; and 2. Hypoemotionality, emotional detachment, and dissociation with decreased sympathetic nervous system activation and increased parasympathetic nervous system functioning usually as a sequela to chronic physical, sexual, and psychological (complex and developmental) trauma where escape was not possible. In addition to the two hyperarousal responses of fight (confronting the threat) or flight (running away from the threat) and the hypoarousal response of freeze (shutting down to block out the threat), some trauma clinicians have added the "fawn" or "appeasement" response, which refers to ameliorating the traumatic threat through pleasing the perpetrator through compliant, servile behaviors (Bailey et al., 2023; Ryder, 2022).

THE BENEFITS OF UTILIZING EXPERIENTIAL THERAPIES

The difficulty with effectively treating trauma with traditional talk therapy is that traumatic situations may result in the blocking of critical cognitive brain processes that are essential for integrating the past, often resulting in the patient reexperiencing rather than resolving the trauma (van der Kolk, 2014). Individuals suffering from the effects of trauma usually report uncontrollable emotions and somatic sensations triggered by reminders of the traumatic situation experienced over and over again in their bodies. The ability to integrate the traumatic memories into a cognitive life narrative are often not available to them, but instead continue to live on somatically, creating a "speechless terror" (Ogden, 2006, p. 28).

Due to the nature of the complex imprint of painful and terrifying unprocessed somatic memories resulting from exposure to traumatic situations, experiential psychotherapies can be particularly helpful as treatment options (Dann, 2022). As many psychotherapy clients who have experienced trauma may not particularly benefit from insight and cognitive-oriented therapies, experiential therapies may be beneficial in enhancing their awareness of their somatic sensations and their physical action patterns (van der Kolk, 2006). Most experiential therapies emphasize a "bottom-up," as opposed to a "top-down" approach to treatment. Top-down processing refers to the prefrontal cortex using current and past information to interpret a situation and involves logic, planning, and problem solving (Reagan, 2021). In traditional top-down talk therapy, the goal of treatment is for the prefrontal cortex to integrate new cognitive perspectives about a difficult situation, which will then result in modification of one's emotions and behaviors. Modalities such as psychodynamic psychotherapy, cognitive-behavioral therapy, dialectical behavior therapy, and solution-focused therapy use such an approach. However, since top-down processing is often impaired in trauma survivors, the experiential therapies incorporate a bottom-up approach that uses bodily sensations and movements to access the trauma and process the impact of it. This is not to say that the experiential therapies do not utilize aspects of a top-down approach as well, but they all emphasize the clients' immediate experiences and bodily sensations.

HISTORICAL OVERVIEW OF THE DIFFERENT EXPERIENTIAL PSYCHOTHERAPIES

The following briefly describes notable experiential psychotherapies in the context of their historical roots. All 15 of these modalities are included as separate chapters in this book. Probably the oldest experiential therapy that is still utilized is *Psychodrama*, developed as one of the first forms of group therapy in the first decades of the 1900s in Vienna, Austria by Jacob L. Moreno, in which participants act out important scenes in group members' lives and process them together (Hough, 2014). However, *Gestalt therapy*, created by Fritz Perls, Paul Goodman, Laura Perls and others in the early 1950s probably had more influence over the early development of experiential therapy than any other modality. Developed as a counterpoint to the reductionist and authoritarian nature of Freudian psychoanalysis, it has been referred to as a "phenomenological" therapy, in which the immediate experiences of clients are focused on in great depth in the here and now of the therapy room (Yontef, 1993). Its theoretical underpinnings were borrowed from many schools of thought such as Gestalt psychology, Lewin's field theory, Reichian body-oriented psychoanalysis, the phenomenological philosophy of Husserl, and the dialogic philosophy of Martin Buber, as well as Zen Buddhism (Bowman & Nevis, 2005). In the Gestalt therapy's use of the "empty chair technique," the influence of psychodrama is apparent.

Strongly influenced by Gestalt therapy, *Hakomi therapy* was developed by Ron Kurtz in the late 1970s and *Emotion Focused therapy* was created by Leslie Greenberg and Sue Johnson in the 1980s. In comparison to Gestalt therapy, Hakomi therapy attends far more to clients' somatic experiences and also emphasizes mindfulness, a concept that was not common-place at the time of its creation (Bageant, 2012; Kurtz, 2020). Emotion focused therapy presents a highly developed theory regarding emotions with an array of techniques to provide adaptive emotional responses to life experiences (Watson, 2018). Gestalt therapy, with its emphasis on clients' experiential exploration of the different parts of themselves, also influenced the creation of *Internal family systems therapy* by Richard Schwartz in the 1980s (Zur Institute, 2023). This modality, which has become increasingly utilized in the past decade, focuses intensely on the client's system of different internal personalities created to keep deep emotional pain at bay (Anderson et al., 2017). *Transformational chairwork*, an experiential therapy developed by Scott Kellogg in the last two decades, expands greatly on Gestalt therapy's use of the empty-chair technique (Kellogg & Garcia Torres, 2021).

Focusing is a very important modality in the history of experiential psychotherapy that was developed by Eugene Gendlin in the late 1960s outside of the influence of Gestalt therapy.

Gendlin worked with Carl Rogers and performed research regarding which clients were more likely to benefit from psychotherapy. He found that when clients were able to intuitively attend to their internal body experiences during the therapy process, which he referred to as a "felt sense," they were more likely to have successful treatment outcomes (Gendlin, 1981).

Consequently, Gendlin developed ways to instruct clients how to develop this "felt sense." This developed into a modality called *focusing-oriented/experiential psychotherapy*. With its focus on attunement to bodily sensations, mindfulness, affect, and emotional self-regulation, Gendlin's work had a major influence on the development of the more somatic-oriented experiential therapies, specifically *Hakomi therapy* and *somatic experiencing therapy*, and furthermore impacted the creation of the concepts of *emotion-focused therapy* (Cornell, 2013).

In regard to the somatic-oriented therapies, Hakomi therapy's focus on clients' bodily sensations led directly to the creation of *sensorimotor psychotherapy* by Pat Ogden in the 1980s, a modality that focuses on working experientially with the physiological manifestations of trauma and early life attachment issues (Fisher, 2019). Another increasingly utilized trauma-focused experiential therapy with a different line of development and conceptual framework is *somatic experiencing therapy*, created by Peter Levine beginning in the 1970s (Brom et al., 2017). There has been a surge of attention to these two somatic therapies in recent years with clinicians emphasizing the need for bottom-up therapy approaches to treatment to counteract the neurological damage incurred by trauma (Bergner, 2023).

A number of experiential therapies were developed mostly apart from the aforementioned influences. The theoretical basis of *intensive short-term dynamic psychotherapy (ISTP)*, developed in the 1970s by Habib Davanloo, is rooted in psychoanalytic psychotherapy. Focusing on the phenomenon of client resistance, Davanloo developed unique experiential interventions to facilitate the client's visceral experiences of underlying defended emotions (Wolff, 2013). Influenced by Davanloo's work, as well as positive psychology, emotion focused therapy, and especially attachment theory, Diana Fosha developed *accelerated experiential-dynamic psychotherapy (AEDP)* in the early 2000s (Ely, 2023; Tunnell & Osiason, 2021). Fosha (2021) describes AEDP as a highly collaborative, transformative psychotherapy that focuses experientially on the processing of overwhelming, traumatic life experiences and through a trusting therapeutic relationship "seeks to engender new experiences of feeling understood, of recognizing and expressing emotional truths that previously have gone unacknowledged and of integrating positive affective experiences linked to healthy action tendencies and resources" (p. 5). *Coherence therapy*, created in the 1990s by Bruce Ecker and Laurel Hulley, is an experiential therapy in which the emotional truth of the client's disturbing symptom is strongly validated in the immediacy of the therapist-client relationship and then later juxtaposed with an alternative emotional truth experienced by the client that is not in synch with that symptom (Ecker & Hulley 2015; Rice, Neimeyer & Taylor, 2011). *Compassion focused therapy*, developed by Paul Gilbert in the early 21st century, focuses on the client being able to develop affiliative rather than hostile emotions toward the self. Recognizing that clients are often cognitively aware of the lack of truth in their self-attacking thoughts associated with previous trauma without being able to internalize more positive feelings about themselves, this modality incorporates experiential methods to enhance self-compassion (Gilbert & Irons, 2015; Irons & Lad, 2017). Perhaps the most widely used experiential psychotherapy for treating trauma is *eye movement desensitization and reprocessing (EMDR)*, which was created in the late 1980s by Francine Shapiro outside of the influence of many of the other modalities. As originally formulated, this modality involves a methodical treatment approach where the clients focus on the emotions and cognitions that arise when they recall a traumatic situation as they follow the back-and-forth motions of the therapist's finger that alternatively stimulates the right and left hemispheres of the brain (Leeds, 2009). More recently, other forms of bilateral stimulation, such as auditory tones and other electronic devices are commonly utilized.

Expressive arts therapy has a totally different history of creative development than the other therapies in this book. Art, music, drama, dance, and poetry have been used throughout the history of humankind as a method for individuals and communities to heal from emotional pain. The contemporary field of expressive arts therapy was created in the 1970s by Shaun McNiff and Paulo Knill at Leslie College in Cambridge, Massachusetts, with later important contributions by Natalie Rogers (Leslie University, 2023; Malchiodi, 2020).

As traumatic experiences are encoded in the brain as memories in the form of imagery and bodily sensation, this modality can be an invaluable approach to the integration of traumatic experiences (Gantt & Tripp, 2016).

It is important to note that two major schools of psychotherapy approaches are not considered to be experiential by the editors of this book: *Humanistic therapies* and *third wave cognitive behavioral therapies*. Humanistic approaches, such as person-centered and existential psychotherapies, have been included as experiential modalities by some authors (Watson et al., 1998). These therapies certainly emphasize the clients' perceptions of their existence and the development of an authentic partnership between therapist and client. However, they tend to focus more on discussions of content related to the client's reality, rather than attending to the moment-by-moment tracking of the client's total mind and body perceptions in the room.

Some might also consider third wave cognitive behavioral therapies that focus on mindfulness and acceptance of one's negative thoughts and difficult emotions, such as dialectical behavior therapy (DBT), acceptance and commitment therapy (ACT), and mindfulness-based cognitive behavioral therapy (MCBT), to be forms of experiential treatment. Whereas mindfulness certainly includes a strong focus on the client's whole-body experiences in the moment, the emphasis of these therapies is directed more toward teaching clients skills in order to live a more fulfilling life and less on experiential therapies' focus on the innate healing process of self-discovery of the client's inner world in the context of an authentic healing relationship with the therapist.

Whereas the purpose of this book is to demonstrate how the different experiential psychotherapies can be useful in the treatment of trauma, it is not the intent of the editors to claim that these forms of therapy are necessarily the preferred treatment for those suffering from the aftermath of trauma. There are certainly a wide range of therapies with a significant evidence base for treating trauma, including different forms of cognitive behavioral therapy, exposure therapy, dialectical behavior therapy, and narrative therapy. Every human being is different, and what works for one person may not necessarily work for someone else. However, it is hoped that the reader of this book will gain an understanding of the unique contribution that experiential therapies offer for those suffering from posttraumatic difficulties.

REFERENCES

American Psychiatric Association [APA], (1980). *Diagnostic and Statistical Manual of Mental Disorders* (DSM), 3rd Edition. Washington, D.C.: Author.

American Psychiatric Association [APA], (2013). *Diagnostic and Statistical Manual of Mental Disorders* (DSM) 5th Edition. Washington, D.C.: Author.

American Psychiatric Association [APA], (2022). *Diagnostic and Statistical Manual of Mental Disorders* (DSM) 5th Edition, Text Revised (DSM-5-TR). Washington, D.C.: Author.

Amir, M., & Lev-Wiesel, R. (2003). Time does not heal all wounds: Quality of life and psychological distress of people who survived the Holocaust as children 55 years later. *Journal of Traumatic Stress, 16*, 295–299.

Anderson, F., Sweezy, M., & Schwartz, R. (2017). *Internal family systems skills training manual: Trauma-informed treatment for anxiety, depression, PTSD, and substance abuse.* Eau Claire, WI: PESI.

Atwoli, L., Stein, D.J., Koenen, K.C., & McLaughlin, K.S.A. (2015). Epidemiology of post-traumatic stress disorder: Prevalence, correlates and consequences. *Current Opinion in Psychiatry, 28*(4). https://www.ncbi.nlm.nih.gov

Bageant, R. (2012). The Hakomi method: Defining its place within the humanistic psychology tradition. *Journal of Humanistic Psychology, 52*(2), 178–189. doi: 10.1177/0022167811423313

Bailey, R., Dugard, J., Smith, S.F., & Porges, S.W. (2023). Appeasement: Replacing Stockholm Syndrome as a definition of a survival strategy. *European Journal of Psychotraumatology, 14*(1), 2161038. https://www.tandfonline.com/doi/full/10.1080/20008066.2022.2161038

Benjet, C., Bromet, E., Karam, E.G., Kessler, R.C., et al. (2015). The epidemiology of traumatic event exposure worldwide: Results from the World Mental Health Survey Consortium. *Psychological Medicine 46*(2), 1–17. Doi:10.1017/S0033291715001981

Bergner, D. (2023, May 18). Want to fix your mind? Let your body talk. *The New York Times Magazine.* https://www.nytimes.com/2023/05/18/magazine/somatic-therapy.html

Bowlby, J. (1969). *Attachment and Loss: Attachment.* London: The Hogarth Press

Bowman, C.E., & Nevis, E.C. (2005). The history and development of Gestalt therapy. In A.L. Woldt & S.M. Toman (Eds.), *Gestalt therapy: History, Theory, and Practice* (pp. 3–20). Thousand Oaks, CA: SAGE Publications.

Brave Heart, M.Y. (1999). Gender differences in historical trauma response among the Lakota. *Journal of Health and Social Policy, 10*(4), 1–21.

Bremner, J.D., & Wittbrodt, M.T. (2020). Chapter One - Stress, the brain, and trauma spectrum disorders. *International Review of Neurobiology, 152,* 1–22. doi: 10.1016/bs.irn.2020.01.004

Brom, D., Stokar, Y., Lawi, C., Nuriel-Porat, V., Ziv, Y., Lerner, K., & Ross, G. (2017). Somatic experiencing for post-traumatic stress: A randomized controlled outcome study. *Journal of Traumatic Stress, 30,* 304–312. doi: 10.1002/jts.22189

Carrion, V.G., & Wong, S.S. (2012). Can traumatic stress alter the brain? Understanding the implications of early trauma on brain development and learning. *Journal of Adolescent Health, 51*(2) Supplement S23–S28. doi: 10.1016/j.jadohealth.2012.04.010

Cornell, A.W. (2013). *Focusing in Clinical Practice: The Essence of Change.* New York & London: W.W. Norton & Company.

Danieli, Y. (Ed.). (1998). *International Handbook of Multigenerational Legacies of Trauma.* New York: Kluwer Academic/Plenum Publishing Corporation

Dann, J. (2022). *Somatic Therapy for Healing Trauma: Effective Tools to Strengthen the Mind-Body Connection.* Emeryville, CA: Rockridge Press

DeGruy, J. (2017). *Post Traumatic Slave Syndrome: America's Legacy of Enduring Injury and Healing.* New York: HarperCollins.

Ecker, B., & Hulley, L. (2015). *Coherence Therapy Tool Kit for Focused, In-Depth Effectiveness.* https://coherencetherapy.org/files/CT_Toolkit.pdf

Ehlers, A. (2015). Understanding and treating unwanted trauma memories in post-traumatic stress disorder. *Zeitschrift für Psychologie/Journal of Psychology, 218*(2), 141–145. doi: 10.1027/0044-3409/a000021

Ely, P. (2023). Diana Fosha on Accelerated Experiential-Dynamic Psychotherapy (AEDP). *Psychotherapy.net*. https://www.psychotherapy.net/interview/AEDP-Diana-Fosha#section-the-origins-of-aedp

Felitti, V.J., Anda, R.F., Nordenberg, D., Williamson, D.F., Spitz, A.M., Edwards, V., et al. (1998). Relationship of childhood abuse and household dysfunction to many of the leading causes of death in adults. The adverse childhood experiences (ACE) study. *American Journal of Preventive Medicine, 14*(4), 245–258.

Fisher, J. (2019). Sensorimotor psychotherapy in the treatment of trauma. *Practice Innovations, 4*(3), 156–165. doi: 10.1037/pri0000096

Ford, J.D., Grasso, D.J., Elhai, J.D., & Courtois, C.A. (2015). Social, cultural, and other diversity issues in the traumatic stress field. In *Posttraumatic Stress Disorder: Scientific and Professional Dimensions*, (2nd Edition, pp. 503–546). Cambridge, MA: Elsevier Academic Press. doi:10.1016/b978-0-12-801288-8.00011-x

Fosha, D. (2021). Introduction: AEDP after 20 years. In D. Fosha (Ed.), *Undoing Aloneness & The Transformation of Suffering into Flourishing; AEDP 2.0.* (pp. 3–18). Washington DC: American Psychological Association.

Galea, S., Nandi, A., Stuber, J., Gold, J., Acierno, R., Best, C.L., et al. (2005). Participant reactions to survey research in the general population after terrorist attacks. *Journal of Traumatic Stress, 18*(5), 461–465.

Gantt, L., & Tripp, T. (2016). The image comes first: Treating preverbal trauma with art therapy. In J.L. King (Ed.), *Art Therapy, Trauma, and Neuroscience* (pp. 67–99). New York, NY: Routledge.

Gendlin, E.T. (1981). *Focusing.* New York, NY: Bantam Books.

Gilbert, P., & Irons, C. (2015). Compassion focused therapy. In S. Palmer (Ed.), *The Beginner's Guide to Counselling and Psychotherapy* (2nd Edition) (pp. 127–139). London, UK: SAGE.

Geoghegan, N. (2019). *Introduction To Experiential Psychotherapies. Experiential Psychotherapy Institute.* https://www.experiential-psychotherapies.com/

Goldstein, R.B., Smith, S.M., Chou, S.P., Saha, T.D., Jung, J., Zhang, H., Pickering, R.P., Ruan, W.J., Huang, B., & Grant, B.F. (2016). The epidemiology of DSM-5 posttraumatic stress disorder in the United States: Results from the National Epidemiologic Survey on Alcohol and Related Conditions-III. *Social Psychiatry and Psychiatric Epidemiology, 51*(8), 1137–1148. doi: 10.1007/s00127-016-1208-5

Herman, J. (1992). *Trauma and Recovery.* New York, NY: Basic Books.

Hough, M. (2014). *Counseling Skills and Theory* (4th Edition). Abingdon, Oxon, UK: Hodder Education.

Howie, H., Rijal, C.M., & Ressler, K.J. (2019). A review of epigenetic contributions to posttraumatic stress disorder. *Dialogues in Clinical Neuroscience, 21*(4), 417–428. doi: 10.31887/DCNS.2019.21.4/kressler

Idsoe, T., Dyregov, A., & Idsoe, E.C. (2012). Bullying and PTSD symptoms. *Journal of Abnormal Child Psychology, 40*(6), 901–911.

Irons, C., & Lad, S. (2017). Using compassion focused therapy to work with shame and self-criticism in complex trauma. *Australian Clinical Psychologist, 3*(1), 47–54.

Jones, E. (1918). War shock and Freud's Theory of the Neuroses. *Proceedings of the Royal Society of Medicine, 1*(Sect Psych), 21–36. PMID: 19980291; PMCID: PMC2066212. https://www.ncbi.nlm.nih.gov/pmc/articles/PMC2066212/

Kellogg, S., & Garcia Torres, A. (2021). Toward a chairwork psychotherapy: Using the four dialogues for healing and transformation. *Practice Innovations, 6*(3), 171–180. doi: 10.1037/pri0000149

Kessler, R.C., Sonnega, A., Bromet, E., Highes, M., & Nelson, C.B. (1995). Posttraumatic stress disorder in the National Comorbidity Survey. *Archives of General Psychology, 52*(12), 1048–1060. doi: 10.001/arcpsyc.1995.03950240066012

Kiser, L.J. (2007). Protecting children from the dangers of urban poverty. *Clinical Psychology Review, 27*(2), 211–225.

Krystal, H., & Niederland, J. (1968). *Massive Psychic Trauma.* New York: International University Press.

Kurtz, R. (2020). History of Hakomi method. *Ron Kurtz Hakomi Educational Materials.* https://hakomi.com/history

Lahousen, T., Unterrainer, H. F., & Kapfhammer, H-P. (2019). Psychobiology of attachment and trauma—Some general remarks from a clinical perspective. *Frontiers in Psychiatry, 10,* 914. doi: 10.3389/fpsyt.2019.00914

Leeds, A.M. (2009). *A Guide to the Standard EMDR Protocols For Clinicians, Supervisors, and Consultants.* New York, NY: Springer.

Leslie University (2023). The rise of expressive therapies. https://lesley.edu/article/the-rise-of-expressive-therapies

Lewis, L.M. (2012). *Dickens, His Parables and His Reader.* Columbia, MO: University of Missouri Press

Lifton, R.J. (1968). *Death in Life: Survivors of Hiroshima.* New York: Random House.

Malchiodi, C.A. (2020). *Trauma and Expressive Arts Therapy.* New York, NY: Guilford.

Ogden, P. (2006). *Trauma and the Body.* New York, NY: W.W. Norton and Company.

Osei-Boamah, E., Pilkins, B.J., Steven R., & Gambert, S.R. (2013, June). Post-Traumatic stress disorder: A historical perspective of an evolving. *DiagnosisConsultant360, 21*(6).

Oxford Dictionaries (2013). *Trauma.* Retrieved from http://oxforddictionaries.com/definition/english/trauma

Pizarro, J. Silver, R.C., & Prause, J. (2006). Physical and mental health costs of traumatic war experiences among civil war veterans. *Archives of General Psychiatry, 63,* 193–200.

Purcell, R., Pathé, M., & Mullen, P.E. (2005). Association between stalking victimisation and psychiatric morbidity in a random community sample. *British Journal of Psychiatry, 187,* 416–420.

Qassem, T.D., Aly-ElGabry, D.A., Alzarouni, A.K., Abdel-Aziz, K., & Arnone, D. (2021). Psychiatric co-morbidities in Post-traumatic Stress Disorder: Detailed findings from the adult psychiatric morbidity survey in the English population. *Psychiatric Quarterly, 92*(1), 321–330. doi: 10.1007/s11126-020-09797-4

Rakoff, V. (1966). A long-term effect of the concentration camp experience. *Viewpoints, 1,* 17–22.

Reagan, R. (2021, October 22). Trauma treatment modality series: "Top-down" and "Bottom-up" approach to therapy. *Trauma Therapist Network.* https://traumatherapistnetwork.com/trauma-treatment-modality-series-top-down-and-bottom-up-approach-to-therapy/

Rice, K.G., Neimeyer, G.J., & Taylor, J.M. (2011). Efficacy of Coherence Therapy in the treatment of procrastination and perfectionism. *Counseling Outcome Research and Evaluation, 2*(2), 126–136. 10.1177/2150137811417975

Roberts, A.L., Gilman, S.E., Breslau, J., Breslau, N., & Koenen, K.C. (2011). Race/ethnic differences in exposure to traumatic events, development of post-traumatic stress disorder, and treatment-seeking for post-traumatic stress disorder in the United States. *Psychological Medicine*, *41*(1), 71–83. doi: 10.1017/S0033291710000401

Ryder, G. (2022). The fawn response: How trauma can lead to people-pleasing. *PsychCentral*. https://psychcentral.com/health/fawn-response

Straussner, S.L.A. & Calnan, A.J. (2014). Trauma through the life cycle: A review of current literature. *Clinical Social Work Journal*, *42*(4), 323–336. doi: 10.1007/s10615-014- 0496-z . http://link.springer.com/article/10.1007%2Fs10.15-014-0496-z

Straussner, S.L.A., & Phillips, N.K. (2004). Social work interventions in the context of mass violence. In S.L.A. Straussner & N.K. Philips (Eds.), *Understanding Mass Violence: A Social Work Perspective* (pp. 3–19). Boston: Allyn and Bacon.

Terpou, B.A., Harricharan, S., McKinnon, M.C., Frewen, P., Jetly, R., & Lanius, R.A. (2019). The effects of trauma on brain and body: A unifying role for the midbrain periaqueductal gray. *Journal of Neuroscience Research*, *97*(9), 1110–1140. doi: 10.1002/jnr.24447

Tran N.M., Henkhaus, L.E., & Gonzales, G. (2022). Adverse Childhood Experiences and mental distress among US adults by sexual orientation. *JAMA Psychiatry*, *79*(4), 377–379. doi:10.1001/jamapsychiatry.2022.0001

Tunnell, G., & Osiason, J. (2021). Historical context: AEDP's place in the world of psychotherapy. In D. Fosha (Ed.), *Undoing Aloneness & The Transformation of Suffering into Flourishing; AEDP 2.0.* (pp. 83–105). Washington DC: American Psychological Association.

U.S. Department of Veterans Affairs. (2022). *Complex PTSD*. National Center for PTSD. https://www.ptsd.va.gov/professional/treat/essentials/complex_ptsd.asp

VandenBos, G.R. & American Psychological Association (2015). *APA Dictionary of Psychology* (2nd Edition). Washington DC: American Psychological Association.

van der Kolk, B.A. (2006). Foreword. In P. Ogden, *Trauma and the Body* (pp. 17–26). New York, NY: W.W. Norton and Company.

van der Kolk, B.A. (2014). *The Body Keeps The Score*. New York, NY: Penguin.

van der Kolk, B.A., Roth, S., Pelcovitz, D., Sunday, S., & Spinazzola, J. (2005). Disorders of extreme stress: The empirical foundation of a complex adaptation to trauma. *Journal of Traumatic Stress*, *18*(5), 389–399.

Watson, J.C., Greenberg, L.S., & Lietaer, G. (1998). The experiential paradigm unfolding: Relationship and experiencing in therapy. In L.S. Greenberg, J.C. Watson, & G. Lietaer (Eds.), *Handbook of Experiential Psychotherapy* (pp. 3–27). New York: The Guilford Press.

Watson, J.C. (2018). Mapping patterns of change in emotion-focused psychotherapy: Implications for theory, research, practice, and training. *Psychotherapy Research*, *28*(3), 389–405. doi: 10.1080/10503307.2018.1435920

Wolf, D.M. (2013). Intensive Short-Term Dynamic Psychotherapy in the private practice of psychiatry. *Psychiatric Annals*, *43*(11), 491–495. doi: 10.1176/appi.psychotherapy.2002.56.2.225

World Health Assembly, 72. (2019). *Eleventh Revision of the International Classification of Diseases*. World Health Organization. https://apps.who.int/iris/handle/10665/329357

Yehuda, R., Halligan, S.L., & Grossman, R. (2001). Childhood trauma and risk for PTSD: Relationship to intergenerational effects of trauma, parental PTSD and cortisol excretion. *Development and Psychopathology, 13*(3), 733–753.

Yehuda, R., & Lehrner, A. (2018). Intergenerational transmission of trauma effects: Putative role of epigenetic mechanisms. *World Psychiatry, 17*(3), 243–257. doi: 10.1002/wps.20568. PMID: 30192087; PMCID: PMC6127768.

Yontef, G.M. (1993). *Awareness, Dialogue, & Process*. Highland, NY: Gestalt Journal Press.

Zur Institute (2023). *Internal Family Systems*. https://www.zurinstitute.com/clinical/

2

CHAPTER 2
TRAUMA-FOCUSED PSYCHODRAMA

Scott Giacomucci and Haydn Briggs

INTRODUCTION

Trauma-focused psychodrama is a powerful and effective method for healing different forms of trauma. Psychodrama was created over 100 years ago and has evolved over the years into a versatile and potent modality. The embodied, relational, and creative aspects of psychodrama promote healing within the body, brain, and self. The inclusion of trauma-informed principles and strength-based roles help to promote containment and safety throughout the treatment. Psychodrama provides an avenue for participants to act out inner conflicts, develop new strengths to face trauma, revisit and undo painful memories, practice for future scenarios, and embody post-traumatic growth. This chapter outlines the history, research, theories, and methodology of trauma-focused psychodrama while providing an overview of the treatment process and a case example. Strengths and limitations of the model are discussed.

BRIEF HISTORY

The history of psychodrama is rich and complex and can only fully be understood within the larger context of the ideas of its founder, Jacob L. Moreno, MD. Psychodrama was developed as part of Moreno's triadic system – sociometry, psychodrama, and group psychotherapy. However, psychodrama was the last of the major methods that Moreno created, and its underlying philosophy and practice were directly connected to Moreno's prior ideas and approaches including his mysticism and existential philosophy, the Theater of Spontaneity, sociatry, sociometry, and group psychotherapy. Moreno largely rejected Freud's ideas of psychoanalysis and created his own approaches in opposition to it. He harshly critiqued psychoanalysis, the passive stance of a psychoanalyst, and the idea of *the talking cure*. Instead, he promoted action and healing through relationships. His ideas were unconventional at the time. In attacking the psychoanalytical community, his own ideas ended up largely marginalized within the mainstream treatment and psychology communities. Moreno was a Romanian psychiatrist who believed that the suffering in the world warranted healing on larger scales than individual treatment. His mysticism led to a vision of *sociatry*, or healing for society, which fueled his experimentation with theater as an avenue for promoting change in large audiences. His Theater of Spontaneity and sociometry ideas both also emerged in the early 1920s before he immigrated to New York City in 1925. The Theater of Spontaneity (which later evolved into Impromptu Theater in New

DOI: 10.4324/9781003455851-2

York) involved regular sessions where role-players enacted stories from the audience or the newspaper to promote catharses or new perspectives. He declares the birthday of psychodrama to be April 1st, 1921, when he facilitated a session in Vienna using an empty chair to represent a future leader of the new world order in Europe.

Moreno's sociometric ideas emerged through his work in a refugee camp in Austria and later as a researcher for the state of New York. The basic premise of sociometry is that the primary problems within communities and groups could be resolved through the restructuring of individuals within the group in ways that they would be positioned to support each other. His experimentation of this idea in Sing Sing Prison was presented in 1932. This was the first time the terms "group therapy" or "group psychotherapy" were used (Giacomucci, 2021). Moreno's ongoing sociometric work, outlined in *Who Shall Survive?* (1934), laid the foundation for later research in social network theories, group dynamics, and participatory action research.

In 1936, Moreno founded his mental health hospital in Beacon, New York where the culmination of his previous ideas and approaches merged to create psychodrama as a psychotherapy approach. Jacob Moreno met Zerka Toeman in 1941, they married in 1949, and together they refined, taught, translated, and published for multiple decades. By the early 1950s, at least one third of all mental health hospitals were using psychodrama in their programming (Borgatta, 1950). Throughout the 1950s to the 1970s, Moreno's work continued to grow in popularity and was taught in many universities, integrated into countless inpatient hospitals (especially the Veterans Administration hospitals), multiple branches of the US military, various organizations in diverse industries, and influenced many other psychotherapy leaders. The Morenos traveled around the world teaching psychodrama and collaborating with the international community. Psychodrama became further popularized through the Human Potential Movement, Encounter Groups, T-Groups, sensitivity training, and humanistic psychology. Many leaders in the field have suggested that Moreno directly or indirectly influenced nearly all experiential or active therapies (Berne, 1970; Schultz, 1971). As he grew older, Moreno was upset that his work had been "cannibalized," as many were using interventions from sociometry or psychodrama while disregarding the underlying philosophy and theories from which they came. Jacob Moreno died in 1974 after a long illness.

After his death, Zerka Moreno and other leaders in the psychodrama community continued to refine the methods and promote them around the world. Zerka died at the age of 99 in 2016. As psychodrama's popularity in the United States declined throughout the latter part of the 20th century, it grew in popularity in other countries. This decline seems to have been influenced by various systemic forces including deinstitutionalization, the medicalization of mental health treatment, managed care, evidence-based practice trends, the development of new experiential therapies, the absence of psychodramatists in academia, and the mixed reputation that psychodrama developed due to its use by professionals without proper training/supervision or in ways that contributed to retraumatization or harm (Giacomucci, 2021). While psychodrama and Moreno are rarely mentioned in US graduate programs, in multiple other countries one can get an entire masters or doctorate degree specifically in psychodrama (Giacomucci, 2021). Psychodrama continues to be very popular in various countries in South America, Europe, and Asia and appears to be growing in demand in the United States in the past decade.

ASSESSMENT OF RESEARCH EVIDENCE

The evidence base for psychodrama as a trauma treatment encompasses nearly 100 years of literature and continues to grow. The research on psychodrama highlights its effectiveness while more recent neuroscience findings highlight the importance of body-based and action methods for treating trauma. Current research points to psychodrama as an effective treatment approach for various mental health diagnoses including PTSD and trauma-related issues, but more research with higher quality research designs is warranted (Orkibi & Feniger-Schaal, 2019; Orkibi, Keisari, Sajnani, & de Witte, 2023). In psychodrama-specific research on PTSD, various studies highlight its effectiveness with various populations including war veterans, patients in substance use treatment, men with various histories of trauma, adolescents who experienced abuse in childhood, and survivors of mass shootings, relational trauma, and natural disasters (Giacomucci, 2023). Psychodrama has been included in the meta-analyses and systematic reviews of other larger research bases which demonstrate effectiveness for PTSD treatment – such as experiential psycho-therapies, creative arts therapies, and body- and movement-oriented interventions (Baker et al., 2018; Elliott et al., 2013; Orkibi, Keisari, Sajnani, & de Witte, 2023; van de Kamp et al., 2019). Psychodrama was developed many decades before PTSD was recognized as a diagnosis. While there are several decades of psychodrama studies available highlighting its effectiveness, including research on trauma and PTSD, there remains a need for additional research with diverse populations and with additional randomized controlled trials.

FUNDAMENTAL CLINICAL CONCEPTS

Psychodrama is one of the most complex modalities of psychotherapy. While an exhaustive list of clinical concepts is beyond the scope of this chapter, the myriad fundamental clinical concepts can be broadly organized into theoretical concepts, and then interventions.

THEORETICAL CONCEPTS

Moreno's *spontaneity-creativity theory*, inspired by his mysticism and existential philoso-phy, describes spontaneity as the energy that allows an individual to "respond with some degree of adequacy to a new situation or with some degree of novelty to an old situa-tion," with creativity being the "arch substance" catalyzed by spontaneity (Moreno, 1964, p. xii). Put succinctly, Moreno's triadic system – sociometry, psychodrama, and group psychotherapy – is the mechanism by which people can stimulate and access the process of spontaneity-creativity, through which all intrapsychic, intrapersonal, and social change occurs (Giacomucci, 2021).

The next significant theory important for understanding psychodrama is Moreno's *role theory*. Within psychodrama, role theory is the basis for understanding both personality and development. A person's self or personality is the composition and aggregate of the roles that a person occupies. "Roles do not emerge from the self, but the self emerges from roles" (Moreno, 1934). Roles can be somatic, psychodramatic, and social. The cul-mination of the roles in each category comprises our somatic, psychodramatic, and social selves, respectively. Roles follow a staged process of role development and are influenced by role dynamics such as role training, role conflict, role reciprocity, and so on. Within role theory, wellness is measured by the breadth and depth of one's *role repertoire*, and the ease with which they move between those roles.

Psychodrama's *action theory* – the concept that talking alone cannot effect the best change and, in fact, limits it – is fundamental to psychodrama and Moreno's theories. One's role isn't just cognitive or emotional, it's behavioral and action based, too. The Morenos observed how their patients, through action in *surplus reality* – the enactment of fantasy or subjective reality that happens during a psychodrama – increased their spontaneity and experienced change through action. The spontaneous, autonomous, and healing nature of this process inspired Zerka Moreno to coin the term *autonomous healing center* to describe the healing inside of an individual or group that psychodrama aims to access (Giacomucci, 2021). The Morenos also observed two types of catharses. *Catharsis of abreaction* describes the experience of tension release related to the issue, providing a sense of relief and resolution, often through what psychodrama became known for in the late 20th century – tears and anger. *Catharsis of integration*, the ultimate goal of psychodrama, describes the reordering or transformation of intrapsychic structures (Giacomucci, 2021).

Finally, any discussion of psychodrama is incomplete without a discussion of *sociometry*. In practice, many use the word "sociometry" interchangeably with "warm-up." While sociometric group action methods are one of the primary warm-up processes used in psychodrama, sociometry itself describes the study of social relationships and interactions, while warm-up itself describes the internal and external process of preparing for the action portion of a psychodrama. In addition to group action methods based on sociometry, warm-up also includes group screening and intake processes, introductions, norms, and more. Sociometry often includes the use of various pen-to-paper or experiential processes including social atoms, sociograms, sociometric tests, spectrograms, locograms, floor checks, step-in sociometry, and others, which are beyond the scope of this chapter.

PSYCHODRAMA INTERVENTIONS

While the theory behind Moreno's triadic system forms the foundation of psychodrama, there are specific interventions used during the psychodrama itself to help guide the *protagonist* (the group member with the primary role in a psychodrama, around which the psychodrama is formed) toward their *contract* (agreed-upon goal with the psychodrama director/therapist), often including one of the catharses. The protagonist is the center and primary role in a psychodrama. Selected by the group, the protagonist's topic and goal becomes the central focus of the group.

One of the initial steps in a psychodrama is *scene setting*, done collaboratively between the protagonist and the director, and can involve a variety of interventions to create the scene. A protagonist may *concretize* intrapsychic qualities, figures, or anything else in their life through the assignment of an item (often an empty chair or scarf) or person to act as a physical symbol or occupy that role. The protagonist may *sculpt* the scene through the intentional placement of multiple concretized people or items in the space (Giacomucci, 2021).

Sometimes interwoven into the process of concretization or done separately, often following scene setting, a protagonist and director may enroll other group members into various roles important to the psychodrama. These other group members, in roles, are called *auxiliary egos*. Auxiliaries are chosen by the protagonist and/or director to hold and play various roles within the protagonist's psychodrama. Role reversal describes the process of switching roles with another player in a psychodrama (whether it be played by a human or concretized with an object). Through role reversal (two group members switching roles with each other), auxiliary egos can observe how the role is best played for the protagonist *(role training)*, and the protagonist gets a new perspective by seeing the situation from the point of view of someone else. *Doubling* is another way the group can help role train an auxiliary and contain and deepen the protagonist's experience in the psychodrama. While there are many different types of doubles and doubling, the action of doubling describes another group member or the director offering a statement (from the "I") for the protagonist to repeat if it fits and change if it doesn't. The double can be done by group members spontaneously, or can be a specific role (Giacomucci, 2021). At any point in a psychodrama, the director may invite the protagonist into the *mirror position*, where the protagonist exits the stage and observes the drama from a new perspective, helpful in creating new insights and perspective on whatever is being enacted (Giacomucci, 2021). This survey of fundamental concepts in psychodrama is merely an introduction to systems of much greater complexity. Further resources for learning will be referenced later in the chapter.

DESCRIPTION OF THE THERAPY PROCESS

The five elements of a psychodrama are the stage, the director, the protagonist, the auxiliary egos, and the audience. Each is equally important. The stage is wherever the psychodrama takes place. The director leads the protagonist and the psychodrama, maintaining an awareness of the protagonist, the contract and movement toward the contract, the group members, and management of the space and auxiliaries. The protagonist is the primary role in the psychodrama, whose life is enacted and who contracts with the director for the psychodrama. The auxiliary egos are those others in the group who play roles in the protagonist's psychodrama. Finally, the audience are all those who witness the psychodrama. Through the various interventions and processes described previously, and to be elaborated on in a case example, the psychodrama proceeds toward a climax, catharsis, and/or fulfillment of the contract with the protagonist. In an individual psychodrama, auxiliaries are replaced by objects or empty chairs used to concretize roles, and there is no audience (Giacomucci, 2021).

As mentioned previously, all psychodrama work follows a three-phase structure: Warm-up, action, and sharing. While psychodrama is applicable to both groups and individuals, group psychodrama is the preferred method for its nuance and richness (Giacomucci, 2021). The warm-up phase of a psychodrama can involve anything that helps prepare the group or individual for action. Warm-up ends with the selection of a protagonist through various methods. In an individual psychodrama, the patient or client is the protagonist, though this doesn't discount the importance of adequate warm-up. While the action phase is where most of the change happens in psychodrama, the quality of warm-up is one of the greatest determinants for key factors of the session including the success of the psychodrama, the group or individual's connection to the work being enacted, the safety and containment, and overall quality of the group (Giacomucci, 2021). The psychodrama begins with the selection of the protagonist and ends when the contract – the goal of the session – between the director and protagonist is fulfilled. Through various methods, the director and protagonist decide on a contract for the session that fits their treatment progress, treatment context, and is attainable within the constraints of the group.

The final phase of the psychodrama is sharing. At this point, the protagonist is free from the spotlight and can rest. Moreno referred to psychodrama as "psychic surgery" (Moreno, 1934). As such, the protagonist is in the proverbial recovery room during the sharing phase. There are two types of sharing. First, auxiliaries, as part of their process of de-roling, share what came up for them in the role (either somatically, emotionally, cognitively, or interpersonally). In this process, group members who were auxiliaries can deepen their own experiences of related roles, and the protagonist can gain valuable interpersonal or intrapsychic data about their work. Second, everyone in the group has an opportunity to share about how they connected to the content and process of the drama. It is important to note that sharing is not a time to give feedback, either positive or constructive, to the protagonist. The sharing portion of the group is a chance for audience members to join with the protagonist in vulnerability, and for the protagonist to be brought back into being part of the group. In an individual psychodrama, a protagonist may share about their experience with the therapist (Giacomucci, 2021).

The preceding process for a single individual or group psychodrama session parallels the structure of treatment over time, and is analogous to phase-oriented trauma treatment. The warm-up phase of psychodrama matches the focus on safety and containment with trauma survivors that precedes work with defenses, trauma processing, grief, and other more challenging work, which itself parallels the action phase of a psychodrama group. The final phase of treatment with trauma survivors focuses on integration and post-traumatic growth, similar to the sharing phase of a single session of psychodrama (Giacomucci, 2023). This process, both in a single session and treatment over time, will be demonstrated in case example vignettes later in this chapter.

CASE EXAMPLE

The following is a fictional account of a psychodrama group session within the context of a treatment center focusing on trauma and addiction.

WARM-UP

Jane enters the group and takes a seat. She and 11 others are seated around the room, waiting for the group session to begin. Jane is in both individual and group trauma-focused psychodrama treatment. The director, who is the psychodrama group facilitator, begins the group discussing rules and norms around confidentiality, choice, physical touch, and breaks. Specifically, the director specifies the importance of confidentiality, emphasizes that everything in group is voluntary with levels of chosen engagement, reminds people to ask permission before any physical touch, and reminds folks to remain in the room for the duration of the group session if they can. The director invites clients to embody their commitment to the rules and norms by standing up. They all do so.

Jane and the others observe a pile of scarves in the middle of the room, around which they stand in a circle.

DIRECTOR: Take a look at the person to your left. Think about the strengths you've seen in them since you first began working with them in the group. If it's your first time in the group or their first time in the group today, just think of a strength you've seen even in this brief time. When you feel ready, come to the center of the circle, choose a scarf to represent that strength, and return to your place in the circle.

Group members enter the center, sift through the scarves, and choose one at a time. Jane chooses a red corduroy scarf.

DIRECTOR: Now we'll go around the circle and present them to your person, telling them how this strength can help them heal from trauma. When you finish accepting your scarf, place it on the floor and we'll form a circle of them. This circle of strengths will be our stage today.

One by one, individuals present the strengths to one another. Jane gives a strength to Matt.

JANE: Matt. I chose this scarf to represent your passion. I see such a fire in you to recover and grow every time we're together here.

Jane hands Matt the scarf. Matt places the scarf in the circle. Other group members continue to present strengths to each other. After the Circle of Strengths, the director invites group members to step forward if they would like to volunteer themselves and a topic for the psychodrama.

Jane and one other group member, Nina, step into the center of the room. Jane articulates her topic related to her struggle with committing to her trauma recovery. Nina expresses her topic as being related to having a conversation with a deceased loved one. After both topics are named, the director instructs the other participants to identify which topic would help them the most today – emphasizing that the choice is between topics, not based on the person proposing it.

Group members make their way to the center of the room choosing Nina or Jane's topics. There's a clear majority of choice for Jane's topic, so she becomes the protagonist.

ACTION

DIRECTOR: Jane, come and walk around this circle with me and tell me a bit more about your topic and your goal. Go ahead and share whatever feels important.

JANE: Okay. Well, I guess it's sort of hard to admit, but all the talk about not being able to decide stuff had me feel okay admitting some of the stuff that's happening inside me. I mean, I'm here and I'm doing the work. Even as protagonist. But there's a big part of me that wants to not to do this at all, and that actually likes all the stuff I'm trying to get help with. I like getting into intense relationships, I like feeling crazy and wild and manic. A really big part of me likes that feeling. But obviously I also really want to get better and heal from my past trauma too. Just feels like something I should deal with, I guess.

DIRECTOR: Can anyone else in the group relate to that feeling? Raise your hand if so.

Nearly everyone in the room raises their hand.

DIRECTOR: Take a look around, Jane. Looks like this is the group's work too. So it sounds like you're caught between this part of you that really wants to recover from trauma and "do the work," and one that isn't ready to let some of these other things go. Is that right?

JANE: Yes, that's right, but it's more than that too. It's a part of me that doesn't want to let things go but also really enjoys them in some ways, really values them in some ways.

DIRECTOR: Got it. So, I'm thinking we could have a conversation with one or both of those parts today. How does that sound?

JANE: Sounds good to me. Sounds sort of scary. I'm not really sure what it will be like.

DIRECTOR: We can figure it out as we go. First, can you pick someone in the group to play the role of your double, sort of like your positive and wise inner voice?

JANE: Yeah sure. Matt, will you be my double?

MATT: Sure.

DIRECTOR: Okay, Double, come on over here next to Jane. I'd like you to just repeat positive and true statements, from the "I," that you know to be true about Jane. Jane, if they fit, repeat them, if not, change them to make them fit.

MATT/DOUBLE: I'm courageous

JANE: I'm courageous.

MATT/DOUBLE: I can do this.

JANE: I'm going to try to do this.

DIRECTOR: Great. Double, you'll stay with Jane the whole time and you can speak out messages as you feel like it. Jane, same thing goes for you. You can repeat them, change them, or leave them. So, Jane, you

	said it sounded sort of scary. Is there a person in your life, a strength, figure, anything that helps when you're struggling with trauma?
JANE:	Well, the first thing I thought of was my dog, Philo.
DIRECTOR:	Great. Can you pick someone to be Philo? Just trust your gut and your choice.
JANE:	Sure. Nina, will you be Philo?
NINA:	Sure.
DIRECTOR:	Come on up, Nina. Jane, where should Philo be?
JANE:	I guess maybe here in front of me on the floor, facing me. Perfect, thanks Nina.
DIRECTOR:	Go ahead, Jane. What do you want to say to Philo?
JANE:	You're a good boy, Philo. Thanks for always being there.
DIRECTOR:	Okay, Jane, reverse roles with Philo.

Nina (Philo) and Jane switch physical locations.

DIRECTOR:	Jane [Nina] will you repeat that last message to Philo [now Jane].
NINA (JANE):	You're a good boy, Philo. Thanks for always being there.
DIRECTOR:	Go ahead and respond, Philo.
JANE (PHILO):	Of course, Jane. I love being your buddy.
DIRECTOR:	Philo, can you remind Jane of a time where she was brave?
MATT/DOUBLE:	I'm brave.
JANE (PHILO):	Yeah. You were so brave when that other dog was barking at us and running towards me. He was bigger than both of us and you got in front of me to keep me safe.
FACILITATOR:	Reverse roles. Repeat that back.

Jane and Nina reverse roles, switching physical locations and switching roles.

NINA (PHILO):	You were so brave when that other big dog was coming after us. You kept me safe.
JANE:	Yeah. That was scary.
DIRECTOR:	Reverse roles.

Jane and Nina reverse roles, switching physical locations and switching roles, again.

DIRECTOR:	Philo, it seems like Jane here is having trouble with ambivalence related to her trauma recovery. Can you remind her of a time you've seen her face hard decisions that didn't have a certain direction?
JANE (PHILO):	Yeah. Well, I guess when you left Steve. He wasn't nice to me either. But he really was abusive to you. And one day you took me and we just left there and lived somewhere else even though you didn't necessarily have a whole plan.
DIRECTOR:	And can you tell Jane how that was for you, Philo, and how it made you feel?
JANE (PHILO):	I felt safe with you. I'm always happy to be with you no matter what you want to do. I love you.
DIRECTOR:	Reverse roles.

Jane and Nina switch roles and physical locations again.

DIRECTOR (TO NINA):	Okay, Philo, repeat back the important stuff you said.
NINA (PHILO):	Steve was so mean to you. And he was mean to me, too. You took me and we left there and were safe. I know that was hard for you. You made me feel so safe the whole time. I love you.
JANE:	I love you, too, Philo.

Jane and Nina take a pause and take in the messages both in the roles and for themselves.

DIRECTOR:	Okay, Jane, earlier we talked about these two sides of you that you wanted to get to know more. Can you pick people from the group to be each of them?
JANE:	Yeah. Stacy, will you be the part of me that's not sure about trauma recovery? Mark, will you be the other one?
DIRECTOR:	Go ahead and place them where they need to be in the room.

Jane directs each to a space in front of her, moving Philo to her side.

DIRECTOR:	So, we have a couple of options here, Jane, and I'll encourage you to just trust your gut here. One option is we can continue speaking to and getting to know these roles, these parts of you. Another option is sculpting. We can manage how we want these to relate to each other. Which are you pulled towards?
JANE:	You know, I think I want to do the sculpting thing to see what happens.

Jane, with the director's support, places the auxiliary roles (the "not-recovery one," "trauma recovery one," and Philo) around the room and in specific positions to represent how she feels in relation to them. After observing, she shifts their positioning and location to what she aspires to inside of herself. First, she places the "not-recovery one" in a feet-planted, halt sign out, shaking fist forward, and making an angry sound. She gives this role the line, "you can't make me. I won't let you." Next, she places the "trauma recovery one" across from the "not-recovery one" in a pleading position, making frustrated motions, noises, and prayer hands towards the "not-recovery one." She gives this role the line, "please! You have to!" The director has Jane watch both roles cycle through their positions, lines, sounds, and movements. Jane shares what it feels like to watch. She shares it seems crowded, frustrating, and uncomfortable. The director checks with Jane to see if anything is missing from the scene. Jane gives further direction for the "trauma recovery one" to chase the "not-recovery one" around the room while they continue their other actions. The director brings Jane's attention to Philo, the other role, and asks where he belongs in this scene. Jane surprises herself, realizing Philo is guarded by the "not-recovery one." She places Philo behind the "not-recovery one" and directs him to follow that role wherever he goes. Jane begins to cry as she watches the scene play out, having an insight into the deeper role each of these parts of her play.

The director invites Jane to shift the scene to how she'd like it to be. She places both the "trauma recovery-one" and "not-recovery one" side by side, in relaxed positions, facing Philo, who is facing away from them. They're now behind him. She gives the line "I can let Philo see me be vulnerable. He already knows" to the "not-recovery" one, and the line "I'm not alone. I don't have to do this alone" to the "trauma recovery one." Jane watches the scene play out again. The director invites her to watch as long as she'd like, until the scene feels complete and integrated.

One by one, each role approaches Jane, de-roling by brushing off their shoulders and shaking their limbs. Each repeat their name and return to their seats.

SHARING

DIRECTOR: Now's the time for sharing. Remember that sharing is talking about how we connected to the protagonist's work, not giving feedback to the protagonists, or the folks who played other roles, even if it's positive feedback. Jane, you get to rest and take it all in. For those of you who played a role, you can share what came up for you in the role as well as how you connected to the role. Does anyone want to start?

NINA: I can start. Thanks for choosing me to play Philo, Jane. I noticed right away in the role I was just happy to see you, be near you, and be close to you. And I really did feel safe, protected, and prioritized by you. As far as how I connect to the drama? Pretty much in every way. I have my own Philos in my life and my own not-recovery and trauma recovery parts that I'm constantly in battle with. I'm actually usually scared to admit it at all, so it helped me a ton to see you name it and do your work with it.

MARK: I can go next. It felt good to be able to fully embody your trauma recovery and sort of my own recovery. Like Nina said, I have the same struggle constantly. A huge part of me wants to give up and keep doing what I'm used to. I felt a lot of calm in the role even though I expected to feel a little more frenzied or powerful. Especially when you shifted us.

Others share the ways in which they related to the psychodrama or benefited from participating or observing. The director brings the group session to a close.

PSYCHODRAMA FOR THE TREATMENT OF TRAUMA

Psychodrama is a viable treatment option for survivors of trauma including acute trauma, complex and developmental trauma, traumatic loss, and collective trauma. The research on psychodrama demonstrates its effectiveness in treating post-traumatic stress disorder (PTSD), interpersonal issues, unresolved emotional situations, anxiety, depression, and other mental health conditions (Giacomucci, 2023). Psychodrama is not a manualized treatment with a step-by-step formula; instead, each session is tailored to the group, protagonist, goal, and issue at hand. The process-oriented nature of psychodrama psychotherapy allows for its adaptation to various conditions and disorders as well as the resolution of varied past traumatic experiences. Psychodrama treatment is based in the here and now and affirms the client's subjective reality, which makes it easily adaptable for any trauma-related issue. This is employed through the specific contracting or goal setting with the protagonist and the director's use of an array of psychodramatic interventions based on the client and the group's here-and-now presentation.

The psychodramatic treatment of trauma is achieved through various psychodrama interventions and group psychotherapy dynamics within the process which directly and indirectly address PTSD, complex post-traumatic stress disorder (C-PTSD), and other trauma-related symptoms. The use of sociometry and the warming-up process before the psychodrama is essential as it begins the process of accessing spontaneity while promoting safety and group cohesion. Sociometric warm-ups also offer group members opportunities for practicing social skills and titrating in and out of trauma-related emotions. Many warm-ups include an element of playfulness or humor, which helps to promote safety and connection. The warm-up helps to solidify group and individual goals while normalizing experiences and symptoms, which is particularly helpful for trauma survivors who may feel broken or alone. A sense of mutual aid, peer support, and collaboration are achieved in the warm-up while emphasizing autonomy and consent. After the warming-up process, a topic and protagonist are established from the group and a clear goal or contract is articulated between the protagonist and the director.

In trauma-informed psychodrama practices, the psychodrama scene will often begin with strength-based or supportive roles to stabilize the protagonist before enrolling trauma-based or antagonist roles. It is also quite helpful for participants new to psychodrama as it familiarizes the protagonist and the group with the psychodrama process before including more difficult roles. The use of strength-based roles promotes a sense of safety, strength, confidence, and support for the protagonist and the group while effectively offering new insights into addressing the trauma through dialogue with strength and supportive roles. For example, a client struggling to make sense of childhood neglect and trauma might choose resilience, empathy, and God as supportive roles to help them; through dialogue and role reversals with these roles, they are likely to access new action insights and meaning making related to their past trauma. Strength-based roles help to resource the protagonist and approach the trauma from a position of safety and containment which can help desensitize discussions of the trauma and renegotiate one's emotional relationship to the traumatic memory. The use of strength-based roles promotes spontaneity (developing a new response to the memory or symptoms) and mitigates symptoms of reexperiencing, avoidance, arousal, reactivity, negative cognitions or moods, emotional dysregulation, interpersonal difficulties, and negative self-concept. Some trauma-focused psychodrama sessions, especially in inpatient settings or with groups earlier in their trauma recovery journey, might only include strength-based roles in the psychodrama scene, yet still provide a very cathartic and meaningful experience for all involved. By nature of PTSD, clients are already reexperiencing and reenacting the trauma in their lives, mind, and body, therefore it is not always necessary to also reenact it with psychodrama in order to heal.

Trauma-focused psychodrama does often include revisiting roles or moments from a traumatic memory, but this must be done carefully to prevent retraumatization or harm. The use of interventions such as doubling, the mirror position, and concretization can help stabilize a protagonist (and the group) when enrolling trauma-based roles or scenes in psychodrama. It is important that the facilitator be aware of the group's capacity to tolerate discomfort and that the psychodramatic process be contained to prevent pushing the group outside of their window of tolerance (Giacomucci, 2023). One sequenced structure for trauma-related scenes is "Do-Undo-Redo," during which an aspect of the traumatic memory would be concretized in a scene, then interrupted by the protagonist, and the scene would evolve into something new with a different ending than what actually happened in the protagonist's life (Schreiber & Giacomucci, 2024). For example, a client who experienced sexual abuse might first sculpt a scene related to the memory by positioning role players to in the room to symbolically represent themself as a child, their mother who sexually abused them, and their father who did not protect them (Do). Doubling and other interventions could be used to help the protagonist express emotions related to the scene. Then, the protagonist could be supported to interrupt the scene to protect and nurture themself as a child at the time of the trauma (Undo). Scenes to follow could include standing up to their mother, confronting their father for not protecting them, and even enrolling other parent-like figures to promote a corrective emotional experience (Redo). This "Do-Undo-Redo" structure, when used carefully, is quite effective in desensitizing and reprocessing a traumatic memory while offering a new corrective experience. The re-doing aspect of this sequence can also be used without reenacting a trauma scene. This is particularly useful for clients who have experienced traumatic loss. For example, in a psychodrama focused on traumatic loss, after building up strength-based roles, the protagonist could then have a conversation with their loved one who died. This psychodramatic dialogue would give them the opportunity to say anything that was left unsaid before the death to promote closure. Next, the protagonist would role reverse and become their deceased loved one and speak to themself to promote acceptance, forgiveness, healing, closure, and meaning making.

Trauma-focused psychodrama also might involve role training to manage future situations that might be triggering or to practice implementing new growth into one's life and relationships. For instance, a client who has experienced ongoing discrimination based on their identity and developed a sense of helplessness and disempowerment joins a psychodrama group and becomes the protagonist. Their goal is to feel more empowered and not be frozen when experiencing microaggression in their workplace. One option for the psychodrama scene is to identify common scenarios of microaggressions in the workplace and use role playing to practice responding to them in new and empowered ways. Role training new responses and behaviors is an effective way to help clients integrate healing and post-traumatic growth into their lives beyond the therapy session. In psychodrama theory, PTSD or C-PTSD (or any mental illness and most social problems) would be attributed to a deficiency in spontaneity as well as an inability to access the role or role behavior associated with an adequate or new response to the internal, relational, or societal problem. Psychodrama creates change by helping clients cultivate spontaneity and new roles that promote new and suitable responses to the problems at hand.

Psychodrama allows clients to explore trauma recovery–related symptoms, memories, roles, goals, and behaviors in action instead of simply talking about them. The experiential nature of the process offers a matrix of healing for all involved. Although a psychodrama may appear to be individual therapy with a group audience, when it is facilitated by a skilled director, guided by sociometry, it maintains a group-as-a-whole focus. Participants who play roles for the protagonist or observe the psychodrama are encouraged to see themselves in the protagonist's experience and/or the other roles on stage, which prompts catharses and insight for all.

STRENGTHS AND LIMITATIONS

Sociometry, psychodrama, and group psychotherapy as outlined by Moreno and built upon by many are uniquely equipped for the treatment of trauma. Psychodrama is comprehensive, holistic, and fun. The comprehensive nature of psychodrama lends itself well to use as a metamodel, or delivery system, of many other theories, models, and approaches. It is adaptable to nearly any population, any number of people at a time, with any approaches. For example, it has been well documented as a useful approach in psycho-education, relapse prevention, and integration with other theoretical approaches including cognitive behavioral therapy, dialectical behavioral therapy, internal family systems therapy, psychoanalytic and Jungian modalities, a 12-step approach, and more (Giacomucci, 2021). Additionally, it has many more nonclinical applications (education, advocacy, social justice work, and more) than other modalities, and is regularly applied in other spaces beyond psychotherapy (Giacomucci, 2021).

Like most therapeutic approaches, it's not without its shortcomings and risks. The same spontaneity, adaptability, and freedom of psychodrama that creates healing and safety also has the potential to be unpredictable and harmful. Because it is nearly impossible to manu-alize, becoming competent in psychodrama takes many more hours of training than other models, and is not easy to integrate until one becomes a more advanced director. The complexity of choices and interventions from moment-to-moment create high potential for retraumatization and harm if a director doesn't have a firm basis in trauma-informed care principles, safety, and containment within group work. Encounter group culture, T-groups, therapeutic communities, and other psychodrama-adjacent groups run by lay-men in the 1980s and 1990s became infamous for an overemphasis on catharsis and anger, creating a negative reputation of psychodrama. The long training process can be daunting, complicated, and expensive for the average clinician to pursue full certification as a psy-chodrama practitioner (which requires 780 training hours), especially within the managed-care landscape of treatment where quicker models are preferred by agencies. As a result of this, it's hard to find both psychodrama groups for clients and psychodrama trainings within the United States as compared to other countries. There's much speculation around why this is, but most conclude it's a result of the direct challenges from psychodrama to the dominant cultural medicalization of psychotherapy and individualism that is present in American culture and modern treatment contexts (Giacomucci, 2021).

The continued growth and application of this model will depend on its continued integration by creative and daring clinicians and trainers across the country, integration with trauma-informed and trauma-focused psychotherapeutic principles, and subtle, slow paradigm shifts toward more collectively minded healing. This shift matches the trends on the cutting edge of therapy practice where experiential models are undergoing a resurgence and rediscovery.

ADDITIONAL RESOURCES FOR LEARNING (ALSO SEE REFERENCE LIST)

SUGGESTED BOOKS

- Chesner, A. (Ed.). (2019). *One-to-one psychodrama psychotherapy: Applications and technique*. Routledge.
- Dayton, T. (2022). *Sociometrics: Embodied, Experiential Processes for Relational Trauma Repair*. Central Recovery Press.
- Giacomucci, S. (2023). *Trauma-informed Principles in Group Therapy, Psychodrama, and Organizations: Action Methods for Leadership*. Taylor & Francis.
- Hudgins, K., & Durost, S. W. (2022). *Experiential Therapy from Trauma to Post-traumatic Growth: Therapeutic Spiral Model Psychodrama*. Springer Nature.
- Moreno, J. D. (2014). *Impromptu Man: J.L. Moreno and the Origins of Psychodrama, Encounter Culture, and the Social Network*. Bellevue Literary Press.

SUGGESTED WEBSITES

- American Society of Group Psychotherapy & Psychodrama – www.ASGPP.org
- American Board of Examiners in Sociometry, Psychodrama, & Group Psychotherapy – www.PsychodramaCertification.org

SUGGESTED VIDEO RESOURCES

- Action Explorations online psychodrama courses – www.actionexplorations.education
- YouTube channels with free psychodrama educational content include the following:
  - Action Explorations – https://www.youtube.com/@ActionExplorations
  - American Society of Group Psychotherapy & Psychodrama (ASGPP) – https://www.youtube.com/@asgpppsychodrama9847/videos
  - Phoenix Trauma Center & Dr. Scott Giacomucci – https://www.youtube.com/@PhoenixTraumaCenter
  - Sergio Guimaraes – https://www.youtube.com/@sguimaraes100
  - Tian Dayton – https://www.youtube.com/@tiandayton6150

REFERENCES

Baker, F.A., Metcalf, O., Varker, T., & O'Donnell, M. (2018). A systematic review of the efficacy of creative arts therapies in the treatment of adults with PTSD. *Psychological Trauma: Theory, Research, Practice, and Policy, 10*(6), 643.

Berne, E. (1970). A review of gestalt therapy verbatim. *American Journal of Psychiatry, 126*(10), 164.

Borgatta, E. (1950). The use of psychodrama, sociodrama and related techniques in social psychological research. *Sociometry, 13*(3), 244–258.

Elliott, R., Watson, J., Greenberg, L.S., Timulak, L., & Freire, E. (2013). Research on humanistic-experiential psychotherapies. In M.J. Lambert (Ed.), *Bergin & Garfield's Handbook of psychotherapy and behavior change* (6th ed.) (pp. 495–538). Wiley.

Giacomucci, S. (2021). *Social Work, Sociometry, and Psychodrama: Experiential Approaches for Group Therapists, Community Leaders, and Social Workers* (p. 435). Springer Nature.

Giacomucci, S. (2023). *Trauma-informed Principles in Group Therapy, Psychodrama, and Organizations: Action Methods for Leadership*. Taylor & Francis.

Moreno, J.L. (1934). *Who Shall Survive? A New Approach to The Problems of Human Interrelations*. Washington, DC: Nervous and Mental Disease Publishing Co.

Moreno, J.L. (1964). *Psychodrama, first volume* (3 ed.). Beacon, NY: Beacon House Press

Orkibi, H., & Feniger-Schaal, R. (2019). Integrative systematic review of psychodrama psychotherapy research: Trends and methodological implications. *PloS One, 14*(2), e0212575.

Orkibi, H., Keisari, S., Sajnani, N.L., & de Witte, M. (2023). Effectiveness of drama-based therapies on mental health outcomes: A systematic review and meta-analysis of controlled studies. *Psychology of Aesthetics, Creativity, and the Arts*.

Schreiber, E. & Giacomucci, S. (2024). Psychodrama, Sociodrama, Sociometry, and Sociatry (Section 32.2). In B.J. Sadock, V.A. Sadock, & P. Ruiz (Eds.), *Kaplan and Sadock's Comprehensive Textbook of Psychiatry* (11th ed.) Wolters Kluwer.

Schultz, W.C. (1971). *Here Comes Everybody*. New York: Harrow Books.

van de Kamp, M.M., Scheffers, M., Hatzmann, J., Emck, C., Cuijpers, P., & Beek, P.J. (2019). Body-and movement-oriented interventions for posttraumatic stress disorder: A systematic review and meta-analysis. *Journal of Traumatic Stress, 32*(6), 967–976.

3

CHAPTER 3
GESTALT THERAPY AND TREATMENT OF TRAUMA

Alan Cohen

INTRODUCTION

This chapter discusses the theoretical premises and clinical interventions of Gestalt therapy, as it is applied to working with trauma victims. Through attending to experiential elements of creative adjustment, present centered contact ("contact boundary"), self/world construction, contact interruption, somatic experience, field theory, and organismic self-regulation, this chapter will illustrate both how trauma experiences are processed and how they result in symptomatic experience. This will be the basis for exploring a treatment approach for treating individuals impacted by trauma utilizing Gestalt therapy. Verbatim case examples will be provided to illustrate the relational implementation of this experiential approach for two major forms of trauma (acute "shock/incident" trauma, and "complex/developmental" trauma) with four progressive stages of treatment demonstrated.

BRIEF HISTORY

Gestalt therapy was developed by Fritz Perls, MD, PhD and his wife, Lore Perls, PhD, in the late 1940s, and appeared in publication in the book *Gestalt Therapy: Excitement and Growth in the Human Personality* by Fritz Perls, Ralph Hefferline, and Paul Goodman (1951). Fritz Perls originally trained as a Freudian psychoanalyst and shared a background in Gestalt psychology (a research-oriented approach that sought to understand how human perception works) with Lore. These two approaches to human experience formed a basis to their new approach. Other strong influences were body oriented psychoanalysis (Wilhelm Reich), existentialist philosophy (Husserl, Heidegger, Merleau-Ponty, and Sartre), social field theory (Kurt Lewin), relational dialogue (Martin Buber), psychodrama (Jacob Moreno), and Zen Buddhism (Bowman, 2005). All of these influences were synthesized into an approach that emphasized experiential awareness in the present as the foundation of mental health and the interruption of this process of present-centered contact as the basis of psychopathology.

Fritz Perls was particularly dissatisfied with psychoanalysis, due to its rigidity of thought, its authoritarian/hierarchical relationship between patient and therapist, and its neglect of the present (the only point in time in which change is possible) while exploring the past (Yontef, 1993). In the 1940s Fritz and Lore developed another approach, which kept some of the important contributions of psychoanalysis but integrated thought and technique

DOI: 10.4324/9781003455851-3

which would focus more on awareness than insight; highlight experience over under-standing; create a more horizontal, less hierarchical therapist/client relationship; and focus on the human capacity to grow and self-regulate given sufficient awareness and support. Fritz initially called this approach concentration therapy in his first book, *Ego, Hunger, and Aggression*, and later Gestalt therapy, with the publication of his second book (Bowman & Bowman, 2022).

During the counterculture movement of the 1960s, Gestalt therapy flourished in the United States, where a focus on growth, freedom, and unlimited possibilities was part of the zeitgeist. It allowed and encouraged people to cast off their "shoulds" as a way of navigating and seek a sense of their own personal meaning in order to find a fulfilling way of living. But by the late 1960s, some of the "no holds barred" approach in some Gestalt therapy workshops began to give Gestalt therapy a bad name in the therapeutic commu-nity (Winitsky, 2022). This has diminished the popularity of this approach in the United States, despite Gestalt therapy having readjusted to its initial ground of phenomenological and relational investigation. But, while Gestalt therapy has been relegated to the back-ground in the United States, it has become a primary approach in Europe, Asia, South America, and the Middle East (Bowman, 2005). Ironically, this is largely the result of Fritz having initiated Gestalt therapy trainings in Europe beginning in 1969. These training conferences have continued to the present and trained thousands of therapists, who have in turn opened training institutes in many countries. In Europe, therapists can earn university degrees in Gestalt therapy and be licensed as such.

FUNDAMENTAL CLINICAL CONCEPTS

The basic unit of awareness is *Contact*. Gestalt therapy defines Contact as the awareness of some element of the Environmental Field, or the world. Where the person and the world engage is referred to as the *Contact Boundary*. This is where the person's awareness "meets" their needed aspect of the environment (Mann, 2021). This boundary is constantly chang-ing and defines how the person experiences their "self." This includes our bodies (sensa-tions, emotions, needs), as well as the world outside our skin. In healthy circumstances this Contact is always changing, is focused on the present, and allows us to navigate according to our needs for comfort and growth, and our concern for danger. When we are aware of a need, we can then engage the world in a manner that can satisfy the need. When we are in contact with danger, we can mobilize our energies to flee or fight (take action) in order to preserve ourselves.

The choices of action that we make in meeting our needs or preserving our safety are what Gestalt therapy calls *Creative Adjustment*. This is defined as the way in which the person chooses to engage, defend, or flee such that the situation is resolved and the need is satisfied (Wheeler, 1991). Some examples would be noticing the sensation of thirst and reaching for a cold glass of water; feeling lonely and reaching out to a friend; feeling too hot in the blazing sun and finding some shade; or being aware of an upcoming exam and sitting down to study. All of these examples indicate the person's capacity to notice a need and "take care of it" so that it is resolved: The thirst is quenched, the loneliness is replaced by a feeling of warmth and connection, the body temperature is regulated, and the person assimilates the knowledge that will prepare them for the test. Once taken care of, the person can move on to the next emerging need or interest, without concern for what had been "figural" (the *figure* being the object of awareness that represents the need). This process allows us to preserve ourselves and to grow, since growth involves the capacity to notice ourselves, notice the current resources of the world that would add to our capacity, and to engage in a manner that allows us to take what is new and make it a part of ourselves. Likewise, the figure of a mosquito buzzing in our ear is resolved by an artful swat. The need is resolved and dissipates, no longer a figural concern. This process can only occur in the present, where there is Contact and Creative Adjustment. In Gestalt therapy theory, we consider that a healthy person ("organism") thus self-regulates, and orients toward growth (Latner, 1986). Growth is seen as the contact with that which is not yet part of the person (an experience, a capacity, knowledge, etc.) in a manner that deepens or expands the person's capacities and their sense of self. We seek to find what we need to maintain ourselves, but then also what we need to grow. Gestalt therapists posit that growth is an innate drive, from the moment of birth, and continues throughout life, unless contact with the person's own experience, or elements of the external world are interrupted – or the actual conditions require a heightened focus on survival (e.g. war, famine, abuse, or natural disaster).

When we are unable to Creatively Adjust, to resolve the need or the danger in the situation, we do two things: We take whatever action we are capable of to "manage" the situation in the absence of our capacity to "resolve" the situation; and we interrupt contact with ourselves (our bodily feelings and emotions) and/or with the environment. That is, we take emergency action. For example, if we are unable to stand up to a bully (in the family or in the schoolyard), we may become skilled at humor in an attempt to "deflect" attention. Or we may turn our aggression against ourselves (i.e. physically tighten or have self-attacking thoughts) rather than risk expressing our aggression to our antagonist. (This turning against the self is referred to as *retroflection*.) Or we may diminish our awareness of our pain by deadening or dissociating from our bodily sensations. So, in the absence of being able to remove the source of pain, we remove our capacity to notice the pain. When we need to make these maneuvers in acute situations or chronic situations, these strategies tend to become ongoing ways of being and relating, largely out of our awareness. They become interruptions to contact, and are habitual, unaware, and acontextual (i.e. they persist long after the situation that required this way of managing has passed). They are "adjustments" or "adaptations" rather than Creative Adjustments. The accumulation of these fixed ways of orienting and acting restrict our lives, since our fluid ongoing contact with ourselves and the world is interrupted without our awareness and is substituted with chronic ways of "managing" and numbing. The "emergency measures" that were taken in the absence of the capacity, support, or resources to resolve a problem become preserved and repeated, as if the person is still managing the original situation with limited resources (e.g. being a child who does not have the strength and/or the cognitive capacities to comprehend and/or defend themselves). This is a rigidified way of being without awareness – either of the elements in the actual present, or of the repetition of the "unfinished" past.

A basic premise of Gestalt psychology and of Gestalt therapy is that situations or experiences that have not been resolved remain "unfinished" and keep pressing for completion (Sills et al., 2012). This is seen as a healthy drive to find need satisfaction, completion, and wholeness. So, the "adjustment" someone makes to manage a situation does not resolve it, and the situation and the need keep "pressing" for completion (via a new Creative Adjustment). But this healthy process (i.e. the need seeking completion and satisfaction) is interrupted by the old adaptations, or "*fixed gestalts*," leading to a repetition of the historic failure (Mann, 2021). Therefore, themes keep emerging and repeating, only to be dealt with as one had to when one was less capable and the world was less supportive and/or more hostile. The past keeps "intruding" into the present. This creates the symptoms that generally bring the person into the therapy situation: Anxiety, depression, and difficulty satisfyingly managing our interactions with others and the world.

DESCRIPTION OF THE THERAPY PROCESS

Gestalt therapy is what is referred to as an "experiential" therapy. Gestalt therapists distinguish between cognition (thinking about something, often from a somewhat removed point of view), and *contact*, which is an immediate experience in the present, usually involving the senses. While cognition involves generalizations based on past learning and future forecasting, contact is open to the novelty and specificity of the present moment. So, the Gestalt therapist will seek to draw the patient's attention to the present. An example might be:

PATIENT:	"My son fell this week and slammed his head. We had to rush him to the ER."
THERAPIST:	"That sounds frightening. But I notice that as you are telling me, you seem fairly expressionless, and you are looking away. Could you tell me while looking at me?"
PATIENT:	Looks at therapist and sees a look of compassion, and bursts into tears.
THERAPIST:	"Can you say what just happened?"
PATIENT:	"When I saw the concern on your face, I felt surprised. I've been holding myself together, but your caring allowed me to let go. I always feel like I'm in it by myself."

In this vignette, we see that the description of the emergency alone would not have changed the patient's emotional state. Contact with the therapist's expression, however allowed for the experience of support, so the patient no longer needed to "hold herself together." This was not a cognitive decision, but rather a felt response to the experience of the therapist's compassion. It also highlighted for the patient her belief that she has to live in the absence of support.

The Gestalt therapist is therefore engaged in being with their patient in a way that can support them in noticing their present experience while bringing awareness to ways in which they are inhibiting contact. And since fixed beliefs (*introjects*) like "I have to be in it by myself" interfere with the person's ability to see the support that may actually be available, the Gestalt therapist may want to explore how this may be related to earlier life experiences:

THERAPIST:	"How old were you when you first remember having that thought?"
PATIENT:	"I remember being four when my brother Jake was born. He had a lot of medical problems, and my parents were completely focused on him. I guess I learned to take care of myself and not be a bother. That's what I got praise for. As I grew up Jake's problems continued and I became more practiced at being self-sufficient, and was told that made me special."
THERAPIST:	"You were so very young to have to learn to not need anyone's support! Could you visualize the scene you just described and tell me what you see?"
PATIENT:	"There's a machine by Jake's bed. I think it's to help him breathe. And my parents are huddled over him."
THERAPIST:	"And where are you? I don't hear you in the picture."
PATIENT:	"Oh. I almost didn't notice. I see myself standing in the doorway."
THERAPIST:	"What would you want to say to yourself?"
PATIENT:	"Don't be a bother."
THERAPIST:	(seeking to enhance contact with this historical self) "Can you see what her expression is when you say that to her?"
PATIENT:	Pauses to look. "She looks so sad!"
THERAPIST:	"What happens to you when you see that?"
PATIENT:	"I want to comfort her." Imagines holding her, feels tearful.
THERAPIST:	"From this place, what do you now want to say to her?"
PATIENT:	"You are a little girl and you deserve to be held, even if Jake is sick. You still need to be taken care of."
THERAPIST:	"Can you see what it's like to be that little girl now?"
PATIENT:	(cries while feeling held) "I'm sad, but I'm not alone now."

In this piece of experiential work, the patient and therapist return to a point in time that was imprinted on the patient. In the original circumstance the patient had to "make do" with being praised for her self-sufficiency. But in this work the patient was able to bring resources (i.e. her adult understanding and her compassion) that weren't present or available at the time. And that led to a different experience of what was possible. As one more step, returning to the situation with her son, the Gestalt therapist might ask the patient to look at him again and try on saying: "I'm very sad and still scared about my son, and your caring helps me not have to feel alone." When a Gestalt therapist suggests that a patient "try on" a statement, it is not for the sake of giving an interpretation or an explanation; it is for the patient to notice viscerally what resonates as true and, perhaps, what doesn't. So, the patient may try on the statement and then say "I still feel alone, but much less alone."

With respect to human functioning, Gestalt therapists posit that change can only occur through contact with direct experience. Contact is seen as essential to healthy functioning (i.e. awareness of a need and the current environmental conditions). In Gestalt therapy, fluidity of self is conceptualized as a healthy capacity to respond to internal needs or external circumstance in a manner that accounts for the actual current situation. Rigidly fixed ideas and unaware interruptions to contact are seen as a basis for unhealthy functioning. A Gestalt therapist is, therefore, interested in understanding the person's difficulties, while also being interested in helping them to notice (become aware of) how they are or aren't in contact with themselves and with the world. For example, the patient might begin by telling the therapist about a fight with his spouse.

PATIENT:	"Joanne and I had a bad fight last night. She's always worrying about money, and asking if I remembered to pay all the bills. I just had it and went off on her. Are all women so critical? Anyway, it didn't end well."
THERAPIST:	"Sam, I notice that when you tell me about your fight you are clenching your jaw. Are you aware of this?"
PATIENT:	"Huh, no."
THERAPIST:	"Well, could you notice now?"
PATIENT:	"Yeah, I'm clenching pretty tight!"
THERAPIST:	"Could you see what it's like for you to tell me again 'Joanne and I had a bad fight' and relax your jaw?"
PATIENT:	(does so and states) "I feel sad."
THERAPIST:	"Could you visualize Joanne and imagine telling her that you're sad about what happened between you?"
PATIENT:	Closes his eyes and does so. After a minute he opens his eyes and says to the therapist "I really love her and maybe I have to learn to not take her worry so personally."

The experience of feeling his sadness and bringing it into contact with his partner shifts the experience from one of detachment and intellectualization to one of noticing "how" he is holding his emotion out of awareness (keeping himself from being in contact with his felt emotion), and then to feeling the emotion (releasing the "retroflection"), and finally, bringing the emotion into relational contact with the partner. The emotion of sadness can then lead to contacting the need to repair the relational rupture and to opening a dialogue that offers and asks for vulnerability. Further, the Gestalt therapist may consider that this clenching against feeling or revealing sadness may be an old adaptation ("failed" creative adjustment). The therapist might be curious about the observed habitual response and ask: "Is this clenching against your sadness familiar?" or "How old do you feel when you have to clench your jaw to hide your vulnerability?" Remember that two principles of Gestalt therapy are operative here: 1) that situations that are not resolved or completed live on in their emotional valence; and 2) the strategies that one was forced to utilize become habitual and reified (frozen and out of awareness). If we help our patient to take the time to notice the feeling of clenching against sadness (deepened awareness, since in the therapy session the clenching is now connected to its purpose) along with the accompanying bodily sensations and any imagery or memories that arise, our patient might then say "I feel like a seven-year-old boy whose father expected him to 'toughen up' and 'be a man.'" Whereas that might be something to discuss and analyze in more cognitive or analytic approaches, in Gestalt therapy we prefer to re-engage in the contact that was unresolved. So, we might ask our patient:

THERAPIST:	"Could you visualize your father as he was then and see what you might want to say to him now?"
PATIENT:	(With eyes closed) "I can begin to get an image, but I'm starting to feel afraid."
THERAPIST:	"What do you see that's scary?"
PATIENT:	"Dad looks very stern."
THERAPIST:	"Could you say 'Dad, you frighten me?"
PATIENT:	"He looks confused!"
THERAPIST:	"What might he say about his confusion?"
PATIENT:	(As father) "I don't want to frighten you, but I don't want you to get hurt. The world can be hard, and I want to teach you to protect yourself."

Now we want our patient to notice his response. He may feel surprised by the caring that his father could not show him directly, or angered that his father expected this of him before it was needed or could make sense to him. In either case, the Gestalt therapist would support the patient to continue the dialogue until there was some more clarity and resolution, therefore helping the patient complete the unfinished situation, derive more meaning (or revise the meaning that a seven-year-old boy could decipher), and to find a new relationship to his own vulnerability. Gestalt therapy posits that the direct experience in a session of the "wounding situation" has a more profound affect than helping the person to cognitively understand the possible causes of his patterns. This allows the patient to bring their current resources and supports to the wounding situation, relationship, or circumstance. Likewise, we might help the person orient to a healing situation or relationship that they have lost contact with. A question like "Who comforted you when you were young?" might bring back a memory of a grandparent who died when the patient was five. But the memory can be re-engaged in a similar way by asking "How did he/she comfort you?" The patient may recall a warm lap and being read to or the smell of a flannel blanket. In any case, re-engaging these sensory memories experientially can help our patient to find a capacity to comfort themselves, and to revive a feeling of a safe, loving relationship.

UTILIZATION OF THIS METHOD FOR TREATING TRAUMA

While Gestalt therapy with a less psychologically wounded population is relatively unstructured – working with the process of what becomes figural for the patient and helping them become aware of how they deal with their experience – working with victims of trauma calls for a more structured application of Gestalt therapy principles. The severity of their symptoms, their dissociation from sensory experience, and their heightened sense of danger require a sequence of steps in the repair and restoration of healthy self-regulation. Trauma is seen as an experience that is so severely frightening, painful, or damaging that the person cannot "creatively adjust" (i.e. deal with the situation in a manner that resolves the problem). As we have seen in the preceding section, the inability to creatively adjust can be part of most peoples' experience. The feeling or need keeps pressing for completion, but remains largely out of awareness and dislocated from the origins of the experience. The same mechanism is at work with victims of trauma: The original situation is too severe or massive to be negotiated or "metabolized," and the person automatically (i.e. largely without conscious thought or intent) takes emergency action. This includes disassociating from bodily feelings (if the source of the pain cannot be managed the mechanism for feeling the pain is to "shut off" – akin to a circuit breaker), as well as a feeling of detachment and/or hyper-vigilance (including chronically heightened levels of "stress hormones" secreted in the fight/flight/freeze situation). Thus, the survival mechanisms seek to block the experience of pain and detach from the dangerous situation, while maintaining a heightened awareness of a recurrence of the danger. It can be seen in this that these survival maneuvers are remarkably healthy reactions to a severely threatening and overwhelming situation. But these responses remain locked in place, even when the original situation has passed.

There are two basic subtypes of trauma victims: Acute "shock trauma," and "developmental/complex trauma." Shock trauma refers to having been exposed to horrendous one-time situations like being present at the World Trade Center on 911, being in a car crash that killed one's child, being assaulted, experiencing a natural disaster, or being in war (the original term given soldiers with these symptoms was "shell shock," later replaced by PTSD). Developmental/complex trauma refers to having experienced ongoing physical, sexual, and psychological abuse or abandonment as part of one's early childhood development.

Both sub-types of trauma are debilitating, cause ongoing suffering, and prevent one's ability to move forward with their lives. They are literally stuck, repetitively re-experiencing the horrendous feelings and seeing no respite in the present. Victims of developmental/complex trauma have been denied the possibility of developing a healthy personality, marked by caring relationships, a strong sense of self, and a capacity to navigate the world in a nuanced way. Also, their perpetrators are most often family members, who developmentally represent the world and are seen to be sources of empathy, comfort, and protection. Victims of acute/shock trauma (when the trauma occurs in adulthood) have often been able to develop a relatively healthy sense of themselves and the world prior to the trauma, but also get stuck in the lockdown and disassociation common to both groups.

Both groups, while needing somewhat different consideration, are well treated by Gestalt therapy. Gestalt therapists value the authenticity of the "I-Thou" relationship; the empathic, grounding relationship with the therapist is essential to this work, particularly with people who have never been able to develop stable, trusting relationships with another person. But with the "acute" victim as well, the chronic experience of fear and danger is well served by the presence of an emphatic, safe other. Both types of trauma survivors are living in a state of constant fear and (paradoxically) detachment. Both need to go slowly, in developing a feeling of safety in the therapeutic relationship, as well as finding ways ("tools") for creating a bodily feeling approaching calm. Without this emphasis early in the therapeutic process, the patient will either not be available (shut down), or will engage prematurely, leaving their automatic responses to take over (fight/flight/freeze). Gestalt therapists use a variety of interventions such as attention to the breath, developing soothing bodily sensations, guided imagery of nature in which the senses are engaged ("can you smell the salt water and feel the breeze on your face?"), noticing the safety of the therapy room, and learning to meditate, as well as other creative approaches.

Gestalt therapy was influenced by Zen Buddhism, with its emphasis on present centered awareness. Many Gestalt therapists utilize a form of mindfulness meditation, involving noticing the breath and allowing thoughts to pass while taking a position of observing the thoughts rather than reacting to them. This develops a capacity to notice without reactivity. It can be particularly helpful to utilize Transcendental Meditation, in which the process is one of "following" a mental/sub-vocal sound and letting thoughts pass unobserved. This tends to lead to an experience of being present with no particular thoughts and can promote a pleasant experience of calm and openness. This also allows the nervous system to "reset," replacing stress-based brain wave patterns with increased alpha wave production, reducing cortisol production, and allowing the mind to be alert while the body is at rest.

In all of these interventions, helping our patient to learn how to reorient to the safety available in the present is an essential first step in the work. These "tools" can be taught in the therapy session, but also practiced outside of the session. While phases of Gestalt therapy treatment for trauma are delineated in the following sections, it must be remembered that the work will not strictly fit into these categories and must be adjusted to fit the current needs and phenomenology of the individual client at each point in the therapy process.

PHASE 1

In the initial phase of the treatment, we begin to introduce the experience of the senses, primarily sensations in the body. Since many individuals who have experienced trauma have largely dissociated from bodily feelings in an attempt to mitigate the experience of pain, we begin with reintroducing sensory experience. In Gestalt therapy theory, we see the capacity to notice needs and to contact the present as dependent on awareness of sensory cues (e.g. the rumbling in my belly informs me of my hunger; the gentle breeze on my face or the smell of fresh cut grass may elicit feelings of soothing). We refer to this as "Fore-Contact," the attunement to the sensory cues that our body conveys and receives. With dissociated states, there is little or no current experiential information, and so the felt memory of the traumatic situation is preserved. The present, however, is likely safer and more reliable than the traumatic situation, and so contact with the body and the present moment will tend to not only restore healthy self-function, but also convey sensory information which allows for an experience of safety.

An example might be:

THERAPIST: "Can you tell me what you're aware of in your body?"
PATIENT: "Nothing much."

THERAPIST:	"Would you be willing to notice how you are breathing?"
PATIENT:	(pays attention) "I'm hardly breathing at all."
THERAPIST:	"Could you put your hand on your belly and let your breath go deeper?"
PATIENT:	(Does this for a few breaths)
THERAPIST:	"What do you notice?"
PATIENT:	"I feel my body more. And a bit calmer."

Breathing is a primary mechanism for the body to feel sensation, so shutting off feeling involves minimizing breath. When we help people to notice the breathing inhibition (which has become chronic and out of awareness), it allows them the possibility of reinstating contact with the body in current circumstances. Contact with other senses (sight, sound, smell, taste, touch/movement) will also begin to restore the person's contact with the (safer) present.

THERAPIST:	"Could you look around the room and find a pleasing object or color?"
OR:	"Could you rub your hand on your arm in a soothing way (while you breathe)?"
OR:	"Do you notice the chair holding your weight?"

Questions like these that draw the patient's attention to their sensory experience of the present can enable their capacity to experience the support of their body and (gingerly) of the environment. The experience of noticing the chair holding them up may be novel, since there is likely a belief and expectation that "there is no support outside of my skin."

PHASE 2

Once there is some establishment of an *experience* of support in and around the body, the focus can expand to include making the presence of the therapist more figural. The interest, empathy, and reliability of the therapist has been present through Phase 1, but has been more of a background element. Now the explicit awareness of the presence and trustworthiness of the therapist will be essential to doing further work:

PATIENT:	(To the therapist) "I don't even know why I'm coming here, when you're too busy to care."
THERAPIST:	"When you look at me right now as I sit with you, tell me what you see."
PATIENT:	(Refocuses her eyes, and seems confused) "You look very present and warm."
THERAPIST:	"You looked confused when you first looked at me".
PATIENT:	"Yeah. I wasn't seeing you. I was seeing all the folks who were supposed to care but were full of it"
THERAPIST:	"Then what's it like for you to see me?"

PATIENT: "It's confusing, and it's hard to trust this feeling, but I feel safer and less alone."

Helping the patient to have the experience of seeing creates the possibility of a slight shift in her way of predefining things and others (as unsafe and unreliable). Again, this becomes a basis for finding safety in this frightening journey of revisiting the original trauma in a way that can provide healing.

PHASE 3

As the patient begins to develop trust in the therapeutic relationship (based on the consistency, transparency, and empathic responsiveness of the therapist), it becomes possible to revisit the original trauma. This is a delicate process, again, since a premature exposure can re-traumatize the patient. The support of the therapeutic relationship, learning to find safety in one's sensorium, and learning healthy ways to disengage without disassociating need to be "figural" (i.e. present in the foreground) during the next phase of the work.

THERAPIST: "Could we start with noticing your breath and your weight in the chair? (Pause for patient to engage). And could you look around the room while you breathe and say what you see?"
PATIENT: "I see the rug, the lamp, the color of the walls ..."
THERAPIST: "And what's that like for you?"
PATIENT: "The room looks safe, and I feel a little calmer."
THERAPIST: "And as you breathe can you look at me?"
PATIENT: "That feels harder."
THERAPIST: "Could you peek?"
PATIENT: Pauses, then peeks. "You look friendly."
THERAPIST: "From this place – this safe room, your breath and body, my friendly presence – are you ready to look back to what happened? You can just peek and then come back here again."
PATIENT: Pauses, looks at therapist, then closes her eyes for a moment, then opens them.
THERAPIST: "You're back. Look around this room and breathe. Can you tell me what happened when you closed your eyes?"
PATIENT: "I didn't see much ... the color of my old room ... and I felt scared (cries)."
THERAPIST: "It was very scary back then. Now you're here and you're safe. Can you notice that?"

The therapist looks to slowly build a tolerance (i.e. develop sufficient support) to allow the patient to begin to re-contact the original situation. It is very important to develop the experience of safety first, and then to notice (i.e. contact) the experience of safety that awaits upon her return. During this entire process the therapist may make observations or suggestions, but will always defer to the patient's readiness, honoring the capacity to say "no," "not yet," or "not so much." We also have to educate the patient to their capacity to say "no," since this may have been taken away from them early in their traumatic past.

This phase of the treatment is slow and incremental. The powerful painful feelings that were shut down need to be experienced and digested from the safety of the present. Horror, grief, anger, and guilt must be noticed and attended to with the therapist's compassion, so that the patient can begin to learn how to feel that compassion for herself. Meanings that the patient has learned as a result of the trauma (e.g. "I am worthless," "there is no safety," "it's all my fault") must be re-assessed in light of the renewed contact and the context of the present. During this phase the therapist must maintain a heightened attunement to the patient's readiness and capacity to remain in contact and must help the patient to be able to disengage in a manner that allows them to find safety and comfort, rather than fleeing to dissociation.

PHASE 4

As the work in the first three phases begins to consolidate, attention can be directed to the patient's current life circumstances and relationships. The revision of meanings and beliefs that were taken from the traumatic experience will need to be applied and tried out. Coming back into the present with a perspective that includes the pain of the past as well as the possibilities of the present will be necessary to consolidate the work and to allow the patient to create a life that feels true and has meaning and satisfaction.

ASSESSMENT OF RESEARCH EVIDENCE

While therapy modalities that can be systemically manualized (e.g. cognitive behavioral therapy, motivational interviewing, EMDR) tend to attract people in academia who are oriented toward quantitative research, Gestalt therapy tends to attract therapists who are more oriented to focusing on the experiential nature of their work in their clinical settings. Therefore, although there is a significant body of Gestalt therapy research, it is less extensive than some other therapy modalities. In this regard, there is unfortunately a paucity of research regarding Gestalt therapy as a treatment for PTSD. One exception to this is the work of Willi Butollo, a German psychologist, who with his colleagues compared the long-term effectiveness of a modified form of Gestalt therapy called dialogical exposure therapy (DET) to a type of cognitive behavioral therapy called cognitive processing therapy (CPT) in treating individuals with PTSD as a result of acute trauma in adulthood (Butollo et al., 2016; König et al., 2018). At the end of the study period and at two-year follow-up, the two methods were roughly equivalent in their effectiveness. However, at follow-up, the younger patients in the CPT group profited more from treatment than the older ones, whereas there was no such difference in the DET group. Another study in Iran examined the effectiveness of Gestalt therapy on war veterans and found it to be effective in reducing symptoms of PTSD (Nazari et al. 2014). As previously discussed, Transcendental Meditation can be incorporated into trauma treatment in Gestalt therapy as a therapeutic adjunct. Studies with diverse populations have indicated the effectiveness of utilizing Transcendental Meditation for this purpose (Nestor et al., 2023; Nidich et al., 2016; Rees et al., 2013).

CASE EXAMPLE

In this section, a case example of working with acute (shock) trauma from a Gestalt therapy lens is presented. Scott was a 29-year-old man who came to therapy with symptoms of panic attacks, sleeplessness, inability to focus his thoughts, profuse sweating, and loss of interest in eating, social contact, and other forms of pleasure. He had been living alone in a small cottage near a beach when the "superstorm" Hurricane Sandy made landfall. He had not evacuated, not realizing the strength of the storm and the seriousness of the impending danger. When the storm hit, it was too late to leave, and he decided to ride out the storm in his cottage, to near-disastrous results.

THERAPIST:	"Hi Scott. What brings you here?"
SCOTT:	(Body tense and eyes darting around the room) "I've never been to therapy before. But since the storm I haven't been myself. I can't eat, I can't sleep, and a lot of the time I can hardly breathe."
THERAPIST:	(Asks some questions to get a sense of the context and onset of Scott's symptoms, and a brief developmental history) "I see that life was going along pretty well for you before the storm hit?"
SCOTT:	"I had some things I was trying to work out, but for the most part life was good."
THERAPIST:	"Then we can pay attention to what happened, is that ok?"
SCOTT:	"I just want to stop feeling like I'm about to die."
THERAPIST:	"Well, it sounds like you were about to die, but can you look around the room and see if you're safe now?"
SCOTT:	"I know it's safe here, but that doesn't help."
THERAPIST:	"Of course, your body is still back there in the danger. But let's spend some time here, to help your body arrive. Is that okay?"

Therapist works with Scott to develop somatic contact with sensory input. Works with developing awareness of breath, bodily sensation, visual contact, and interpersonal safety.

THERAPIST:	"Would you be ready, from the safety of this room, to return to the scene?"
SCOTT:	"I'm a bit freaked out about returning there in any way. But, how would we do this?"
THERAPIST:	"As you sit in your chair (reference to current sensory awareness) could you envision the inside of your cottage as Sandy is approaching and tell me (anchors Scott to current relationship) what you are experiencing."
SCOTT:	(Closes eyes) "The wind is loud, very loud. I'm thinking I made a big mistake by staying."
THERAPIST:	"Okay, can you open your eyes and look around the room? Can you breathe?"
SCOTT:	"I'm glad to be back (smiles). It's scary there."
THERAPIST:	"You can stay here as long as you'd like. We don't have to do more today, only if you want to and feel ready."

The work proceeds with attunement and consideration on the part of the therapist. Scott is given control over his "dosing," even allowing for sessions that don't involve sensorily returning to the cottage. Trauma victims have experienced a frightening loss of control in the trauma situation, so the therapist strives to reinstate the patient's sense of control in this process.

(SUBSEQUENT SESSION)

THERAPIST:	"All right, if you're ready we can go back."
SCOTT:	"I know I have to if I'm going to get over this."
THERAPIST:	"As you close your eyes to return, could you tell me 'Alan, now I'm experiencing this …'" (The therapist is continuing to anchor the patient in the present through their relationship and by using his name. The patient can feel both anchored to the present and not alone in the past.)
SCOTT:	"Okay. Alan, the house is shaking and I'm scared. Alan, the wind just blew out the glass in the window, and I'm hiding behind the bed."
THERAPIST:	"Okay Scott, could you return to this room now?"

The therapist and patient continue to work through the entire experience in this way. The emotions that are evoked in Scott during this work are acknowledged and given support. Scott is helped to learn how to allow himself to experience his emotions while he comforts himself with his breath, his touch, and with the support of the therapeutic relationship. They arrive at Scott's realization that he endured the terror and that he survived. Deep tears of self-compassion and gratitude emerge, are acknowledged and understood, and are supported empathically. At this point the work can turn more toward consolidation. In a subsequent session, Scott reports: "I drove past the old bungalow a few days ago and for the first time I didn't feel panic. I felt some sadness, but I also felt alive."

STRENGTHS AND LIMITATIONS

Gestalt therapy is a powerful approach to heightening awareness of human experience (phenomenology), and so can be very effective in eliciting change, while some other approaches focus more on eliciting cognitive understanding or relief from particular symptomology. Gestalt therapists believe that experiential change elicits a greater "felt" clarity regarding historical causation and current reinforcement of old dysfunctional "failed" creative adjustments.

Gestalt therapy also helps the person to focus on understanding *how* they deal with their experience, so their learning is not confined to a particular event, symptom, or area of their life – but their heightened awareness of how they operate in the present can become generalized to a greater capacity to be present in their lives in full. The approach is not a collection of techniques or interventions, but a way of understanding and entering in to the patient's way of experiencing themselves and the world, and as such must be approached in a skilled, sensitive, and mindful way. However, for those patients who are averse to an experiential approach and seek treatment that focuses on cognitive understanding or behavioral interventions, Gestalt therapy may not be an optimal fit.

Gestalt therapy has a simple, yet powerful and complex understanding of how to enter a person's experience, and some of those "tools" or "techniques" can be detrimental if not applied with an understanding of the patient's capacity to manage such a heightened experience. Prematurely entering into highly charged experiences without first building a base of internal and external support is problematic and can be detrimental. But Gestalt therapy also offers the capacity to experientially develop those supports in an effective and "grounding" way. In this light, Gestalt therapy can be effectively applied to a broad range of diagnostic and life issues, in the hands of a well-trained, attuned, and empathic therapist. It is for this reason that Gestalt therapists require years of intensive training and supervision before they can be certified to practice as a Gestalt therapist.

RESOURCES FOR LEARNING

READINGS

Mann, D. (2021). *Gestalt therapy: 100 key points and techniques* (2nd ed.). Abingdon, Oxon, UK: Routledge.

Perls, F., Hefferline, R.F., & Goodman, P. (1951). *Gestalt Therapy: Excitement and growth in the Human Personality*. New York, NY: Dell Publishing Co.

Polster, E., & Polster, M. (1974). *Gestalt therapy integrated*. New York, NY: Vintage

Skottun, G., & Krüger, A. (2022). *Gestalt therapy practice: Theory and experiential learning*. London, UK: Routledge.

Taylor, M. (2014). *Trauma therapy and clinical practice: Neuroscience, Gestalt and the Body*. Maidenhead, U.K: McGraw Hill Education.

Van Dusen, W. (1975). Wu Wei, No-mind, and the fertile void. In J.O. Stevens (Ed.), *Gestalt Is*, (pp. 87–93). Moab, UT: Real People Press.

Woldt, A.L. & S.M. Toman (Eds.) (2005) *Gestalt therapy: History, Theory, and Practice*. Thousand Oaks, CA: SAGE Publications.

Yontef, G.M. (1993). *Awareness, Dialogue, & Process*. Highland, NY: Gestalt Journal Press.

VIDEOS

Curtis, R. (2017). Gestalt therapy empty chair with past relative: Counseling role play. https://www.youtube.com/watch?v=-WU4uYYfqs0

Grande, T.L. (2016). Gestalt therapy role-play: Two chair technique with "angry part" or self. https://www.youtube.com/watch?v=ahm-ALEOscce

Letourneau University (2011). Gestalt theory: Michelle and Holly. https://www.youtube.com/watch?v=NwM84AgJFoA

Perls, F. (1970). Madeline's Dream. https://www.youtube.com/watch?v=TFqhPe5DR98 (Begin watching at 5 minutes 20 seconds where the Gestalt therapy dreamwork starts.) https://www.youtube.com/watch?v=TFqhPe5DR98&t=711s

Resnick, R.W., & Resnick, R.F. (2016a). Coming home (trailer). https://vimeo.com/ondemand/gestaltfilms/510014316?autoplay=1

Resnick, R.W., & Resnick, R.F. (2016b). Coming home again (trailer). https://vimeo.com/ondemand/gestaltfilms/510014456?autoplay=1

REFERENCES

Bowman, C.E. (2005). The history and development of Gestalt therapy. In A.L. Woldt & S.M. Toman (Eds.), *Gestalt therapy: History, Theory, and Practice* (pp. 3–20). Thousand Oaks, CA: SAGE Publications. In P. Cole (Ed.). *The relational heart of Gestalt therapy* (pp. 1–11). Abingdon, Oxon, UK: Routledge. doi: 10.4324/9781003255772-

Bowman, C.E., & Bowman, C.A. (2022). A classical beginning and a relational turn: A Gestalt therapy case study. In P. Cole (Ed.). *The relational heart of Gestalt therapy* (pp. 113–125). Abingdon, Oxon, UK: Routledge. doi: 10.4324/9781003255772-11

Butollo, W., Karl, R., König, J., & Rosner, R. (2016). A randomized controlled clinical trial of Dialogical Exposure Therapy versus Cognitive Processing Therapy for adult out-patients suffering from PTSD after Type I trauma in adulthood. *Psychotherapy and Psychosomatics, 85*(1), 16–26. doi: 10.1159/000440726

König, J., Karl, R., Rosner, R., & Butollo, W. (2018). Difficulties in conducting long term fol-low ups in psychotherapy research–Issues in the literature and data from a random-ized therapy comparison study for posttraumatic stress disorder. *Journal of Nervous and Mental Disease, 206*(7), 513–521. doi: 10.1097/NMD.0000000000000844

Latner, J. (1986). *The Gestalt therapy book.* Gouldsboro, ME: Gestalt Journal Press.

Mann, D. (2021). *Gestalt Therapy: 100 Key Points and Techniques* (2nd ed.). Abingdon, Oxon, UK: Routledge.

Nazari, I., Mohammadi, M., & Nazeri, G. (2014). Effectiveness of Gestalt therapy on Post Traumatic Stress Disorder (PTSD) symptoms on veterans of Yasuj City. *Armaghan-e-Danesh, 19*(4), 295–304.

Nestor, M.S., Lawson, A., & Fischer, D. (2023). Improving the mental health and well-being of healthcare providers using the transcendental meditation technique during the COVID-19 pandemic: A parallel population study. *PLOS One, 18*(3), e0265046.

Nidich, S., O'Connor, T., Rutledge, R., Duncan, J., Compton, B., Seng, A., & Nidich, R. (2016). Reduced trauma symptoms and perceived stress in male prison inmates through the transcendental meditation program: A randomized controlled trial. *Permanente Journal, 20*(4). Published online: https://www.thepermanentejournal.org/doi/10.7812/TPP/16-007 doi:10.7812/TPP/16-007

Perls, F., Hefferline, R.F., & Goodman, P. (1951). *Gestalt Therapy: Excitement and Growth in the Human Personality.* New York, NY: Dell Publishing Co.

Rees et al. (2013). Reduction in posttraumatic stress symptoms in Congolese refugees practicing transcendental. *Journal of Traumatic Stress, 26*(2), 295–298. doi:10.1002/jts.21790

Sills, C., Lapworth, P., & Desmond, B. (2012). *An Introduction to Gestalt.* Thousand Oaks, CA: SAGE Publications.

Wheeler, G. (1991). *Gestalt Reconsidered.* New York, NY: Gardner Press.

Winitsky, M. (2022). Introduction: The emergence of the relational perspective in Gestalt therapy. In P. Cole (Ed.). *The Relational Heart of Gestalt Therapy* (pp. 1–11). Abingdon, Oxon, UK: Routledge. doi: 10.4324/9781003255772-1

Yontef, G.M. (1993). *Awareness, Dialogue, & Process.* Highland, NY: Gestalt Journal Press.

4

CHAPTER 4
THE USE OF EXPRESSIVE ARTS THERAPY FOR THE TREATMENT OF TRAUMA

Jennifer Byxbee

INTRODUCTION

Expressive arts therapy (EXA) is an experiential approach utilizing creative expression through visual arts, dance/movement, music, drama, poetry, and play to enhance emotional, psychological, and physical well-being. The expressive arts have been recognized for centuries for their unique healing capacities. Before the establishment of psychology as a formal science and well before psychotherapy became a recognized means of healing and health, individuals have employed the expressive arts, and various forms of imagination, as responses to experiences of joy, trauma, and loss. EXA uniquely combines sensory and expressive elements, recognizing that verbal communication alone is insufficient. When used as a modality for treating post-traumatic stress disorder (PTSD) and complex post-traumatic stress disorder (C-PTSD), EXA aligns with current trauma research acknowledging that traumatic memory is a somatic experience – a bodily event (Levine, 1997; van der Kolk 2014). Trauma-informed EXA adopts a holistic "whole-brain approach, with a focus on the qualities associated with the right brain, which serves as the primary storage site for traumatic experiences. This chapter discusses the integration of sensory and expressive elements EXA uses to address the complexities of trauma experiences and their impact on the brain.

BRIEF HISTORY

Expressive therapies gained prominence alongside the development of psychiatry in the late 1800s and early 1900s. Although the therapeutic benefits of artistic expression have been recognized for centuries, the formal application of expressive arts therapy in psychotherapy emerged in the 20th century, gaining particular popularity in the 1970s. Initially, creative arts therapies, as they were called, were used as separate modalities with their own methodologies, theoretical frameworks, and credentialing boards. The six modalities that make up expressive arts therapies are: Art, music, dance/movement, dramatic enactment, creative writing/poetry, and play. Expressive arts therapy differs from traditional single-modality approaches by integrating and combining various art forms within a single session.

Shaun McNiff (2009) who founded the first expressive arts therapy graduate program at Lesley College (now Lesley University), began his career in the early '70s by creating an art studio within a psychiatric hospital. Inspired by the pioneering work of psychiatrist

DOI: 10.4324/9781003455851-4

Maxwell Jones, Rudolf Arnheim's understanding of art psychology, and psychiatrist Hans Prinzhorn's book "Artistry of the Mentally Ill," McNiff developed an approach highlighting the "presence of a universal urge within the psyche to express and heal itself" and connect through creative expression (p 47).

At Lesley, McNiff worked closely with Paola Knill, the originator of the term "intermodal expressive therapy," collaborating to develop the fundamental principles of the field. Expressive arts therapy drew insights from contemporary education studies, particularly integrated arts methods, emphasizing the significance of sensory activities and diverse modes of expression in learning. EXA was also influenced by both Gestalt psychology and Gestalt therapy in its improvisational, phenomenological, experiential approach, incorporating the "here and now" and principles that underscore the interconnectedness of mind, body, and expression as well as Jungian psychology (McNiff, 2009).

As mental healthcare has moved toward more integrative approaches, practitioners have become increasingly interested in applying sensory-based, action-oriented methods like EXA. McNiff (2009) states, "When art and psychotherapy are joined, the scope and depth of each can be expanded and when working together, they are tied to the continuities of humanities history of healing" (p. 259). Today EXA continues to garner attention as it can be used alone or employed as a complement to traditional therapeutic methods to enhance the overall therapeutic process.

FUNDAMENTAL CLINICAL CONCEPTS

Expressive arts therapy is an experiential, improvisational, holistic, humanistic, and phenomenological approach to therapy. Engaging in an expressive arts process is multifaceted and encompasses various aspects of emotional, cognitive, and psychological well-being. Cathy Malchiodi (2020) explores two fundamental principles inherent in the application of expressive arts in psychotherapy. First, the arts serve as modes of self-expression, contributing to the therapeutic process and illuminating the potential for change, repair, and growth within the therapeutic context. Second, the integrated utilization of the arts for health and well-being, encompassing the alleviation of trauma, is not a recent phenomenon; rather, it is ingrained in humanity's collective history. Throughout time, people have employed arts, music, sound, movement, dance, dramatic enactment, and various forms of imagination as responses to experiences of joy, trauma, and loss (Malchiodi, 2020).

One of the distinctive aspects of expressive arts therapy is its emphasis on nonverbal communication. Clients are encouraged to use the arts as a means of conveying emotions and experiences that may be difficult to express verbally. Regardless of the specific art form used in a session, the expressive arts process offers individuals a means of communication, enabling them to explore their inner thoughts creatively and symbolically. In his description of "intermodal expressive therapy," Paolo Knill (1995) discusses the importance of using all of the arts in therapy. Rather than a focus on the product of the specific modality, the focus should be on "the basic human need or drive to crystallize psychic material; that is, to move towards optimal clarity and precision of feeling and thought" (Knill 1995, p. 30).

Freud spoke of the transformative power of creative expression in sublimating our repressed emotions and desires (Freud & Richards, 1991). Sublimation can be defined as the redirection of taboo or forbidden impulses toward socially valued activities, particularly creative endeavors, thereby serving as a mechanism for self-control (Kim et al., 2013). Stephen Levine's (1992) approach to using all of the arts in therapy trusts that in the sometimes difficult and disintegrating movements of creative imagination "lies the cure" to our psychic ills (p. 69). The creative imagination unifies the multiplicity of experiences that often cause our emotional fragmentation, proving especially beneficial within the context of trauma recovery (Levine, E. & Levine, S., 1999).

In *The Principles and Practice of Expressive Arts Therapy* (Knill, Levine, & Levine, 2005), Knill discusses the experiential and improvisational aspects of the work, recognizing the value of providing *a range of play* for clients that helps clients to stay in the here and now that is connected to all alternative world experiences. Decentering, as conceptualized by Knill, involves moving away from the " patterns of thinking and behavior that contribute to the feeling of being "stuck experienced by many clients. Through a focus on artistic expression, clients are invited into a realm of boundless potential, spontaneity, and the unforeseen elements inherent in the realm of imagination. The provision of a range of play serves to juxtapose the constraints of the limitations imposed by current circumstances and the habitual thought patterns in which individuals may find themselves (Knill, Levine & Levine, 2005). For instance, in an expressive arts therapy session, a client who perceives a lack of agency or control in their everyday life can experience a sense of mastery and authority over the artistic materials. Similarly, an individual struggling to assert themselves in real-life situations can explore and express assertiveness by embodying assertive characters in a drama session or play with volume and bigness in a music experience. Moreover, a client feeling trapped in a stagnant job with few prospects can physically manifest the desired movement and freedom during a dance/movement experience, providing a dynamic contrast to their perceived stagnation in reality.

The use of EXA in treatment supports clients in having a sense of control over difficult material as well as a natural titration of difficult material. By alternating between verbalizations and creative expression, the client and therapist can alternate between content and the here-and-now grounding of the experience. Clients are encouraged to use art, movement, and other creative expressions as a means of conveying emotions and experiences that may be difficult to express verbally. Artistic creations in EXA often involve imagery and symbolism. Clients may use symbols, colors, and metaphors to represent their internal experiences, enabling a deeper exploration of their subconscious.

Expressive arts therapy is often practiced in group settings, which encourages collaboration, relationship building and fosters connection to community. EXA can honor diverse cultures and traditions within its therapeutic framework by drawing inspiration from the history of artistic expression and ritual found in every culture throughout time. EXA also prioritizes individuals' sense of mastery by providing support as needed in the execution of expression, while empowering clients by centering their preferences in materials and modalities.

DESCRIPTION OF THE THERAPY PROCESS

This section delineates the structure of an expressive arts therapy session, dividing it into five key segments: Pre-session, check-in, assessment, directive or body of the session, and processing or closing. The aim is to present a foundational structure, inspired by Knill's methodology outlined in his chapter "Foundations for a Theory of Practice" (Knill, Levine, & Levine, 2005).

The following is a case example from a group therapy session for adolescents in an inpatient psychiatric unit of a hospital.

PRE-SESSION: Before every session, the therapist must carefully consider the potential materials or props to be used. This process can be more spontaneous for certain art forms like drama, play, and poetry, and more deliberate for others, such as visual arts and music. When working with a new client, having a range of materials readily available proves beneficial in supporting the improvisational nature of expressive arts therapy.

In the case illustrated by the following inpatient group example, the therapist was well prepared as the session took place in an art room equipped with an extensive array of materials and props. Acknowledging the specific needs of the identified population, the therapist keeps on hand "supportive, grounding supplies," including wood for building, and a collection of bases and adhesives.

CHECK-IN: At the beginning of the group session, the therapist led members in a self check-in. She invited them to make a mark on a page that would describe how they are feeling today or a mark that felt good to make in this moment. The clients did not move to engage in activity.

A group member expressed frustration, questioning the necessity of attending the group when they were going home soon, a sentiment echoed by several others in agreement. This sparked a brief discussion that revealed to the therapist the commonality of impending discharges for many clients in the following weeks.

The check-in is a brief acknowledgment of the transition into the session. This can be a formal verbal check-in as would take place in any other psychotherapy session or a ritualistic nonverbal check-in that signifies the beginning, such as mark-making, movement, a sound, a facial expression, a written word, or a line in response to a comment such as, "Make a movement to show how you're feeling right now." The rationale of the check-in is to gauge patients' responses and level of interests and to begin to settle into an experimental and experiential atmosphere. In an EXA session, it is not necessary for the therapist to stay with one modality. Shaun McNiff states,

> Within the overall environment of the studio, I adjust and plan according to the unique needs of individuals. One person might need to warm up with body movement in order to paint with more fluidity, whereas another might need to sit down and meditate in order to benefit from stillness and quiet focus.
>
> (McNiff, 2016, p. 474)

Starting the group in this way allows the therapist to take the temperature of the group, thus enabling her to know how to respond. Like the body of the session, it is not meant as an assignment to be graded on participation. It is important to easily be able to pivot and shift your ideas based on what clients are presenting, thus keeping clinicians in the process of creating. The mark-making activity of the check-in process was largely ignored, but this provided important information about the clients' needs at the moment.

ASSESSMENT: Upon assessing the group dynamics, the therapist noted the group's resistance to art making, which stood in contrast to the member's usual level of readiness to participate. This behavior was interpreted by the therapist as a manifestation of the ambivalence and anxiety surrounding the imminent departure from the hospital setting and the overall lack of support in making this transition, as well as a way of taking control or protesting something they could resist. Given that many group members had spent weeks on the unit, the prospect of discharge, either to return home or move to a longer-term facility, generated mixed emotions among them.

In the assessment segment, the therapist connects clients' identified goals with the therapist's assessment of clients' daily reality. Based on this assessment, the therapist introduces the art-expression (visual art, music, dance, movement, writing, and/or play). The therapist guides clients into the experience by using open-ended prompts that highlight the clients' dilemmas or as indicated by the therapist's observation of clients' issues.

DIRECTIVE AND BODY OF SESSION: The therapist addressed the group members' transitional phase, recognizing the dual nature of change – exciting yet intimidating. The group acknowledged this realization through verbal affirmations or nonverbal cues, with some choosing to avoid direct eye contact with the therapist. The therapist offered the idea that "the transition out might evoke frustration or anger," which prompted more of a reaction by the clients. Following this acknowledgment, the therapist presented the directive:

> Let's collectively envision the need to cross a bridge on our journey to the next phase. Picture what that bridge might be like – perhaps a suspension bridge, a stone bridge, or a rope bridge. Using the materials available in the art room, let's each make a bridge to help us transition from one place to another.

To support the creative process, each client received a sturdy base made of cardboard or wood, tailored to withstand even the heaviest available materials. The group members predominantly chose wood and immersed themselves in the building task. The therapist needed to be ready to assist with materials or make suggestions that responded to the patient's art choices. This assistance served as a form of relational support intended to help each patient feel seen and an implicit relational expression that help is available, possibly in contrast to their self-world constructions. The therapist attentively observed the materials selected by each member, particularly noting those who opted for flimsier or softer options. In response, the therapist offered reinforcements for their structures. For instance, the therapist addressed Sara, "I see you're constructing your bridge out of felt; would you like some cardboard to affix your cloth shapes?" In another instance, with Jay, "Your bridge seems to be extending beyond the base; would you like me to attach another base to continue building?" With a third member who appeared to be struggling to keep things standing up as he worked, the therapist inquired, "Would you like me to hold that for you while it dries so you can keep going?"

During the core segment of the session, typically lasting as short as 30 minutes, the therapist undertakes the responsibility of guiding the clients in creating or enacting something inspired by the given prompt. In this crucial phase, the therapist takes on the roles of both studio assistant and scene partner. While observing the distinct needs of the client and recognizing the thematic undertones of each expressed or unspoken requirement, the therapist remains in-role without explicitly naming or interpreting the unfolding process.

In this section, based on the population and context of the theme, it is important to foster an environment of success not for aesthetic reasons but rather to help each member gain a sense of mastery and control. In order to achieve this environment with visual art therapy the therapist would need to thoughtfully arrange materials around the room in an organized and easily accessible manner before introducing the EXA directive. Had the therapist introduced this bridge-building directive without proper preparation, the clients would have been "set up" to not complete their bridges or to have them collapse, thus highlighting the old fixed narrative of this population not having control over their lives, not having the tools they need, and/or lacking support to help them go on to the next phase of life. Instead, with the pre-session considerations adhered to, the therapist can go into the role of helper or what Edith Kramer referred to as "the third hand" (Kramer, 2000). The concept of "the third hand" in art therapy refers to an assisting force in the creative process that operates without intruding or altering the client's intended meaning. The central task of art therapy involves facilitating the transformation of emotions into visual expressions, which may not be easily articulated in words. Art therapists must strive to empower each client to create visual communications that authentically convey their experiences, within the constraints of the client's abilities and circumstances. In parallel with specific therapeutic interventions, art therapists should aim to provide the support that nurtures the creative process without imposing external ideas or preferences, ensuring that the client's artistic expressions remain genuine and meaningful (Kramer, 2000):

> Art therapists must also command a "Third Hand," a hand that helps the creative process along without being intrusive, without distorting meaning or imposing pictorial ideas or preferences alien to the client. The Third Hand must be capable of conducting pictorial dialogues that complement or replace verbal exchange.
>
> (p. 48)

PROCESSING OR CLOSING OF THE SESSION: The therapist, observing the group thus far in the session, took note of clients' interest in speaking but their reluctance to speak directly about the feelings evoked. Whether this was because the feelings were unknown or the clients did not feel safe or interested in verbalizing them does not matter. Choosing to stay in the metaphor, the therapist was able to highlight the theme and meaning of the session in a safe contained way that invited reflection without demanding it.

The therapist facilitated group processing by suggesting,

> "Let's take a walk around and observe all the bridges created this week. What stands out to you? When you look at your bridge, what do you see? Would you feel comfortable driving or walking across it? What surrounds the bridge, and do you know its starting point? What about its destination?"

Prompting the group, the therapist inquired, "How was the experience of creating your bridge?" One member shared, "It was great. I liked working with the big pieces of wood; mine was so heavy that I needed three bases from you and Jay's help to glue it down." Acknowledging the additional support required, the therapist responded,

> "It sounds like you enjoyed working with the materials and creating the bridge, but needed some extra support to stabilize it. With that help from Jay, you were able to construct a secure structure capable of taking you from one place to another."

During the processing phase, the therapist adopts one of two approaches. The first approach involves examining the artwork in connection with the earlier discussed theme of the session. The second approach focuses solely on the present moment, emphasizing the sensory aspects of the artwork and the session, which can remain nonverbal. To determine how to lead in verbal processing, the therapist must evaluate how the clients interacted throughout and be curious to see how the clients respond to the ending. If the therapist stays in the here and now and in the senses, the clients may make connections to the theme on their own, inviting a deepening of the dialogue. The clients may also be unable or uninterested in speaking about the work, instead choosing to observe with the therapist and utilize a sensory approach to examine and summarize what just happened. The therapist assesses the clients, looks for cues, and holds on loosely to any expectation, remaining in the "play" of the session, creating and improvising based on the clients' said or unsaid needs.

When processing the work of the session, it is beneficial to follow a sequence outlined by Knill, Levine, & Levine. (2005) that progresses from the most tangible aspects to the underlying meaning. Begin by exploring the "surface" of the work or piece, delving into the observable elements. Then, examine the "process of shaping," focusing on how the artwork was created and the techniques involved. Move on to explore the "experience of doing it," considering the emotional and sensory aspects of the artistic process. Finally, culminate the observation by questioning "what does the work say?" – seeking to understand the deeper meanings and messages conveyed by the work. In the session, the therapist may touch on all of the ways to process the work or stay in the exploration of the surface of the work or piece depending on the needs of the clients.

Mala Betensky, child psychologist and art therapist, offered a deliberate, impartial, and open way of inviting EXA clients to look at what they have created that places "each person's inner reality as a fact of paramount importance" (Betensky, 2001, p 26). The phenomenological approach involves visual display, distancing, and intentional looking. By asking, "What do you see?" the therapist emphasizes the significance of individual perception and meaning. This question encourages the creator to explore their unique way of seeing, highlighting the importance and merit of subjective reality. Similarly, in processing a music improvisation, "What do you see?" becomes "Did you notice?" Did you notice the loud sharp bang of the cymbal followed by a slow rhythmic beat of the drum? Or with movement, poetry, or play, "What did you notice?" "What worked?" and "What happened next?" are all open-ended questions that point out the "characteristics" or "qualities" of the work or materials, and/or the "experience" of creating it. By the therapist staying in metaphor, she was able to speak to themes of support necessary to help the clients transition out of the hospital setting, but highlighted their ability to resource and obtain external help in the moment that added to a successful project.

UTILIZATION OF THE MODALITY FOR THE TREATMENT OF TRAUMA

Expressive arts therapy presents some distinctive attributes that make it particularly effective in trauma work. It has an emphasis on play and imagination and is sensory focused, experiential, improvisational, phenomenological, and relational. As Judith Herman (1997) states in her book *Trauma and Recovery*, "Helplessness and isolation are the core experiences of psychological trauma. Empowerment and reconnection are the core experiences of recovery" (p. 197). The relationship between therapist and client is paramount to the success of the treatment. It is through the relationship that a "holding environment" is created to instill a sense of safety and that Kramer's (1986) "therapist's third hand" is employed to lend ego strength and to co-regulate.

Trauma experts highlight the significance of imagination, creativity, and play in promoting overall well-being and how important they are in healing from trauma. Famous analyst and pediatrician, D. W. Winnicott (1971), stressed the importance of having clients engage in imaginative play to facilitate successful therapy. Stephen Levine (1992) states, "Healing must be understood as the restoration of a person's imaginative capacity" (p 41). In his book *The Body Keeps the Score*, Bessel van der Kolk (2014), names imagination as, "absolutely critical to the quality of our lives." He continues,

> "When people are compulsively and constantly pulled back into their past to the last time they felt intense involvement and deep emotion they suffer from a failure of imagination, a loss of mental flexibility. Without imagination, there is no hope, no chance to envision a better future, no place to go, no goal to reach".
>
> (p. 17)

Expressive arts therapy is a modality that uniquely centers imagination and play to encourage clients to create a new narrative about what's possible or empower them to find a new outcome that centers their agency. Recognizing the power to understand, integrate, and gain a sense of control of our history is crucial to healing.

Sensory-based approaches are ideal for working with trauma because of how trauma affects our sensory experience. By looking at the concepts of exteroception and interoception, we gain insight into how expressive arts can assist in managing traumatic stress. According to Malchiodi (2020), exteroception involves sensing external stimuli through the five senses, aiding in the identification of environmental elements. This sensory input is crucial for trauma survivors as it influences their perception of safety in various situations. Exteroceptive experiences are integral to all forms of expressive arts. Interoception, on the other hand, encompasses the perception of internal bodily sensations including pulse, breathing, and pain, along with proprioception, which relates to one,s sense of position, space, and orientation. Interoception is likened to "gut feelings" within the polyvagal system and a "felt sense" within the body (Gendlin, 1982; Malchiodi, 2020).

Interoception helps one notice and understand what is being felt inside the body. The arts include interoceptive moments. The sense of "being moved" by a piece of art is an example of this, but such internal feelings are not always easily articulated with words. People with PTSD learn to shut down the brain areas that transmit feelings and emotions. Expressive arts therapy is believed to address the lack of interoception in individuals with post-traumatic stress by attentively considering how specific materials, movements, and artworks evoke feelings (Malchiodi, 2020; van der Kolk, 2014).

Trauma impacts the brain and body in complex ways. Emotional experiences linked to trauma as well as memories of sounds, smells, touch, and, visuals are stored in the limbic system and the right hemisphere of the brain (van der Kolk 2014). It is important to use interventions that address the right-brain dominance in order to best process and express trauma (Steele & Malchiodi, 2011). While trauma-informed EXA focuses on the qualities associated with the right brain, there is plenty of room for language and traditional talk therapy within a session to adopt a holistic "whole-brain" approach. Malchiodi (2020) states,

> "It is speculated that because childhood trauma affects the integration of both sides of the brain, sensory and body-based interventions such as expressive arts and play are thought to be effective because they do not strictly rely on the individual's use of language for processing".

(p. 66)

Estrella (2006) suggests viewing EXA as a sensory-based intervention. The therapist is encouraged to consider what will best aid the client's expression in the moment, whether they need distance or embodiment. For instance, visual arts can be used if the client refers to an image, while music can be employed for references to sound (Estrella 2006). Malchiodi (2020) states, "Even when individuals become more aware of their body's sensations, they still often need a process to access a felt sense" (p 159). The central focus of the session becomes how the therapist can help the client create, imagine, and play in order to create access to and support their inner worlds. While it is generally accepted that trauma is both stored in the body and sensory approaches are important when it comes to treating trauma, any intervention that focuses on the body tests a traumatized person's "window of tolerance" (Ogden et al., 2006). Expressive arts therapy is improvisational and flexible, which allows for a natural titration (Malchiodi, 2020). This involves a gradual exploration of traumatic experiences and movement between different modalities that can be less activating for clients than a purely sensory or embodied approach (Levine, 2015). By employing Levine's concept of "pendulation," similar to Knill's "intermodal transfer" (shifting from one modality to another based on a client's needs), clinicians can navigate clients through various levels of embodiment in the expressive arts, starting with less-embodied forms, such as visual art and writing/poetry, that rely on projection (Levine, 2015, Knill, Levine, & Levine, 2005, p 147–153). They can then engage in partially cerebral and sensory elements found in music and drama, eventually progressing to completely embodied experiences like dance/movement and play. This adaptability allows for the gradual introduction of challenging material and a rhythmic movement between such material and resourcing. By slowly introducing difficult material and pendulating between that material and resourcing, the client can establish a sense of safety and stability while integrating them at a manageable pace (Levine, 2015).

In working with this population, it is important to take concrete steps to increase their sense of power and control (Herman, 1997). Herman states, "Many survivors have such profound deficiencies in self-protection they can barely imagine themselves in a position of agency or choice" (p 122). The choice of modality, materials, process, and execution of product are all available for the client in an EXA session. The therapist can highlight the client's agency metaphorically by championing their choicefulness throughout. Expressive arts therapists take on a responsibility to help clients succeed, not in creating a great or beautiful work, but in motivating the artistically untrained client to participate in a process that moves them toward the creation of a work of art or a ritual play (Knill, Levine, & Levine, 2005). As Knill, et al., reminds us, "To achieve this we must consider the skill level of the client and find culturally relevant manifestations of art which are best suited to the client" (p. 97).

ASSESSMENT OF RESEARCH EVIDENCE REGARDING EFFECTIVENESS IN TREATING TRAUMA

Expressive arts therapies are widely acknowledged for their effectiveness in trauma treatment, supported by numerous clinical accounts and positive outcomes demonstrated in meta-analyses (Malchiodi, 2020). van der Kolk (2014) emphasizes the power of art, music, and dance in addressing the speechlessness associated with trauma, suggesting a global cultural use of these modalities in trauma treatment. However, he acknowledges the logistical and financial challenges hindering comprehensive scientific validation. Insufficient research, compounded by the lack of a clear distinction between an expressive arts therapy approach and a mere art experience, contributes to the ongoing debate about its efficacy. Malchiodi (2020) summarizes:

> Although cumulative findings are not strong enough to say that expressive arts therapy or any single form of creative arts therapy demonstrates an acceptable level of evidence and outcomes, there is certainly enough data to say that we know that something probably is working for at least some individuals when it comes to trauma.
>
> (p. 24)

The lack of evidence-based research is a limitation of this modality. Although many studies show a positive outcome from the use of EXA in the treatment of trauma, there is still a lack of clarity on what specifically is helpful. Because engaging in the expressive arts, in general, is thought to improve overall mental health, it is difficult to tease out how the therapeutic model is effective in the treatment of trauma versus how much the act of creation alone is helpful.

CASE EXAMPLE OF USING EXA FOR THE TREATMENT OF TRAUMA

The following case study describes a therapist's long-term work with Lee. The therapist worked with Lee in individual therapy, and Lee was also a member of an art therapy group facilitated by the therapist. Over the years, the therapist used a combination of multiple expressive arts therapy modalities including art therapy, movement, dreamwork, symbolism, and ritual.

Upon completing college, Lee, a 24-year-old white queer cis-gendered woman, sought therapeutic support to address struggles with depression and anxiety. At the time of the intake, she was employed as an art studio assistant to a local painter and had a desire to have a career as a painter herself. Lee revealed a tumultuous and abusive childhood home environment, describing her mother as agoraphobic and depressed, recounting instances of cruelty and humiliation. Her father, driven by political motivations, exhibited controlling behaviors. Lee felt like the black sheep of the family and had aligned with her parents' view of her as a "difficult" child. Lee reported disordered eating and substance misuse starting at the age of 11, as well as a history of self-harm, depression, and suicidality. Lee shared that although she had spoken to many therapists over the years, she had not found the therapy effective in making any changes in her emotional state.

During the first therapy session, Lee was dressed in a long, shapeless black dress and had her dark hair covering her face. She sat hunched on the couch, offering minimal eye contact, and spoke in a soft, often unintelligible whisper. Her thoughts trailed off frequently, making it difficult to understand her. Lee expressed a significant lack of social interactions and support in her life. Lee visibly recoiled when asked about potential romantic relationships, saying, "I am repulsive. I wouldn't want anyone to have to deal with me." Lee consistently expressed self-loathing and engaged in negative self-talk. Lee harbored a profound belief in her intrinsic "badness," and attributed this self-concept as a primary factor contributing to her depression. Her self world view and her identity seemed to be that of, "I am bad, therefore I feel bad" versus what the therapist suspected, "Something bad happened to me to make me feel bad."

Lee was unable to articulate any clear goals or any strengths. Her motivation for bringing herself to therapy was solely because she had recently been experiencing a block in her artmaking. She was also unable to name any feelings and appeared to struggle to stay in the present for more than a few moments. She described herself as having a balloon for a head and feeling that she might float away at any moment. Her word choice frequently revealed dissociative experiences, using words like fuzzy, floaty, confused, hazy, blurry, and detached. Although she couldn't directly articulate her needs, the therapist interpreted her consistently perfect attendance and punctuality each week as an expression of her desire for help.

Because Lee's dissociation was so pronounced, the therapist initially experimented with various body movement-based grounding techniques. It quickly became apparent however that Lee's dissociation was so significant that it presented a very limited window of tolerance for inhabiting her own body. Even simple invitations to feel her feet on the floor, or her back against the chair, were challenging for her. Lee's profound dissociation hindered the comprehensive sensory bottom-up approach and, because her thoughts appeared fragmented due to the trauma, a top-down cognitive approach such as a narrative story was equally challenging. Considering these factors, along with Lee's clear comfort with and affinity for visual arts, the therapist opted to engage with art therapy. The rationale was to titrate her activation levels by utilizing the safety of distance in art, along with its projective nature and grounding elements in the present moments of the process of making and the resulting products.

During one of her earlier sessions, the therapist gave a directive to Lee to draw how she was feeling as she was unable to describe her state with words. The table was laid out with a variety of brightly colored art supplies including pens, pencils, markers, pastels, paint, collage materials, ribbon, tape, stamps, stickers, and different colored paper. After giving the instructions, Lee gazed at the table filled with supplies, slowly rummaged through her bag, and tore out a piece of lined notebook paper from a tattered journal. She sat and manipulated the paper silently until, after about 10 minutes, she handed the therapist the crumpled paper smudged with debris from her bag. When asked for a title she responded in a soft barely audible tone without looking up, "It's origami gone wrong." She continued with a mumble, "It's folded in on itself, having some form, but not permanent." Shrugging to any further exploration, she reached her hand out for the piece and went to throw it in the waste bin. When the therapist asked if she would consider letting her keep it. Lee looked perplexed, "But it's trash," she said. "Well, is it okay if I keep it anyway?" the therapist asked. Lee shrugged and handed it back to her. The gesture of "holding" onto the work symbolized the therapist's offer of care, responding to the part of Lee that longed to be cared for and cherished. This began a ritual that would be the throughline in their work together. Rituals, such as this one, can reinforce consistency. Lee would hesitantly share a piece of herself that she attacked or dismissed, and the therapist would ask to hold onto it, collecting a variety of unfinished colorless objects, fragments of a feeling, thought, or memory, and placing them safely in a container in an attempt to hold and honor what she felt the need to discard. "Repetition not only is the foundation of self-regulatory processes but also instills a sense of safety within oneself and the environment" (Perry, 2009, as cited in Malchiodi, 2020, p. 161).

Lee disclosed about a year into her treatment that she had been cutting herself. Lee was able to find the words to tell the therapist and acknowledged for the first time that she wanted to stop self-harming. When the therapist asked Lee about how she felt sharing this with her, Lee responded: "I don't know. I feel numb mostly. Maybe a little scared that you'll tell me to stop, but I also want to stop." The therapist reflected that although Lee wanted to find healthier ways to cope with her feelings, perhaps she also was afraid of giving up what had in the past served as an important coping strategy for her, to which Lee responded with a small nod. In the sessions that followed, verbal expression, which had been difficult, became nearly impossible in therapy. Sitting in silence for extended periods, she appeared to find some relief in the therapeutic invitation to communicate through art. Recognizing the need for a consistent outlet, the therapist provided Lee with a sketchbook, a tangible container for her unspoken emotions. In the ensuing months, Lee, initially reticent, immersed herself in the sketchbook, utilizing sharp objects like safety pins and broken pencils to imprint puncture and sketch repetitive, small marks on the blank pages, echoing the scars on her arm.

Throughout this process, the therapist mirrored Lee's actions without intrusion, allowing the art to unfold organically. When prompted to verbalize what she noticed in her work, Lee described it plainly, "It is a blank white page with cuts." Encouraging personal owner-ship, the therapist requested Lee to rephrase the statement using the first-person pronoun "I." Stoically, she responded, "I am a blank white page. I am torn. I have cuts," Lee paused and met the therapist's gaze, acknowledging the stark truth within her art and her eyes welled with tears.

As therapy progressed, Lee intermittently introduced dream material, revealing a grow-ing connection to the therapist. In one dream, she recounted an anxiety-inducing sce-nario where she arrived late with balloons, fearing the therapist's displeasure. The dreams unveiled a fragile, newly formed trust, suggesting that the therapist's care was both yearned for and perceived as precarious. Concurrently, Lee's artwork evolved to feature the attach-ment of previously detached parts. As her observing ego developed, Lee began to have more awareness of the various parts of herself and began to act as the integrative pres-ence, slowly putting herself together. In one striking piece, she tore out a section of the page's center, reconnecting it with wire to form a laced effect, prompting her to remark, "It looks like a botched surgery."

The therapist offered Lee support to her observing self, as a means of utilizing the thera-pist's "third hand" for co-regulation. If Lee was the surgeon, the therapist assumed the role of operating room nurse, offering tools and anticipating Lee's need for sutures, tape, and other materials that could be used to bandage, connect, bind, or "hold" the disparate pieces together. Dialogue remained confined to the art-making process, allowing Lee's emotions and experiences to manifest through her creations. At the end of each session, the therapist ritually closed Lee's journal, safeguarding it in a drawer, which became a symbolic act mirroring the containment and preservation of the evolving narrative within the therapeutic relationship.

Slowly Lee started to show signs of improvement. Her artwork began to shift from stark jagged disparate shapes to more organic forms. Much like her earlier work of attach-ing detached parts, Lee's drawings showed a progression of fragments coming together to create form and space and in time, she introduced texture, lightness, and finally color. She agreed to take medication and joined an art therapy group, pivotal in fostering connections. Comprising five women with C-PTSD, the group met weekly, creating art inspired by prompts, with the members sharing their work. The group formed safe, close relationships through their process and sharing in their art. In the group, Lee felt seen and understood, earning respect from members who sought her guidance in their own work. Her success in the group mirrored Judith Herman's thesis about reconnection being at the core of recovery (Herman, 1997).

Through the utilization of expressive arts therapy in Lee's sessions, the therapist effectively communicated predominantly through visual art, providing Lee with a safe avenue for making connections. Although Lee was able to verbalize key issues intermittently throughout therapy, it occurred within a broader nonverbal context where symbolism took precedence, often left unspoken. The phenomenological approach of the work placed equal value on carefully tracking the client's words, bodily movements, affects, and dream material as well as the process and content of her artmaking itself.

STRENGTHS AND LIMITATIONS OF THE MODALITY AS A TREATMENT FOR TRAUMA

Expressive arts therapy proves to be a valuable approach in trauma treatment as a primary or secondary modality. The nature of EXA allows for interventions involving the body, but it maintains room for titration, recognizing that approaches solely focusing on the body might challenge the client's window of tolerance. Given that trauma is often stored in the limbic area of the brain, which is preverbal, having nonverbal options becomes crucial in helping clients express and process traumatic experiences. EXA incorporates principles of mastery, control, and choice, providing a therapeutic space where clients can exercise agency in their creative expressions. The concept of coregulation, often referred to as "the third hand," emphasizes the supportive role of the therapeutic relationship and through the lending of ego strength promotes a sense of safety and stability. EXA offers a community-oriented approach, fostering connections and collaboration within group settings. It recognizes the importance of honoring diverse cultural backgrounds. Additionally, the emphasis on play and imagination in EXA aligns with trauma experts' recognition of the significance of these elements in promoting overall well-being and healing from trauma.

There are several limitations to using EXA as a modality. One significant challenge involves financial constraints, as purchasing art materials and instruments can be costly. Additionally, space requirements present another obstacle, as sufficient room is needed to move freely or engage in activities such as dance or dramatic reenactment. For visual arts, access to a sink or a safe area for drying works in progress may also be necessary. Moreover, the suitability of EXA for certain clients can be an issue, as some individuals may be unwilling to engage in expressive activities. As with many of the experiential and embodied therapies, clients experience fears or resistance to the vulnerability of working less cognitively. Some clients may also struggle with working in metaphor, visualization, or developing a "felt sense." Utilizing EXA with such clients can be challenging, but it can also be beneficial in fostering the development of these abilities.

RESOURCES FOR LEARNING

BOOKS

Robbins, A. (1994) *A Multi-Modal Approach to Creative Art Therapy*. London: Jessica Kingsley

Rogers, N. (1993) *The Creative Connection: Expressive Arts as Healing*. Pennsylvania: Science & Behavior Books.

JOURNAL

Levine, S. *Poiesis, A Journal of the Arts and Communication*. https://egspress.com/catalogue/poiesis_vi.php

VIDEOS

Malchiodi, Cathy: youtube channel: https://www.youtube.com/@cathymalchiodi

REFERENCES

Betensky, M. (2001). *What Do You See? Phenomenology of Therapeutic Art Expression*. Jessica Kingsley Publishers.

Estrella, K. (2006). Expressive Therapy: An Integrated Arts Approach. In C.A. Malchiodi (Ed.) *Expressive Therapies* (pp. 183–209). Guilford Press.

Freud, S., & Richards, A. (1991). *New Introductory Lectures on Psychoanalysis*. Penguin.

Gendlin, E. T. (1982). *Focusing*. Bantam.

Herman, J. (1997). *Trauma and Recovery*. Basic Books.

Kim, E.S., Zeppenfeld, V., & Cohen, D. (2013). Sublimation, culture, and creativity. *Journal of Personality and Social Psychology*, 105(4), 639–666. https://doi.org/10.1037/a0033487

Knill, J.P., Levine, E.G., & Levine S.K. (2005). *Principles and Practices of Expressive Arts Therapy. Toward a Therapeutic Aesthetics*. Jessica Kingsley.

Knill, P. J. (1995). *Minstrels of the Soul: Intermodal Expressive Therapy*. Palmerston Press.

Kramer, E. (2000). "The Art Therapist's Third Hand: Reflections on Art, Art Therapy, and Society at Large." *Art as Therapy: Collected Papers* by Edith Kramer and Lani Gerity.

Kramer, E. (1986). *Art as Therapy with Children*. Schocken Books.

Levine, P. (1997). *Waking the Tiger: Healing Trauma*. North Atlantic Books.

Levine, P. (2015) *Trauma and Memory: Brain and Body in a Search for the Living Past: A Practical Guide for Understanding and Working with Traumatic Memory*. North Atlantic Books.

Levine, S. (1992). *Poiesis: The Language of Psychology and the Speech of the Soul*. Jessica Kingsley Publishers.

Machiodi, C. A. (2020). *The Art Therapy Sourcebook*. McGraw-Hill Education.

Malchiodi, C. (2020) *Trauma and Expressive Arts Therapy: Brain, Body, and Imagination in the Healing Process*. The Guilford Press.

McNiff, S. (2009). *Integrating the Arts in Therapy: History Theory and Practice*. Charles C. Thomas.

McNiff, S. (2016). Pandora's Gifts: Using imagination and all of the arts in therapy. In J.A. Rubin (Ed.), *Approaches to Art Therapy* (pp. 468–478). Rutledge.

Ogden, P., Minton, K., & Pain, C. (2006). *Trauma and the Body: A Sensorimotor Approach to Psychotherapy*. W. W. Norton & Company.

Steele, W., & Malchiodi, C.A. (2011). *Trauma-Informed Practices with Children and Adolescents*. Routledge.

van der Kolk, B.A. (2014). *The Body Keeps the Score*. Penguin.

Winnicott, D. W. (1971). *Playing and Reality*. Tavistock Publications.

5

CHAPTER 5
INTENSIVE SHORT-TERM DYNAMIC PSYCHOTHERAPY FOR THE TREATMENT OF TRAUMA

Patricia O'Keefe Monteleone

INTRODUCTION

Davanloo's intensive short-term dynamic psychotherapy (ISTDP), derived from psycho-analytic theory, is a brief experiential treatment with empirical support for its effectiveness with a wide range of patients, including those suffering from trauma. This chapter will provide an overview of the model including the history and development of this approach, along with a more detailed look into the metapsychology, psychodiagnosis, and Davanloo's road map, known as the central dynamic sequence (CDS). A case example will provide further clarity on psychodiagnosis and CDS. Defense analysis and anxiety regulation techniques are also outlined in the chapter, which are both necessary skills to implement ISTDP successfully. Finally, there is analysis of ISTDP's effectiveness in treating trauma along with its strengths and limitations in doing so.

BRIEF HISTORY

ISTDP was developed in the 1960s by Dr. Habib Davanloo, a McGill University, Montreal, Canada psychiatrist. After his completion of residency at Massachusetts General in the 1950s and embarking upon his own practice, Davanloo became disillusioned with the psychoanalytic treatment of the day with lengthy treatment, questionable results and long wait lists for service. In turn, he set out to develop a therapy based on psychoanalytic principles to effect character change in a short period of time (Kieding, 2021a; Kelly, 2021).

Davanloo's primary influences were Freud's second theory of anxiety and Bowlby's theory of attachment. Davanloo believed that "the vast majority of neurosis stem from conflicting feelings within family relationships …" (Della Selva, 2018, p. 12) due to attachment trauma. Davanloo did not feel ISTDP was a new therapeutic model but rather an *addition* to the body of psychoanalytic knowledge (Kieding, 2021a). In his research, he found that interventions by the therapist that helped the patient identify and process feelings activated in the therapeutic relationship corresponded with unprocessed emotions from historical attachment trauma (Abbass, 2015). This model initially focused on the resistant patient with attachment trauma. Over time, Davanloo's ISTDP evolved to address fragile, high-anxiety patients, including those suffering from PTSD (Whittemore, 1996).

DOI: 10.4324/9781003455851-5

FUNDAMENTAL CLINICAL CONCEPTS

ISTDP is a highly effective experiential modality that has yet to be widely used, some speculate, because of its complexity (Della Selva, 2018). For this reason, the following is a limited overview of the critical concepts of this powerful modality. Becoming proficient in the model takes several years of intense audio-visual supervision.

Although simply put but quite challenging to implement, ISTDP assists patients in experiencing a full range of emotions by unlocking the unconscious. Feelings are the fundamental way one makes sense of the world. They mobilize us to act adaptively to pursue our goals in life (Fredrickson, 2013a). When patients use defenses to ignore their feelings, they allow defense and anxiety to guide their actions rather than their feelings (Fredrickson, 2013a). In the case of a traumatized person, anxiety is high and the use of defenses such as projection and splitting are guiding their interactions, preventing them from living authentically and free from the effects of trauma.

ISTDP is a therapy focused on the attachment relationship between the patient and therapist and all the emotions invoked in the patient within that relationship. The modality is aimed on developing the patient's awareness of the present moment with a focus on the emotions that arise within the transference. It is an emotionally intimate therapy whereby the patient and therapist work collaboratively to develop an open and honest relationship where feelings are accessed and experienced in the treatment room. This is what Davanloo calls the conscious therapeutic alliance. This conscious therapeutic alliance is critical to co-creating the desired change (Fredrickson, 2013a). It is important to note that in ISTDP, the therapist is *not* neutral but is instead wholly supportive of the patient's psychological health and against the patient's use of destructive defenses (Della Selva, 2018; Kieding, 2021b). Research has shown that structural change in brief treatment usually occurs during a crisis where defenses are low and emotions are close to the surface (Della Selva, 2018). Knowing that crisis created an opportunity for change, Davanloo developed interventions that led to an intrapsychic crisis in the therapy room.

There are three components of ISTDP that are essential in implementing the model. All three are necessary for achieving treatment success (Kieding, 2021b). *Metapsychology*, which is the overarching ISTDP theory, is deemed critical to the proper use of the ISTDP model (Della Selva, 2018). The remaining two, *Psychodiagnostic Assessment* and the *Central Dynamic Sequence* (CDS), are the step-by-step guides of implementing ISTDP. The following sections describe each of these components.

METAPSYCHOLOGY

Freud's Second Theory of Anxiety, the concept of *Psychopathologic Dynamic Forces*, *Twin Triangles*, and *Therapeutic Mechanism (Twin Forces)* are four basic metapsychological principles of ISTDP, which are now described.

FREUD'S SECOND THEORY OF ANXIETY

One of the core metapsychology assumptions of ISTDP is *Freud's second theory of anxiety*. It is a central concept of human attachment and represents the beginning of object relations theory (Greenberg & Mitchell, 1983). Della Selva (2018) described it as follows:

> Because of the child's dependence and the centrality of human attachments, any thought, feeling, or action which has led to unwanted separation from or loss of an attachment figure or their love is experienced as dangerous, evokes anxiety, and is avoided. Symptoms are considered to be compromises between the competing need to express the feeling and to defend against it. Symptoms and defenses keep the anxiety, and the feelings propelling it, out of awareness.
>
> (p. 5)

PSYCHOPATHOLOGIC DYNAMIC FORCES

Another of Davanloo's assumptions is psychopathologic dynamic forces, which reflects the anatomy of a wounded psyche. At the core is the attachment rupture, which leads to the pain and cascading of emotions and impulses that are too overwhelming/painful for the child to face, so they become repressed, and lead to the development of defenses in order to avoid the pain (Kieding, 2021b).

TWO TRIANGLES

A critically important metapsychology assumption is called the "two triangles": *Triangle of Conflict* and *Triangle of Person*. Davanloo (Della Selva, 2018, Davanloo 1980, 1995) relied heavily on the two triangles as developed by Menninger in 1958 and further developed by Malan in 1979, as a means to understand and conceptualize intrapsychic conflict and to guide interventions. These triangles serve as the ISTDP therapist's *compass*. They serve as both diagnostic tools as well as a guide to systematic intervention. The first triangle, originally identified by Menninger as the *Triangle of Insight*, later renamed the *Triangle of Conflict*, shows "Feelings" (F) residing at the bottom of the triangle. Davanloo later added "Impulses" (I) to the bottom of the triangle, with "Defense" (D) and "Anxiety" (A) occupying each of the top corners.

A second triangle, added by Malan, the *Triangle of Person*, represents the individual toward whom the conflict is directed and reflects the interpersonal element of the conflict. It emphasizes the importance of the attachment relationship in the intrapsychic conflict. This triangle includes the "Current" people in one's life (C), the "Therapist" (T), also referred to as the transference, on the top corners, with a patient's "Past relationships" (P) occupying the bottom corner of the triangle. Understanding the triangles is essential to Davanloo's modality (See Figure 5.1).

THERAPEUTIC MECHANISM (TWIN FORCES)

Last, but certainly not least, of ISTDP's metapsychological principles is ISTDP's *Therapeutic Mechanism*, which Davanloo (Kuhn, 2014) regards as one of his most significant

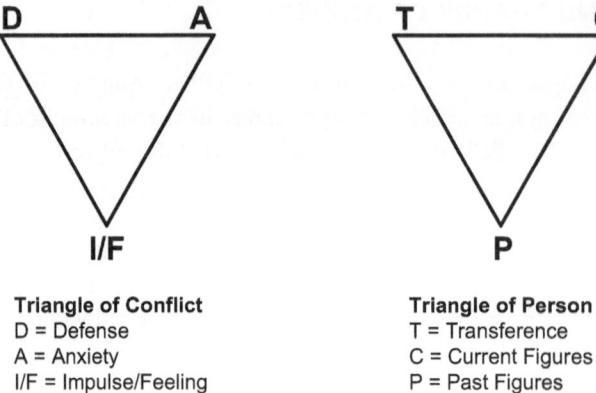

Figure 5.1 Triangles of Conflict and Person

discoveries. Davanloo refers to these as the twin forces of *resistance* and *(complex) transference feelings*. As these twin forces are mobilized, the *unconscious therapeutic relationship* (UTA) increases proportionately (Kuhn, 2014). Davanloo's training and research led him to a paradoxical understanding that, in order to undo the resistance, it is first necessary to increase the resistance in the therapy room. It is the rise of the *complex transference feelings* (CTF) toward the therapist that leads to the undoing of the resistance (Kuhn, 2014, p. 306).

According to the twin forces theory, for all but a few low-resistance patients, attachment trauma leads to the intrinsic *Constructive Part* of a patient (in therapy this is called the unconscious therapeutic alliance, or UTA) being dominated by a corresponding *Destructive Part* (in therapy this is called resistance or defenses) (Kuhn, 2014). Davanloo refers to the UTA as the unconscious part of the patient in the therapy situation that is *constructive* and seeks wholeness or health. The *destructive* part maintains self-punishing actions and suffering as a result of guilt over the complex or mixed feelings (rage, sadness, guilt, positive feelings, etc.) toward early attachment figures. Experiencing these mixed feelings, especially guilt, rather than avoiding them (using defenses), leads to the dismantling of the destructive system and strengthens the UTA (Kuhn, 2014). This concept rests on the idea that as complex emotions are being mobilized in the transference, resistance begins to be reduced while the UTA, the part that knows what is needed to get well, increases. ISTDP effectiveness rests largely on its ability to mobilize the UTA and thereby weaken resistance.

PSYCHODIAGNOSTIC ASSESSMENT

The second essential component of ISTDP is the *psychodiagnostic assessment* and evaluation, which is central to *initiating* and planning ISTDP (Abbass & Town, 2013). This is the process by which the therapist gathers treatment information based on the patient's responses to interventions, particularly during the "trial therapy" period. Therapeutic interventions in ISTDP are used to gather diagnostic information throughout treatment and are deeply intertwined with therapy itself. "This moment-to-moment interweaving of therapeutic intervention and 'diagnostic' feedback is a hallmark of ISTDP, even beyond the initial session" (Kuhn, 2014, p. 28). Such psychodiagnosis reveals a patient's defense structures and anxiety pathways as they shift through the course of therapy (Kuhn, 2014).

Alan Abbass, MD, a leader in the field of ISTDP who studied with Davanloo, went on to develop an algorithm for capturing key psychodiagnostic information with the goal of classifying patients into five psychodiagnostic categories: Three categories of *Classically Resistant Patients* (low, moderate, and high resistance), *High Resistance With Repression*, and *Fragile* (Kuhn, 2014). It should be noted that this component is not part of a DSM diagnoses, but rather a continuing assessment of ego-adaptive capacity, which guides the next intervention and therapeutic task. In essence this assessment determines a patient's ego-strength vs. fragility (Kieding, 2021b). Using the conceptual triangles, the therapist tracks when the patient is experiencing impulses and/or feelings (I-F). The therapist will encourage the patient to continue to feel, facilitating full emotional expression and follow the patient's lead. Davanloo identified three components that must be present for the patient to be fully in touch with their identified feelings: Cognitive, physiologic and motoric (Della Selva, 2018). When the patient is experiencing defense (D), the therapist helps the patient identify and turn away from the mechanisms of the defense. If the defense is deemed syntonic, it requires further intervention to assist the patient in understanding the cost of using such defense and change it from being syntonic to dystonic. When the patient experiences anxiety (A), the therapist will use interventions to regulate the anxiety depending on the anxiety pathway. If anxiety resides in the patient's striated muscles (those muscles attached to the human skeleton that control voluntary movement), it is considered a *green light* and the therapist will continue pressure. If anxiety is present in the smooth muscles (those muscles located in the visceral organs such as the stomach and intestines), this is considered a *yellow light* and the therapist proceeds with caution until the anxiety returns to the striated muscles. Lastly, if anxiety results in *cognitive perceptual disruption* (CPD), the therapist sees this as a *red light* and begins anxiety regulating techniques (Shapiro, 2019).

Additionally, during the psychodiagnostic phase, the motivation and will of the patient are assessed, along with the degree of resistance and ability to self-reflect. The underlying dynamic themes that tend to elicit emotions are noted, as well as the extent to which the patient recognizes their role in their difficulties (Kieding, 2021b).

The psychodiagnosis in any given moment informs the next intervention or therapeutic task. The therapeutic task for a non-fragile patient with attachment trauma is unremitting pressure and challenge, which Davanloo labeled the Vertical Approach, also referred to as the Standard Format. This approach helps the patient rapidly identify their use of maladaptive defenses and turn away from them. The complex feelings that emerge assist in unlocking the unconscious whereby the patient faces the underlying and warded-off feelings and emotions and mobilizes impulses to reexperience the traumatic memory in a new, healing way (Kieding, 2021b).

For the highly traumatized, fragile patient, a graded approach is used, which moves in the same direction as the vertical approach but in a much slower and gentler pace. The therapeutic task for the fragile patient is capacity building, which is achieved by two main interventions. The first is desensitization of intrapsychic material by repeated exposure, and the second is restructuring of defenses to higher order defenses, for example, by replacing projection with intellectualization. While the end goal is the same for each of these patients, the time necessary to complete the goal is longer with the fragile patient (Kieding, 2021b).

CENTRAL DYNAMIC SEQUENCE (CDS)

The third and final component of ISTDP is *the Central Dynamic Sequence (CDS)*, which is used as a "road map" by the therapist. It is a schematic sequence that serves a dual purpose of eliciting psychodiagnostic information, while also being part of the therapeutic mechanism of ISTDP (Kuhn, 2014).

Davanloo developed CDS to begin using in the very first meeting to directly address and break through the defensive barriers to treatment. The initial interview is considered *trial therapy* whereby the therapist identifies, clarifies, and breaks through the defenses to truly know the person's inner experience. It is here that if patients can consciously face their painful feelings that have been previously avoided, they will no longer need to revert to self-defeating and regressive defenses. The ego can then regain its autonomy, allowing for the highest level of functioning (Della Selva, 2018).

The initial interview is highly focused and consists of gentle but relentless questioning and confrontation of a patient's defenses against their true feelings. The therapist repeatedly confronts the patient on their vagueness, avoidance, passivity, and any other defense that gets in the way of conveying their true feelings. The trial has three simultaneous goals: Psychodiagnosis, achieving therapeutic results, and deciding if further ISTDP therapy is desirable. If deemed desirable, the goal widens to creating and maintaining a conscious therapeutic alliance along with identifying goals for treatment and confirming the patient's willingness to work together with the therapist (Kuhn, 2014).

Davanloo identified eight phases in the CDS treatment process. Although outlined sequentially, actual therapy is seen as more of a "spiral" in which the different phases are revisited and interwoven (Kuhn, 2014).

1. **PHASE OF INQUIRY:** In this initial *inquiry* phase, the goal is to identify one or more internally focused problems. During this phase, the therapist rapidly moves to a *dynamic* inquiry, assessing the client's issues based on Malan's two triangles. The therapist monitors the patients' responses and tracks the patients' defenses, unconscious anxiety, underlying feelings, and the various people with whom these conflicts play out by using the triangles as a compass (Kuhn, 2014).
    The therapist will ask an introductory question of the patient such as "What emotionally focused problem would you like my help with?" Or "Can you tell me what seems to be the problem?" (Davanloo, 1995). It is important for the therapist to get a specific example in this phase to avoid intellectualization. The goal of this phase is to get a *headline* with the identified problems and proceed to the Pressure Phase (Kuhn, 2014).

2. **PHASE OF PRESSURE:** Once a thorough inquiry and a list of the patient's presenting problems and symptoms are obtained along with the patient's *will* (the patient's willingness to engage in the therapy process), the next therapeutic task is the examination of the patient's defenses and anxiety pathways. The use of pressure to encourage the patient to identify and experience their underlying emotions helps the therapist to identify the pathways of unconscious anxiety and defense. The pressure to emotionally engage gives rise to complex feelings, which in turn gives rise to anxiety and defense in the treatment room. From this assessment and psychodiagnostic data, the therapist discerns their next intervention. If the client experiences isolation of affect and striated muscle tension, continued pressure and direct mobilization of unconscious is warranted. It the client collapses or goes flat with repression, cognitive perceptual disruption or projective defenses, then capacity building is deemed necessary before returning to the accessing of the unconscious (Abbass & Town, 2013).

   In the pressure phase, the therapist uses any intervention that encourages patients to feel, acknowledge, examine, or otherwise face avoided thoughts, feelings, relationships, or actions. It is one of the essential interventions in ISTDP. An example of pressure is "What are you feeling toward your wife for yelling at you in front of the children?" or "What are you feeling toward X for doing Y?"

   The preceding example demonstrates pressure to feeling, which is a key technique in ISTDP. Pressure is typically posed as questions, and its goal is *not only* to illicit an answer to a direct question but also to explore what ignites the first stages of the rise in complex transference feelings (CTF) which cause anxiety (Kuhn, 2014).

3. **PHASE OF CHALLENGE:** In this phase, the therapist challenges patients' defenses and encourages them to give them up. The challenge is often paired or contrasted with pressure. The pressure intervention encourages the patient to do something that is good for themselves (I/F) (i.e., feeling their feelings) and the challenge intervention is encouraging the patient to stop doing something that is wrong for themselves (D) (i.e., repressing their anger). Challenges include phrases like "I notice you are changing the subject when I ask you what you are feeling towards your wife." Or "I see you are smiling, but you say you are angry" (Kuhn, 2014).

   In some instances, pressure to challenge is useful, an example being, " If you were not smiling over your feelings (challenge), what might you be feeling toward your wife for yelling at you in front of the children (pressure)?" The patient is being challenged to do something differently, a process that is referred to as a *head on collision* with the resistance (Della Selva, 2018, p. 20). When applied correctly, the patient sees the challenge as a collaborative attempt to free them from their defenses (Kuhn, 2014).

   The challenge phase has a purpose beyond encouraging patients to turn against their defenses. It also, like pressure, plays a vital role in the ongoing mobilization of complex transference feeling (CTF) that is essential to the therapeutic mechanism of ISTDP. These complex feelings include appreciation of the therapist for their care and effort, along with irritation that the therapist is pressing against their defenses.

   During the challenge phase, anxiety is already rising from the pressure phase, and defenses become operational, allowing the therapist to engage in defense analysis, which consists of three stages: *Identification and clarification of defenses; Turning the ego against the defenses (syntonic to dystonic); and Pressure and challenge to give up the defenses.*

4. **PHASE OF TRANSFERENCE RESISTANCE:** A key goal of CDS from the start of pressure is "tilting the patient's character defenses in the transference" which is done in this phase (Kuhn, 2014, p. 319). In short, this brings the patient's defenses to resist the therapist and therapy "into the room." This is bringing the maladaptive relationship patterns that the patient enacts in the therapeutic relationship, which are the same maladaptive patterns in the patient's daily life, into full view in the therapy room (Kuhn, 2014).

   This transference allows the therapist to clarify and intervene to disable the unhealthy interaction pattern. The therapist, through intervention, can deactivate the transference, and this is where healing of character pathology occurs. Deactivation of transference is two-pronged. First, the therapist clarifies the therapy-destroying costs of the transference resistance. Second, the therapist discourages the re-emergence of transference resistance by the continual emphasis on the patient-therapist partnership, working toward the patient's goals, and the repeated confirmation of the patient's *will* (Kuhn, 2014).

5. **INTRAPSYCHIC CRISIS/UNLOCKING:** In this phase, the destructive system or defenses are weakened and the constructive system known as the *unconscious therapeutic relationship* (UTA) strengthens and overtakes the defenses, leading to the unlocking of unconscious material (Kuhn, 2014). The unlocking happens when a client's anxiety and resistance are low, and the UTA is mobilized. When the UTA is activated, it allows for direct access to the unconscious, whereby therapeutically beneficial material comes into awareness in the form of memories, images, or links to other material. The importance of this phase cannot be more emphasized. The principal goal of the CDS is to unlock the unconscious so patients can be free from the destructive effects of their defenses (Kuhn, 2014, p. 332; Whittemore, 1996). The patient may experience intense affect in this phase, which is of tremendous therapeutic value (Della Selva, 2018). The therapist facilitates a deepening of the patient's experience by what Davanloo describes as *portraiting the impulse* by asking the patient to use their imagination while expressing the emotion and playing out visually how the body motorically wants to express it (Della Selva, 2018).

6. **ANALYSIS OF THE TRANSFERENCE:** This phase occurs immediately following the unlocking of the unconscious, which encompasses complex feelings (rage, guilt, grief, and loving feelings). It is in this phase that the therapist first begins to use interpretation. In doing so, the therapist recapitulates the utilization of the psychodynamic formulation of the patient's problems using the two triangles (Kuhn, 2014). With the outpouring of affect after removing resistance and defense, meaningful interpretations can occur, especially regarding the triangle of person and conflict. During the recapitulation, the therapist points out the links between current and past experiences, highlighted in what is referred to as *T-C-P links (therapist, current and past)* (Della Selva, 2018). Therapists are careful to point out how the defenses contribute to the patient's symptoms and identified problems. Davanloo stressed the need for and importance of repeatedly highlighting these insights, as research shows a direct relationship between repetition of the process and symptom relief (Kuhn, 2014).

7. **FURTHER INQUIRY INTO DETAILED HISTORY/DYNAMIC EXPLORATION INTO THE UNCONSCIOUS**. As stated previously, history-taking is postponed until after the defenses have weakened. It is here, in the seventh phase, where further inquiry into the patient's developmental history and the process of dynamic exploration into their unconscious occurs (Della Selva, 2018).

8. **PHASE OF CONSOLIDATION**. In this final phase the therapist summarizes the thera-peutic process and recapitulates the insights that were obtained. It can be helpful to have the patient share their experience of the therapy overall and of the therapist (Kuhn, 2014).

One last point to be raised regarding CDS, which is, in essence, the heart and soul of ISTDP, is that the therapist's tone is gentle, but firm. The therapist supports the pa-tient's health and healthy behaviors against their self-defeating defenses. A therapist needs to mindfully remove themselves from any interpersonal struggle by redirecting patients to their internal struggle. This may look like the therapist saying, "I am point-ing out something that I am noticing, but only you know if you are covering your feel-ings with self-attack or minimization." Ultimately, it is the patient's choice to get well, and the therapist is there to assist if they want to move forward. ISTDP recognizes this as the patient's conflict, not the therapist's. The interventions are designed to intensify the patient's internal struggle (Della Selva, 2018).

CASE EXAMPLE

The following is an example of the central dynamic sequence (CDS) using a case example of Mary, a 55-year-old woman who came in for treatment due to issues of depression. Using CDS, it readily led to the processing of early attachment trauma.

THE INITIAL INTERVIEW SESSION

PHASE 1. INQUIRY

THERAPIST:	Hello Mary
PATIENT:	Hello
THERAPIST:	What emotional problem would you like my help with today? (First pressuring question)
PATIENT:	Well, I have been in therapy on and off for most of my life due to depression so I would like to work on my depression.
THERAPIST:	How long have you been depressed? (Pressuring)
PATIENT:	I have been depressed most of my life. I can't remember a time I wasn't depressed.
THERAPIST:	Can we look at a specific time you were depressed? (Asking for specificity)
PATIENT:	I became really depressed when I went through my divorce.
THERAPIST:	Can you tell me more about your divorce and why your marriage ended? (Specificity)
PATIENT:	My husband cheated on me, and after many years, I finally had the courage to divorce him.

PHASE 2. PRESSURE

THERAPIST:	What are your feelings toward your husband for cheating on you? (Pressure to feel)
PATIENT:	I am glad he is gone. (Patient responds with a defense, not a feeling.)
THERAPIST:	But what are your feelings toward him? (Pressure to feel)

PATIENT: I wish I hadn't wasted so many years with him. (Patient responds again with a thought/defense, not a feeling.)

THERAPIST: That is a thought and may be true, but what are the feelings you have toward him? (Defense clarification and pressure to feel)

PATIENT: I am not angry with him; I pity him. (Again, defense, negation)

PHASE 3. CHALLENGE

THERAPIST: Do you notice that when I ask you how you feel about your husband's cheating, you tell me your thoughts or respond with what you are not? If you do not share your feelings with me, how can I help you? (Head-on collision against resistance)

The patient starts to look away and cross her arms. (Tactical defense)

THERAPIST: I noticed you looked away and crossed your arms. Are you having feelings toward me in this moment? (Pressure to feel)

PATIENT: I don't know. (Defense)

THERAPIST: Would you like to know what you are feeling toward me? (Challenge)

PHASE 4. BREAKTHROUGH OF FEELING IN THE TRANSFERENCE

PATIENT: I guess I am feeling annoyed. (Defense, vagueness)

THERAPIST: You guess, or you are? (Pressure)

PATIENT: I am feeling annoyed with you. (Cognitive label of emotion)

THERAPIST: Yes, because I am asking you difficult questions. Where are you feeling this annoyance in your body? (Asking for the physiological component of an emotion)

PATIENTS: I feel some energy in my hands and throat. (Physiological response to emotion)

THERAPIST: How does this energy in your hands and throat want to express this annoyance with me? (Asking for the motoric element of an emotion)

PHASE 5. INTRAPSYCHIC CRISIS/UNLOCKING

PATIENT: I want to scream at you and shake you. (Motoric response or impulse of emotion, I/F)

THERAPIST: Yes, and what would you scream as you shook me? (Facilitating the impulse)

PATIENT: Who do you think you are? Leave me alone! (I/F))

THERAPIST: And what images are coming to you? (Therapist continues to follow and facilitate while in I/F))

PATIENT: I am shaking you and screaming, and you fall to the ground. (I/F))

THERAPIST: How else would you like to express this anger? (Facilitating I/F)

PATIENT: I am kicking you and stomping on you. You are bleeding and cowering. I keep kicking and stomping until you are still. (I/F)

THERAPIST: You kicked and stomped until I am dead? How else would you like to express this anger? (Therapist is following the client while in I/F)

PATIENT:	Now I am feeling bad that I killed you. (Emergence of mixed feelings, I/F))
THERAPIST:	Yes, because you are a nice person. What do you see in my eyes as you see me lying there dead? (Facilitating)
PATIENT:	I see my mother's eyes. [Mary is overcome by a big wave of emotion] (I/F; unlocking of the unconscious)
THERAPIST:	Let the feelings come. (Facilitating I/F)
PATIENT:	Sobbing (I/F)
THERAPIST:	Let them all come. There is a lot of feeling here. Let it come. (Facilitating I/F)

PHASE 6. ANALYSIS OF THE TRANSFERENCE

PATIENT:	(After minutes of deep emotion.) My mother was so horrible to me. She was never there for me in my time of need. All she did was badger me and put me down.
THERAPIST:	And you have a lot of anger and rage towards her. (Interpretation)
PATIENT:	Yes, anger wasn't allowed in my house growing up. I just swallowed it.
THERAPIST:	You just swallowed your anger and it made you depressed. You have had a lifetime of swallowing your anger and a lifetime of feeling depressed. (Interpretation)
PATIENT:	I'm feeling a lot of emotion right now. (Patient is experiencing grief for all the years she spent depressed).

FURTHER INQUIRY INTO DETAILED HISTORY/DYNAMIC EXPLORATION INTO THE UNCONSCIOUS

PHASE 7 & 8. DETAILED HISTORY/DYNAMIC EXPLORATION OF UNCONSCIOUS AND CONSOLIDATION

THERAPIST:	What is coming up for you? Is there a specific memory? (History taking)
PATIENT:	I remember a time when my mother came outside while I was playing with my friends, and she was screaming at me, pulled my hair, and told me to come inside. I didn't even know why she was mad at me. (Another wave of emotion) (I/F)
THERAPIST:	There is a lot of emotion, Mary, for this lifetime of swallowing your anger. Let those feelings come. You do not need to swallow your feelings here. (Facilitating I/F)
PATIENT:	(Sobbing) I spent my whole life swallowing my feelings and wasted my life being depressed. (Waves of emotion) (I/F)
THERAPIST:	You are seeing your lifetime of depression as a result of you swallowing your anger toward your mother for her treatment of you and then again with your husband for cheating on you. Instead of the anger going out on them, you turned it in on you, leaving you depressed. You see? (Recapitulation and C/P/T links)
PATIENT:	I do see. (Consolidation)

THERAPIST: Would you like to continue to work together to take a look at this anger that has left you depressed so you can live a life free from depression; a life of happiness and peace? (Consolidation and confirming patient's will to continue)

PATIENT: Yes. I want to be free of these depressive feelings; to be happy.

THERAPIST: What insights are you taking with you today? (Asking patient to recapitulate)

PATIENT: I didn't realize how much anger I still had toward my mom. Nor did I realize that I have been burying it inside creating my depression. I need to use my voice so I can have peace.

THERAPIST: Yes, you have silenced yourself for a long time. How was it for you to experience this here with me? (Asking patient to recap)

PATIENT: I really appreciate your help and compassion.

THERAPIST: Any other feelings you may be feeling towards me? I recognize this is hard work. (Therapist is looking for mixed emotions)

PATIENT: I am mostly appreciative, but you are right that this is hard! Maybe I'm a little irritated with you for asking these difficult questions. (Consolidation and cognitive label of emotion)

THERAPIST: Of course. How are you feeling the irritation in your body? (Asking for physiological component of emotion)

PATIENT: I was feeling a little bit in my chest but it is gone now. I feel calm and relaxed. And exhausted.

This case example moves seamlessly from phase to phase which sometimes happens, but as Davanloo asserts, more often it looks more like a spiral than a straight line with overlapping phases.

UTILIZATION OF ISTDP FOR THE TREATMENT OF TRAUMA

ISTDP modality was initially developed to treat patients with attachment trauma. It also is an effective trauma therapy for acute trauma and PTSD. The development of the graded format was designed specifically to address the more complex trauma patient, including those with PTSD. The model's use of triangles, anxiety regulation as part of the modality, are essential for the effective treatment of the complex trauma patient who suffers from anxiety discharging into cognitive perceptual disruption (CPD), and whose primary mode of dealing with mixed feelings is through splitting and projecting (Fredrickson, 2018).

ISTDP is also well suited for patients in crisis, or with an acute trauma, as they often have low resistance and are more easily able to access core emotions and impulses. In these cases, defense analysis is often unnecessary, and patients are more readily free to access their emotions as there is little defense operating, and their strong emotions are close to the surface.

ISTDP can be utilized effectively by helping unlock the unconscious feelings/impulses/memories associated with the trauma by regulating anxiety, deactivating projections, and helping patients face their underlying feelings. This in turn leads to integration and strengthening of the ego. Using the eight phases of ISTDP, unlocking these past painful memories allows for the experiencing of the painful and forbidden feelings associated with the trauma. By creating an intrapsychic crisis in the treatment room, when necessary, the unlocking of past painful emotions is brought into consciousness to be fully felt. With that, the defensive self-destructive behaviors in place to avoid such feelings are no longer needed to keep them from surfacing, creating change.

ASSESSMENT OF RESEARCH EVIDENCE REGARDING EFFECTIVENESS IN TREATING TRAUMA

There is a large body of research supporting the use of ISTDP as well as its cost effectiveness. ISTDP was developed by Davanloo's detailed study of a large case series. He used video recording to develop his metapsychology of the unconscious and the resultant techniques for working with the unconscious. Over two decades, 1970–1990, Davanloo included further research on highly resistant, fragile, and somatizing patients. In addition to Davanloo's groundbreaking research, at least 15 process studies have validated various aspects of ISTDP metapsychology (Abbass, 2015).

The most extensive ISTDP case study of 500 patients demonstrated large, significant interpersonal gains and symptom alleviation (Abbass, 2015). ISTDP has been shown to be effective with treatment-resistant patients, somaticizing patients, individuals with personality disorders, and those with mood disorders. Furthermore, research studies have indicated that using ISTDP saves costs through decreased medical service use, hospital use, medication, and disability costs (Abbass 2015).

STRENGTHS AND LIMITATIONS OF THE MODEL AS A TREATMENT OF TRAUMA

ISTDP is an effective treatment for trauma, as it has anxiety regulation built into the model. This is critical as that often is the area that prevents a clinician from processing traumatic material because the patient lacks affect tolerance to withstand the influx of strong emotions. As Jon Fredrickson (2013b) states:

> ISTDP is the only treatment model that understands the pathways of anxiety discharge, has a theory of a threshold for anxiety tolerance, has a theory of differentiating anxiety caused by feeling versus anxiety perpetuated by regressive defenses, and has a theory of anxiety regulation which differentiates anxiety from projective anxiety.
>
> (p. 1)

The graded format of ISTDP creates exposure as well as capacity building, allowing for it to be used with the most severely traumatized of patients.

The limitation of ISTD for treating trauma is that is a very complex modality and mastery of it takes many years of intensive training and supervision. As a result, skilled clinicians and the use of the modality are limited, although momentum is growing in the experiential dynamic therapy (EDT) community.

RESOURCES FOR LEARNING

BOOKS

Della Selva, P. C. (2018). *Intensive Short-Term Dynamic Psychotherapy*. Routledge.
Fredrickson, J. (2013). *Co-creating change: Effective Dynamic therapy techniques*. Kansas City, MO: Seven Leaves Press.

VIDEOS

Kieding, Johannes (2021). Fundamentals of ISTDP. YouTube. https://youtu.be/ApbQ-BCczNI?si=RMge_KAfdby34bVu
Skorman, Marvin (2021). Introductory Presentation on ISTDP. YouTube. https://www.youtube.com/watch?v=90Gp-4cRIJY&feature=youtu.be

INSTITUTES

Many videos, publications, and resources are available at the ISTDP Institute: Istdpinstitute.com.

REFERENCES

Abbass, A. (2015). *Reaching through Resistance: Advanced Psychotherapy Techniques*.
Abbass, A.A., &Town, J.M. (2013). Key clinical processes in intensive short-term dynamic psychotherapy. *Psychotherapy, 50*(3), 433– 437. https://doi.org/10.1037/a0032166
Davanloo, H. (1980). *Intensive Short-Term Dynamic Psychotherapy*. Jason Aronson.
Davanloo, H. (1995). *Unlocking the Unconscious: Selected papers of Habib Davanloo, MD*. John Wiley & Sons.
Della Selva, C.P. (2018). *Intensive Short-Term Dynamic Psychotherapy*. Routledge.
Fredrickson, J. (2013a). *Co-Creating Change: Effective Dynamic Therapy Techniques*. SevenLeaves Press.
Fredrickson, J. (2013b, November 28). "*ISTDP for Traumatized Patients*" ISTDP Institute. https://istdpinstitute.com/2013/istdp-for-traumatized-patients/
Fredrickson, J. (2018, May 1). "*ISTDP and PTSD?*" ISTDP Institute. https://istdpinstitute.com/2018/istdp-and-ptsd/
Greenberg, J.R., & Mitchell, S.A. (1983). *Object Relations in Psychoanalytic Theory*. Harvard University Press.

Kelly, O.P. (Host). (2021, March) Dr. Allan Abbass: Understanding & Navigating Treatment Resistance in Psychotherapy. [Audio podcast episode]. In *Thoughts on Record*. Podcast of the Ottawa Institute of Cognitive Behavioral Therapy. https://open.spotify.com/episode/6FgyfyRAVqSC8KZMBMNKeY?si=xg1vMiOuQ3CITBoDNjNfoQ

Kieding, J. (2021a, February 2). *Marvin* Skorman's introductory presentation on ISTDP [Video]. *YouTube*. https://youtu.be/90Gp-4cRlJY?si=zzUOQvZnkO4vSP3d

Kieding, J. (2021b, March 17). *Fundamentals of ISTDP* [Video]. https://youtu.be/ApbQ-BCczNl?si=RMge_KAfdby34bVu

Kuhn, N. (2014). *Intensive short-Term Dynamic Psychotherapy: A Reference*. Experient Publications.

Shapiro, S. (2019-current). *Core Training*. Malvern, Pennsylvania.

Whittemore, J.W. (1996). Paving the Royal Road: An Overview of Conceptual and Technical Features in The Graded Format of Davanloo's Intensive Short-Term Dynamic Psychotherapy. *International Journal of Intensive Short-Term Dynamic Psychotherapy, 11*, 21–39

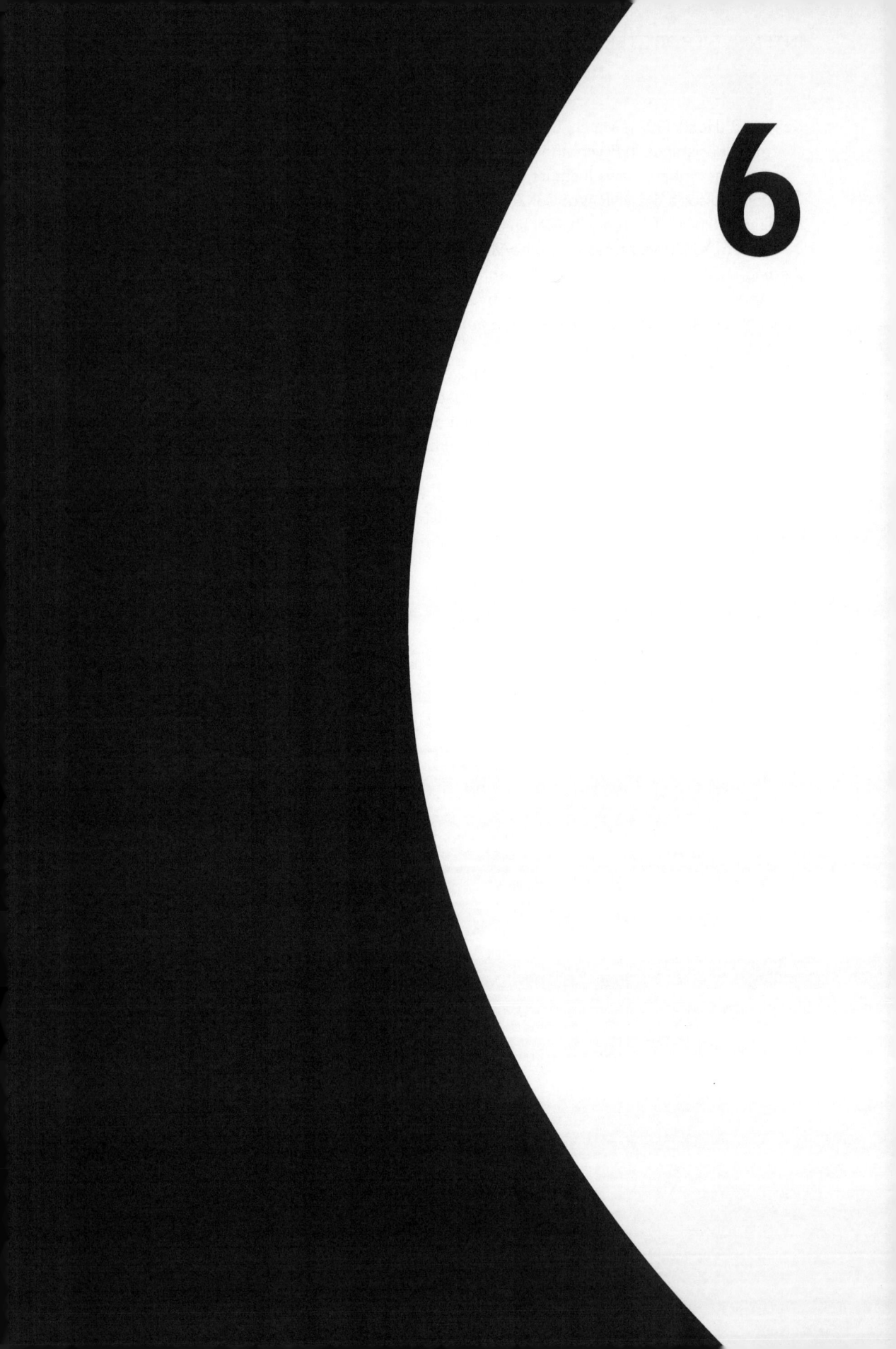

6

CHAPTER 6
SOMATIC EXPERIENCING FOR THE TREATMENT OF TRAUMA

Jordan Dann

INTRODUCTION

Somatic experiencing (SE) is a trauma-informed, body-centered therapy model aimed at resolving the various symptoms that arise as a result of traumatic experience. It was created by Peter Levine, PhD, and is a multidisciplinary intersection of physiology, psychology, ethology, biology, neuroscience, indigenous healing practices, and medical biophysics that has been clinically applied for more than four decades. SE addresses issues related to the mental, physical, and emotional symptoms of trauma, as well as the treatment of syndromes related to patterns in the autonomic nervous system as a result of traumatic stress. SE is founded upon the central understanding of human beings' physiological survival response to any stimulus or event that is perceived as stressful, frightening, or dangerous. An individual's perception of threat activates the preparatory response, which is evolutionary in nature, and triggers the autonomic nervous system to respond by fight, flight, freeze, or fawning. SE provides a framework to assess where a person is "stuck" in the survival response process and offers clinical interventions aimed at resolving fixed physiological states. The primary goal of SE is to assist clients' in "bottom-up" processing of traumatic experience by "tracking" their sensations (interoception, proprioception, and kinesthesis) rather than attending solely to their cognitive or emotional experiences.

BRIEF HISTORY

Dr. Peter Levine, the creator of somatic experiencing, began his career as a scientist in Berkeley, California, in the mid-1960s. While studying the effects of accumulated stress on the nervous system in wild animals, Levine began to focus on animals' physiological release of survival energy in the form of shaking, trembling, or sometimes running after surviving a predatory attack. He observed that animals' ability to mobilize the survival response of fight–flight allowed them to return to homeostasis. He posited that humans also possess the same ability to release physical energy from stress, but that such survival responses are often "overridden" or "thwarted" and remain unresolved and/or uncompleted. This sets the stage for the development of post-traumatic stress disorder (PTSD), other psychological conditions, and autonomic nervous system (ANS) dysregulation syndromes, such as migraines, chronic pain, irritable bowel syndrome, chronic fatigue, fibromyalgia, and others. SE is aimed at releasing this stored energy and turning off the threat of alarm that results in an ongoing state of dysregulation and dissociation.

DOI: 10.4324/9781003455851-6

During Levine's early research, a psychiatrist familiar with Levine's stress research asked him to see a patient of his, referred to as "Nancy," who was suffering from various "psychosomatic" symptoms, such as migraines, premenstrual syndrome, chronic pain, and fatigue, as well as severe panic attacks (Levine, 1997). As Levine began to work with Nancy in an effort to support her awareness of physical tension and engage her parasympathetic nervous system in service of relaxation, she suddenly panicked. Levine saw in his mind's eye the fleeting image of a tiger poised for attack and he blurted out without thinking, "Nancy, there's a tiger coming after you. Run and escape to those rocks. Run for your life!" The patient's body began to spontaneously release energy by sweating, shaking, and trembling, while her breath deepened and her muscle tone softened. After some time, the patient noted a feeling of "profound calm," which accompanied memories of herself at age four as she was being given anesthesia for a tonsillectomy. As she processed these memories, she came into contact with feelings of terror and helplessness. After the session, Nancy reported a dramatic improvement in what had previously been a host of debilitating symptoms (Levine, 2010).

Levine's experience with Nancy and his subsequent research into the nature of stress and trauma deepened his understanding of how trauma affects the body, which eventually led to his Twelve-Phase Healing Program (Levine, 2008). While Levine's work originally focused on shock trauma associated with the imminent threat to life or physical safety (traumas due to combat, catastrophic events, natural disasters, or physical and sexual abuse), he later began to view that developmental trauma consists of similar autonomic nervous system (ANS) disturbance. He has also noted the "intrinsic and wedded relationship between trauma and spirituality" (Levine, 2010, 347). This connection between spirituality and trauma was also observed by researcher and psychopharmacologist Roland Fischer (1973), who provided a schema for showing the association of various parasympathetic nervous system (PNS) and sympathetic nervous system (SNS) activities with mystical and meditative experiences. Because trauma represents an extraordinary depletion of "survival" energy, when this vitality is gradually released and redirected, it is common for individuals to report a "transcendental" or spiritual experience (Fischer, 1973). For some trauma survivors (bearing that they are not recovering from religious trauma), spirituality may mean a relationship with God, faith, or religion. For others, spirituality can mean the ability to cultivate qualities of the spirit such as gratitude, joy, hope, positivity, and connection. For still others, a healthy spirit may be defined as centering one's self in the present moment, understanding that they are part of something bigger than themselves, cultivating healthy interpersonal relationships with others, being a part of a community, or having a connection to the natural world (Russell, et al., 2013).

FUNDAMENTAL CLINICAL CONCEPTS

This section offers a selection of clinical concepts that are fundamental to the SE modality. The most essential clinical concept relates to having a conceptual and experiential understanding of the nervous system.

AUTONOMIC NERVOUS SYSTEM

A foundational understanding of the autonomic nervous system (ANS) is central to somatic experiencing. The ANS governs involuntary aspects of our physical state of arousal and relaxation, such as our heart rate, breath, blood pressure, and chemical signals within the hypothalamic-pituitary-adrenal axis, an internal system that triggers the fight-or-flight response (Gibbons, 2019). The ANS contains two branches: The sympathetic nervous system (SNS) and the parasympathetic nervous system (PNS). The SNS is responsible for increasing our level of alertness in order to respond to environmental or internal stimuli, while the PNS is responsible for signaling rest, safety, digestion, and relaxation.

CO-REGULATION

Co-regulation is the process in which one nervous system influences the nervous system of another. Co-regulation involves various types of responses, including but not limited to: A warm, calming presence and tone of voice, verbal acknowledgement of distress, modeling of behaviors that can modulate arousal, and the provision of a structured environment that supports emotional and physical safety. SE asserts that traumatic experiences can interrupt the development of a person's co-regulatory skills and, out of necessity for survival, the ANS is shaped to independently regulate in the absence of another regulated presence. As Levine states, "Trauma is not what happens to us, but what we hold inside in the absence of an empathetic witness" (Levine, 2010, xii). SE emphasizes the importance of the therapist's ability to serve as an empathetic witness in order for the patient to reestablish their co-regulatory capacities.

RESONANCE

Resonance works in concert with a clinician's visual observations of a patient's behaviors. Empathetic resonance is the clinician's bodily felt sense in response to what the patient expresses, whether it is spoken or through the individual's vocal tone and quality, and/or their nonverbal expression. Resonance requires that the clinician maintains a sensitive awareness of their own ANS regulatory patterns and rhythm in order to effectively observe and sense the patient's ANS states. The clinician's ability to sense when there is excess sympathetic activation in their patient's system, when there is enough parasympathetic tone that allows for relaxation and safety, and when the patient is overwhelmed or dissociated, is key to co-regulatory capacities necessary for helping the patient process traumatic experience.

RESOURCING

Resourcing is the practice of developing an embodied experience of safety, pleasure, and goodness. Even a somatic experience that is reported by the patient as "neutral" or "okay" can be a resource if it serves to engage the PNS when sympathetic activation is present.

Images can also be used as resources, but only when the image can also be felt as a sensation (Kuhfuß, 2021).

BOUND ENERGY

Bound energy is survival energy that was originally mobilized by the system with the intent of fight or flight (SNS charge) or freeze/collapse (dorsal vagal response), but was not able to complete due to the perceived threat associated with the original trauma, hence becoming bound. If the survival response was thwarted then the individual becomes unable to return to a state of relative safety, which is part of the reason why clients with trauma histories can appear "stuck" in the physiological response to the original traumatic event (Levine, 2010). An example of this would be a patient who experienced physical abuse but was unable to fight or flee. A completed survival response means that a person is able to mobilize behavioral response (if necessary), process and integrate the traumatic experience and return to a state of safety and rest.

The survival response cycle partially explains why two people who experience the same traumatic event can present with completely different symptoms and response: Because trauma lives in the body, not the event (Iannotti, 2021). The organismic response to threat involves an initial mobilization to fight or flee; when there is an interruption or non-completion at any part of the threat response cycle energy becomes bound. Bound energy creates a system that is consistently on "high-alert"; the amount of energy required to maintain this state can create trauma- and stress-related symptoms, such as chronic pain, fibromyalgia, migraines, and other low-immunity or autoimmune related syndromes (Gündüz et al., 2018). Over time, bound energy becomes what Levine refers to as "fixity" which, without treatment, limits an individual's ability to respond spontaneously and impedes their ability to respond to present or future threat or danger (Condos, 2020).

PENDULATION

The main goal behind SE is to restore self-regulation and dynamic equilibrium by releasing bound energy in the system. *Pendulation* is the human organism's natural capacity to rhythmically shift between states of distress/contraction (SNS) and states of pleasure/expansion (PNS). Pendulation is an essential ingredient in trauma recovery, since "pleasure and trauma cannot coexist in the nervous system; neurologically, they contradict one another" (Levine, 2010, 175). By assisting the individual to complete healthy active defense responses, one's sense of safety, vitality, and fluidity increases, thereby increasing and expanding their flexibility of functioning (Levine, 2010). Pendulation works in service of releasing bound energy and restoring dynamic equilibrium; SE aims to support healthy pendulation (Levine, 1997) in the autonomic nervous system.

IMPLICIT AND EXPLICIT MEMORY

Implicit memory can be conceptualized as consisting of three categories: 1) learned motor actions (such as riding a bike or dancing); 2) emergency responses (such as fighting, fleeing, bracing, contracting, retracting, setting and maintaining territorial boundaries); and 3) attraction or repulsion (patterns of attraction or avoidance) (Levine, 2015). These three categories of implicit memory are long term and outside of cognitive awareness. In contrast, *explicit memory* is episodic in nature, allowing for chronological organization of events and remembrance of sequence, and it unfolds in narrative formation. While implicit memory is phenomenological and carries the felt-sense, it can accompany explicit memory with narrative or partial narrative. An example may be the warm temperature sensations that spread across our chest and limbs (implicit) as our beloved pet approaches us (explicit), or the pleasant tingling and upward movement in our chest (implicit) as we describe a beloved piece of music to a friend (explicit).

S.I.B.A.M. (SENSATION, IMAGERY, BEHAVIOR, AFFECT, MEANING)

The acronym SIBAM serves as a structure that supports both the patient's and clinician's tracking of the patient's experience (Levine, 2010). The "S" stands for sensations, which include kinesthetic (muscle tension patterns), proprioceptive (awareness of one's body in space), vestibular (balance, acceleration and deceleration), and visceral sensations (of organs and blood vessels). "I" represents image, which Levine uses to refer to all types of impressions that originally come from outside the body and that we have incorporated into the brain as sense memory. Image also includes sight, taste, smell, hearing, and touch. "B" stands for behavior, which is the only element that the clinicians can observe directly, allowing them to infer the patient's inner state. This is done through the clinician's observation of the patient's behavior, including voluntary gestures; postures of the patient's spine and limbs; emotional/facial expressions; autonomic signals (involuntary behavior) such as a change in pulse, blood flow, and breath; visceral behaviors, such as digestive shifts via sounds of the gut; and archetypal behaviors such as involuntary gestures or postural shifts that convey universal meaning. "A" is for affect: Primary human emotions including fear, anger, sadness, joy, and disgust, as well as "contour" feelings which are sensation based and relate to attraction and avoidance, such as disgust or satisfaction. Finally, "M" stands for meaning, the labels we attach to the totality of our experience (Levine, 2015). In many clinical settings, and in general interpersonal dialogue between people, meaning and meaning-making are the primary focuses for interaction. SE holds all dimensions of a patient's experience with equal interest and valiance; SIBAM provides a method for holding the entire phenomenological gestalt of the patient's experience: Sensory, somatic, behavior, emotion, relational, and cognition.

WINDOW OF TOLERANCE

Window of tolerance (Siegel, 2012) describes the optimal state of arousal or stimulation that allows us to function and thrive in everyday life. The patient and clinician's collaboration in identifying the patient's window of tolerance – when they have the capacity for resiliency and integration versus when they are in a state of dissociation or overwhelm – is not only central to trauma processing and renegotiation, but also fundamental in avoiding re-traumatization.

DESCRIPTION OF THE THERAPY PROCESS

A typical session includes "nine building blocks" that are outlined below (Levine, 2010, 74). The clinician may work with these concepts multiple times throughout the treatment hour, which is to say that the building blocks are not necessarily conducted in chronological order but are instead iterative in nature. The following is a description of how these blocks may come together in an SE session. While this is not a description of a specific case, the following narrative portrays what a typical SE session entails, following these nine building blocks.

1) Establish an Environment of *Relative* Safety.
   The SE practitioner might begin by engaging the patient's social engagement system to *establish an environment of relative safety* by saying, "Nice to see you. How are you feeling today?" Or, with the aim of orienting the patient to their immediate surroundings, the practitioner might say, "That's such a vibrant yellow shirt you have on!" For some patients who have experienced trauma, guiding them to "insight" and internal somatic sensation can be quite overwhelming, which is why directing them to "outsight," such as what they see in the office or out the window, can offer accessible stabilization to them so that secure ground can be created before moving to internal sensation.

2) Support Initial Exploration and Acceptance of SENSATION.
   The practitioner explores internal sensation by asking the client, "What sensations are you aware of in your body right now?" or, depending on the patient's expressed need or the clinician's resonance with the patient's current internal state, they might offer, "How would it be for you to take a moment to sense your feet on the ground?" or "Take a moment to bring your awareness to the sensations of your body meeting the chair underneath you." This period of initial sensory exploration is often referred to as "settling" or "settling in."

   The practitioner's resonance is key to their assessment to determine the appropriate intervention to support the patient working inside their window of tolerance. As stated earlier, resonance works in combination with visual observation of the patient's behavior. For instance, if the practitioner observes a heightened sympathetic state, they might spend more time working with grounding techniques in order to further engage the PNS. If the practitioner senses dissociation, they might direct the patient to gently pat their arms and legs in order to create more somatic sensation, and then return to exploring the patient's awareness of their bodily sensation to assess the diminishment of feeling overwhelm.

3) Establish "Pendulation" and Containment: The Innate Power of Rhythm
   Pendulation is a fundamental concept of SE that refers to the "continuous, primary, organismic rhythm of contraction and expansion" (Levine, 2015, 55). People who have experienced trauma are often stuck in chronic contraction, and this fixedness often leaves an individual in a state of helplessness, hopelessness, and despair. The result of this fixedness often means an avoidance of anything that the system perceives as dangerous, which can keep people "stuck" in their trauma. Pendulation allows for gentle, directed guidance to increase tolerance for sensations and experience. This

ongoing practice of moving between expansion and contraction, with the support of the practitioner, begins, in time, to restore a sense of flow and a growing sense of relaxation and safety.

After the initial settling in, the patient might introduce the issue they would like to focus on for the session. For instance, a patient with early developmental trauma who had an emotionally and physically abusive father might say, "My father left me a voicemail this weekend." The practitioner observes the patient catching their breath, a tightening in the throat, and a bracing movement in the chest. This observable behavior demonstrates an increase in sympathetic activation, and the practitioner might begin to work with pendulation in order to engage the PNS by saying, "Let's pause for a moment. Can you bring your awareness to your feet on the floor?" After a few beats of silence to support the patient's somatic awareness, the practitioner might say, "Good, and now sense the chair underneath you. Feel your pelvis, lower back, and upper back meeting the chair."

A few more beats of silence pass as the practitioner observes the patient for indication of PNS engagement. The practitioner observes a softening of the muscles in the patient's neck and face, tracks increased movement of the breath in the upper chest, and reflects this observation to the patient: "It looks like your throat just relaxed and I see your breath just got a little freer. Do you sense that?" Pendulation between polarities of expansion and contraction allows for a continual assessment of safety and ground, develops affect regulation, and supports co-regulation with the therapist. The practitioner's ability to track and verbally reflect a patient's somatic experience develops the patient's capacity for tracking themselves.

4) Titration

Titration is about carefully touching into the smallest "drop" of survival-based arousal, and other difficult sensations, to prevent re-traumatization. For example, the patient may self-report, "My breath feels stable and I feel calmer now." The practitioner now introduces titration before returning to the figure of the patient's father by saying, "How far away from you would you like the voicemail from your father to be? Across the street, across the country …?" The patient smiles a little and responds by saying, "In outer space." The clinician enthusiastically supports the patient's choice, "Great! Outer space. Now, take a moment to let your body really sense how far away the voicemail is." Creative use of imagery that involves distance, size, or invocation of other resources is a method for titration which develops the patient's awareness of their body boundary and increased sense of safety.

The patient takes a few moments and then may say, "I feel safe. He's far away." Practitioner says, "Great. What would it be like to be with 'just a drop' of the experience?" *Titration* involves assisting the patient to touch into the smallest "drop" of traumatic experience. Working with pendulation and titration allows for individuals to safely access and integrate critical survival-based, highly energetic states without feeling overwhelmed, which, as stated earlier can lead to re-traumatization (Levine, 2010). "I feel scared," the patient says as she looks down at the ground. "Is it okay to be with just a little bit of the fear?" asks the practitioner. After a moment, the patient responds, "Yes, it's okay to be with a little bit of the fear …." To continue with titration, the practitioner responds, "Okay. How about taking a moment to look around the room right now? Let your whole head and neck move to take in the space around you. Notice where your eyes are drawn. Notice what feels pleasant to look at right now."

After a little bit of silence to give the patient time to orient to the present environment, the practitioner continues: "How is your body letting you know that it's okay to be with a little bit of the fear?" The patient considers the question and says, "I'm safe right now in this room … and I'm not alone." The patient looks up at the practitioner with a slight smile, some tears emerge in her eyes, and then her chest opens and her head raises a few inches, offering a good indication that the social engagement system is back online; a mark of "safe-enough" and a necessary element of co-regulation.

5) Restoring Active Response
The patient's awareness of the practitioner's presence with her and the observable posture shift from collapse to upright demonstrates a shift from helplessness toward an active, empowered, defensive response. As the patient takes in the therapist's face, her back straightens and her jaw tightens. The practitioner inquires, "What just shifted? You just sat back in your chair and I notice your jaw looks tight." The patient shoots both arms up in the air and shouts, "I'm pissed! What the hell is wrong with him?" The practitioner responds, "Yes! There's some healthy anger. Great! Take a moment to really sense the anger in your body. What does the angry part of you want to say to him?" The patient is energized and steady; she says, "You can't scream at me. If you use that tone of voice with me, I won't engage with you." The patient has a slight smile on her face. "That feels good to say," she offers. The patient's embodied experience of the support of her anger and her ability to express her boundary offers a corrective experience.

6) Uncoupling Fear From Immobility
Animals' immobility response to threat is time-limited, and when they come out of immobility, they have the locked energy available for flight or counter-attack. Human beings on the other hand often find that the energy locked in the immobility response is so strong that it can produce a secondary response of fear. Therefore, a key to releasing bound energy lies in uncoupling fear from the response itself which allows stuck energy to be freed up for use wherever it is needed in the body (Levine, 2008).

The practitioner develops the patient's self-reported enjoyment of her expression by reflecting it back to her: "Yes," the practitioner says, it feels good to say that to him. Can you take a moment to feel your body boundary and sense the limit you just set? Take a moment to notice how you couldn't say that when you were young, but you can say that now, 'You can't scream at me!'

Here the practitioner's use of tense is aimed at "uncoupling" now and then; as a child, the patient felt helpless, but now, with the mobilization of the healthy aggression and the support of the practitioner, the patient has access to something else. The patient says, "I feel like standing up." The practitioner encourages the patient, "Go ahead! Would you like me to stand up with you?" The client nods, "Yes. I would like that," as the patient stands, she begins to tremble slightly, "Oh … I'm shaking a little." The practitioner responds, "Sense your feet beneath you, feel the floor steady underneath your feet, and if it feels okay, just allow your body to shake." The two are now standing together and after a few moments the trembling beings to subside and the patient's breath deepens. She looks up directly into the practitioner's face and says, "Wow, I suddenly feel … powerful."

7) Resolve Arousal Sates by Promoting Renegotiation of Survival Energy

As the client's passive responses are replaced by active ones as she moves out of immobility, a physiological process often occurs: Involuntary shaking and trembling, followed by spontaneous changes in breathing from tight and shallow to deep and relaxed. These involuntary reactions are part of the discharge of bound energy (Levine, 2010).

"Yes," the practitioner says, "take a moment to really sense the feeling of your power." Following this discharge and redistribution of survival energy, and in an effort to integrate creative play with imagery to support the patient's high-level brain functioning, the practitioner says, "You look powerful to me. Is there an image that comes along for you?" The patient considers for a moment. "A superhero with many powers," she says. The practitioner develops this image by saying, "Great. Can you speak as the superhero?" The patient takes a moment and then her voice deepens and she puffs out her chest and says, "I am The Secret Destroyer!" Then her voice softens a bit, "I'm a friendly and a pretty chill superhero. I walk around and do good deeds and laugh with people but," her eyes narrow and nostrils flare and as her voice becomes stronger and louder, she shoots her hands up in front of her chest, "if you mess with me, I can shoot fireballs through my hands and incinerate you!"

8) Restore Self-Regulation and Dynamic Equilibrium

A direct consequence of discharge is the restoration of equilibrium and balance. The 19th-century French physiologist Claude Bernard coined the term *homeostasis* to describe "the constancy of the internal environment as the condition for a free and independent life." However, since equilibrium is not a static process, Levine uses the term "dynamic equilibrium" instead of homeostasis, which describes a restoration of resiliency of a nervous system that can move between states of arousal and relaxed alertness (Levine, 2010).

The practitioner laughs, enjoying the patient's observable self-regulation and relaxed alertness. The patient looks at the practitioner with a relaxed smile, saying, "I'm ready to sit now." The practitioner waits a few moments in silence as the patient looks around the room, naturally orienting to the immediate environment in the present moment.

9) Reorient to the Here and Now and the Present Environment

Trauma is an anachronistic experience occurring in the present moment. Trauma resolution includes restoration of dynamic equilibrium, awareness of the present environment, and our capacity for social engagement. Social engagement engenders a sense of belonging and safety and counters the feelings of fear and danger that are part of trauma.

"What are you noticing now?" the practitioner asks. The patient says, "I like the color of the sky right now." She looks back at the therapist, "and you're smiling. I liked how much you enjoyed my superhero. I like how much you enjoyed my anger. And, I feel good. I feel calm and … like, I'm here." She taps both fists lightly on the arm rests of her chair. Building blocks eight and nine often occur simultaneously following some discharge of bound energy at the end of an SNS activation and PNS settling cycle.

UTILIZATION OF THE SE MODALITY FOR THE TREATMENT OF TRAUMA

Traumatic events and developmental trauma trigger a strong stress reaction in individuals, which may lead to serious psychological and physical illnesses such as post-traumatic stress disorder (PTSD) (Brady, Killeen, Brewerton, Lucerini, 2000). Many people believe that it merely takes time for a person to "get over" their traumatic experience. However, unlike other mental disorders, PTSD has a particularly high rate of persistence and low levels of spontaneous remission (Kessler, Sonnega, Bromet, Hughes, and Nelson, 1995). Moreover, people with PTSD symptoms report high levels of suffering and have an increased chance of developing additional mental disorders, such as major depression or generalized anxiety or substance use disorders (Stewart, Pihl, Conrod, & Dongier, 1998; Straussner & Calnan, 2014). Therefore, the SE model can be used to understand the symptomatology of chronic and complex traumas, including developmental trauma (attachment, bullying), cultural trauma (racism, sexism, micro-aggressions), interpersonal trauma (ongoing domestic or partner-related conflicts), as well as non–life-threatening illness or injury. SE also incorporates specific theory, protocol, and subsequent interventions related to the treatment of high-impact falls, anesthesia, medical trauma, and even surgery preparation, in order to prevent or mitigate traumatic symptoms. Any event experienced as "too much, too fast, too soon" or in the instance of neglect, "not enough, never," can create a traumatic response in the human organism. The SE definition of trauma is not defined by the qualities of the traumatic event, but rather the impact that the stimulus has on the body-mind-system of the person experiencing the event (Iannotti, 2021).

RESEARCH EVIDENCE REGARDING EFFECTIVENESS OF SE IN TREATING TRAUMA

There is limited evidence regarding SE's efficacy as a treatment modality. Kuhfuß et al. (2021) conducted a literature review of studies of the effectiveness and key factors of SE, finding initial evidence that SE has a positive impact on affective and somatic symptoms and measures of well-being in both traumatized and non-traumatized samples. Out of the 16 selected SE studies that fit the inclusion criteria, four studies demonstrated positive effects of SE treatment on post-traumatic stress symptoms for up to one year following treatment. Two studies provided a sufficient data basis for a quantitative analysis of the effect of SE on depressive symptoms, which were absent in the control group. Regarding anxiety symptoms, two out of three studies found a significant reduction in anxiety symptoms due to an SE intervention in the follow-up measurements. With respect to specific symptoms related to natural disasters, two of the three studies demonstrated a reduction in stress-related symptoms. While there has not been enough research to date to advocate for SE as a first-line treatment method, preliminary research demonstrates SE's promise. Beginning research has also pointed to the successful use of SE as a complimentary modality when used with CBT, EMDR, and other modalities.

CASE EXAMPLE

Amelia was a 27-year-old Albanian woman who came to treatment to address a general feeling of "identity loss." After spending the first part of her life in Albania, Amelia attended college in the United Kingdom. She reported a series of abusive and manipulative intimate partners in her life and, while she was very accomplished and intelligent, she felt that she didn't know who she was or what she wanted in life.

Amelia described her parents as unemotional, pre-occupied, and unaffectionate. This affect desert, void of any mirroring, attunement, or positive regard, was replaced by her father's relentless criticism, control, and over-sexualization of her, and her mother's absence of protection or nurturance of her. Amelia had an extraordinary love of literature and she shared a devastating story of a time she received a low test grade. Upon learning of her grade, Amelia's father entered her room unannounced, swiping every beloved book from her shelf into a trash bin as he screamed at her, "No more books until you meet my expectations of what a daughter should be!" This crystalized memory was one of hundreds of other instances of Amelia's father overriding her sense of safety and pleasure with extreme aggression, while her mother stood by offering no protection.

Throughout Amelia's life, for Amelia to express enjoyment about anything that fell outside her father's narcissistic image of what she "should be," to say "no," or to express a need, was to put herself directly in the line of fire. During one of our first sessions, Amelia looked up at me and said,

> "My father told me if I was too fat or too thin. He told me who I could date, where to go to school, and what to do professionally. I have no idea who I am, what I want, what I like, or what I don't like."

These early developmental traumatic experiences with her father explained the strong over-coupling of attachment and fear that Amelia had continued to replicate in her other intimate partnerships.

When I discovered Amelia's love of books, I asked her to name one of her favorite characters with a hope that the feeling of safety she felt from books, and the creativity she experienced inside literary worlds, might be developed somatically as a resource. Amelia named Queen Daenerys Targaryen, also known as the "Mother of Dragons" from the book *Game of Thrones*. I made a note that Daenerys might serve as a competent protector, often an important somatic resource and essential to the resolution of trauma. People who have no experience of competent protection need help building it before they are willing to try connecting with past trauma as we tend not to venture into threatening memories without any hope of competent protection.

In our next session, Amelia began to share a memory of being 11 years old and her father insisting that she sit on his lap. Her body began to constrict as she recounted the event, and I noticed her eyes drop to the floor. I sensed that she was entering into a state of immobility. I asked her if it would be okay if she looked at me, again hoping that her ability to see my face would anchor her in her social engagement system. "Can you tell me what you're aware of in your body right now?" I asked. "My chest feels very tight. Like I'm frozen." This self-report of a frozen feeling was confirmation of the immobility. "What would it be like if Daenerys Targaryen were here right now?" I asked. I saw her chest expand and heard an intake of breath. "Nice breath," I confirmed, supporting the spontaneous physiological sigh that signaled a change in her state and an increase in regulation. "It would be really great," she said. "Yes, that would be great," I confirmed. "Now what are you noticing in your body?" I asked. "I just started to feel my legs ... a little," she said. "Great. What would it be like to push your feet into the floor?" I was curious to see if engagement of the musculature might allow for an increase in sensation and if the assertive movement of pushing might support some healthy aggression in her system. I used my voice to express the invitation for her to push, "really push." As she pushed into the floor, I observed an increase of tension in her jaw, her eyes widen, and her spine extend as she sat more upright. "What would Daenerys say to your father?" I asked. Her posture collapsed again and she began to shake and tremble, "I'm so ashamed," she wept quietly, "He's so powerful. And ... my body on his lap and his hands on me ... I couldn't protect my sister from him, how could anyone protect me?" I had moved too quickly from the emerging competent protector resource and the glimmer of healthy aggression; Amelia had gone straight into the fear and back into immobility.

We spent the next several sessions developing the resource of her healthy aggression in service of protecting her. I employed some boundary work, placing a thick rope on the floor that made a circle around her body. I invited Amelia to stand across from me in the room and, when she said she was ready, I would very slowly take steps toward her, stopping after every step until she sensed in her body that she didn't want me to come any closer. I gave her some boundary language and mirrored her as she forcefully practiced saying, "No!" and "Stop!" as she extended her arms in front of her chest with her palms facing outward toward me.

Initially, Amelia struggled with the boundary exercise. As I found myself at about six feet from her, I tracked an impulse of movement in her shoulders, but I also noticed that Amelia did not move her arms nor did she use her voice to stop me. I reflected my observation of this behavior and asked her if she sensed an impulse to stop me before she actually said, "Stop." She said, "I wanted to say 'stop' but I don't want to hurt your feelings." This bind continued to repeat throughout our early boundary work, demonstrating an overcoupling: To assert herself was dangerous and could mean a loss of connection with me. For months, we started every session with our "boundary ritual" as she began to refer to it, and in time we had begun to uncouple her capacity to assert herself and feel safe. She also began to notice my enjoyment of her "no," my willingness to yield and respond to her "no," and in time she reported an embodied sense that she could say "no" and have limits with me and still be attached.

One day she came into session and said, "I'd like to go back to that memory with my father. I feel ready now." I asked her if it would be okay if we worked really slowly. She agreed, and I invited her to take a moment to feel her body boundary. I began to move my arms around the entire of perimeter of my own body and in a moment, Amelia had joined me in the same movement. She moved her outstretched arms slowly, her palms extended flat. As she swept her arms above her head and to the sides of her body, her eyes, head, and neck followed the movement of her arms. "This feels good," she sighed. "Yes," I confirmed, "that feels really good to you. Take a few moments to notice how your body is letting you know 'this feels good.'" She continued, "I feel … safe. I feel at ease. I can move and I feel like, I can't explain it exactly, but like I'm here." "That's great. Now, can you offer me just a headline of the memory, a few words as if this were a chapter in a book."

A "trauma snapshot" is in essence a titration device, a way to allow for a small "drop" of survival-based arousal to emerge in the patient's system. She looked directly at me and said, "Daddy's icky lap." Initially, a shut-down similar to that of before began to occur; I noticed her body stiffen, her breath become shallow, her chest cave, and her posture slumped, I stayed with my attention on her interoception, and asked, "What are you sensing in your body, Amelia?" "My shoulders feel slumped and it's hard to breathe," she whispered. "Great noticing. Let's pause right here together. Take a moment to really sense the shape of your body. Feel your legs on the ground. Can you feel your pelvis on the couch?" She nodded.

"Good. How would it be to really, really slowly begin to let the vertebrae in your spine stack, and your shoulders to drop down your back. Can you do that really slowing, so that you can sense every part of the movement?"

I wanted to add as much time, space, and support to this experience.

As she began to balance her head on top of her neck spine, I noticed a slight pivot to the left with her sternum leading her chest and her eyes, while fixed, followed the same arc. In my own body, I suddenly felt as if I were on someone's lap and I quickly hypothesized that Amelia was gauging the threat of her father on the left side of her body. I also became aware of not being able to feel my feet in that moment and I spontaneously said to Amelia, "Amelia, what would it be like for you to put your feet on the floor, stand up, turn around and say, 'No!'" I heard an audible intake of breath as she stood up and stepped back away from the couch. She put her arms up in front of her as a somewhat choked, "No" emerged from her throat. "Great, Amelia," I confirmed with warm-chest resonance in my voice to celebrate her courage, "There's some wonderful healthy aggression in your body. Really feel your body boundary now. Daenerys is flying above on her dragon if you need her, and I'm here too if you need me. Now, imagine your voice is a vibrant color – any color you want. Can you imagine your 'no' like you were a dragon breathing fire and that fire was coming up through the earth, through your legs, through your core, and into you throat?" I saw her eyes move toward me a bit and then her face muscles softened slightly. "No!" she said, her voice strong this time as she pushed her arms out away from her body. She looked at me directly. Her face, while flush, was relaxed. "I want to do that again. It feels so good," she said. I invited her to see her father there on the couch and to feel the strength of her entire body and her voice and to notice the protective power that she had beneath the earth, in the sky, and with me beside her. "No! You can't touch me. This is my body. It's my life. I make my own choices and I've had enough!" She turned to me and smiled broadly; a small, gleeful giggle began to bubble up as she said through her laughter, "I'm so fierce right now!" I smiled broadly back at her. "Yes! You are," I said. "It's really beautiful to witness." When she sat down on the couch, she said, "I feel powerful … and calm."

STRENGTHS AND LIMITATIONS OF THE SE MODALITY AS A TREATMENT FOR TRAUMA

The main limitations of SE are that this method of therapy is still considered to be relatively "new" and more long-term research needs to be conducted in order to determine its efficacy. Although there is strong evidence to support the effectiveness of body-based therapies, attending to sensations and inner experience can be overwhelming, abstract, or simply unpleasant for many patients. Therefore, it is important that the practitioner is able to properly diagnose each patient's dominant entry point in order to slowly introduce and titrate somatic work. For instance, if a patient tends to organize cognitively, the SE practitioner should develop their cognitive resource as the primary ground with an intention to slowly expand into sensation, affect, and image. For clients that experience dissociation, developing the ground with image and meaning can eventually create a greater foundation of safety to begin to titrate sensation. While the SE model provides a strong theoretical framework for understanding the autonomic nervous system, affect, behavior, and trauma, ultimately SE is about helping patients gain an appreciation for their body as the home for their experience of the world.

RESOURCES FOR LEARNING

Somatic Experiencing International is a nonprofit 501c3 based on the teaching of Dr. Peter Levine dedicated to transforming lives through healing. https://traumahealing.org

Levine, A. (1997). *Waking the Tiger: Healing Trauma: The Innate Capacity to Transform Overwhelming Experiences*. North Atlantic Books.

Levine, A. (2010). *In an Unspoken Voice: How the Body Releases Trauma and Restores Goodness*. North Atlantic Books.

Levine, A. (2015). *Trauma and Memory: Brain and Body in a Search for the Living Past: A Practical Guide for Understanding and Working With Traumatic Memory*. North Atlantic Books.

Levine, A., Blakeslee, A., and Sylvae, J. (2018). Reintegrating fragmentation of the primitive self: Discussion of "somatic experiencing". *Psychoanalytic Dialogues*, 28(5), 620–628. https://doi.org/10.1080/10481885.2018.1506216

Somatic Experiencing International (2019). "What Is Pendulation in Somatic Experiencing with Peter A. Levine?" https://www.youtube.com/watch?v=LiXOMLoDm68

REFERENCES

Brady, K.T., Killeen, T.K., Brewerton, T., & Lucerini, S. (2000). Comorbidity of psychiatric disorders and posttraumatic stress disorder. *Journal of ClinicalPsychiatry*, 61(Suppl7), 22–32. https://www.psychiatrist.com/wp-content/uploads/2021/02/24280_comorbidity-psychiatric-disorders-posttraumatic-stress.pdf

Condos, D. (2020). Dr. Peter Levine on How Trauma Changes Our Minds and Bodies (S2 E13). https://beyondtheorypodcast.com/dr-peter-levine-on-how-trauma-changes-our-minds-and-bodies/

Fischer, R. 1973. "A cartography of the ecstatic and meditative states." *Leonardo*, *6*(1), 59–66. https://doi.org/10.2307/1572429

Gibbons, C.H. (2019). Chapter 27—Basics of autonomic nervous system function. In K.H. Levin and Chauvel (Eds.), *Handbook of Clinical Neurology*, 407–418. https://doi.org/10.1016/B978-0-444-64032-1.00027-8

Gündüz, N., Polat, A., Erzincan, E., Turan, H., Sade, I., & Tural, Ü. (2018). Psychiatric comorbidity and childhood trauma in fibromyalgia syndrome. *Turkish Journal ofPhysical Medicine and Rehabilitation*, *64*(2), 91–99. https://doi.org/10.5606/tftrd.2018.1470

Iannotti, L. (2021). *The Routledge International Handbook of Social Work and Sexualities* (1st ed.). https://doi.org/10.4324/9780429342912

Kessler, R.C., Sonnega, A., Bromet, E., Hughes, M., & Nelson, C.B. (1995). Posttraumatic stress disorder in the national comorbidity survey. *Archives of General Psychiatry*, *52*(12), 1048–1060. https://doi.org/10.1001/archpsyc.1995.03950240066012

Kuhfuß, M., Maldei, T., Hetmanek, A, & Baumann, N. (2021). Somatic experiencing – effectiveness and key factors of a body-oriented trauma therapy: A scoping literature review. *European Journal of Psychotraumatology*, *12*(1), 1929023. https://doi.org/10.1080/20008198.2021.1929023

Levine, P. A. (1997). *Waking the Tiger: Healing Trauma: The Innate Capacity to Transform Overwhelming Experiences*. North Atlantic Books.

Levine, P.A. (2008). *Healing Trauma: A Pioneering Program for Restoring the Wisdom of Your Body*. Sounds True.

Levine, P. A. (2010). *In an Unspoken Voice: How the Body Releases Trauma and Restores Goodness*. North Atlantic Books.

Siegel, D. J. (2012). *The Developing Mind: How Relationships and the Brain Interact to Shape Who We Are* (2nd ed.). The Guilford Press.

Stewart, S. H., Pihl, R. O., Conrod, P. J., & Dongier, M. (1998). Functional associations among trauma, PTSD, and substance-related disorders. *Addictive Behaviors*, *23*(6), 797–812. https://doi.org/10.1016/S0306-4603(98)00070-7

Straussner, S. L. A., & Calnan, A. J. (2014). Trauma through the life cycle: A review of current literature. *Clinical Social Work Journal*, *42*(4), 323–335. https://doi.org/10.1007/s10615-014-0496-z

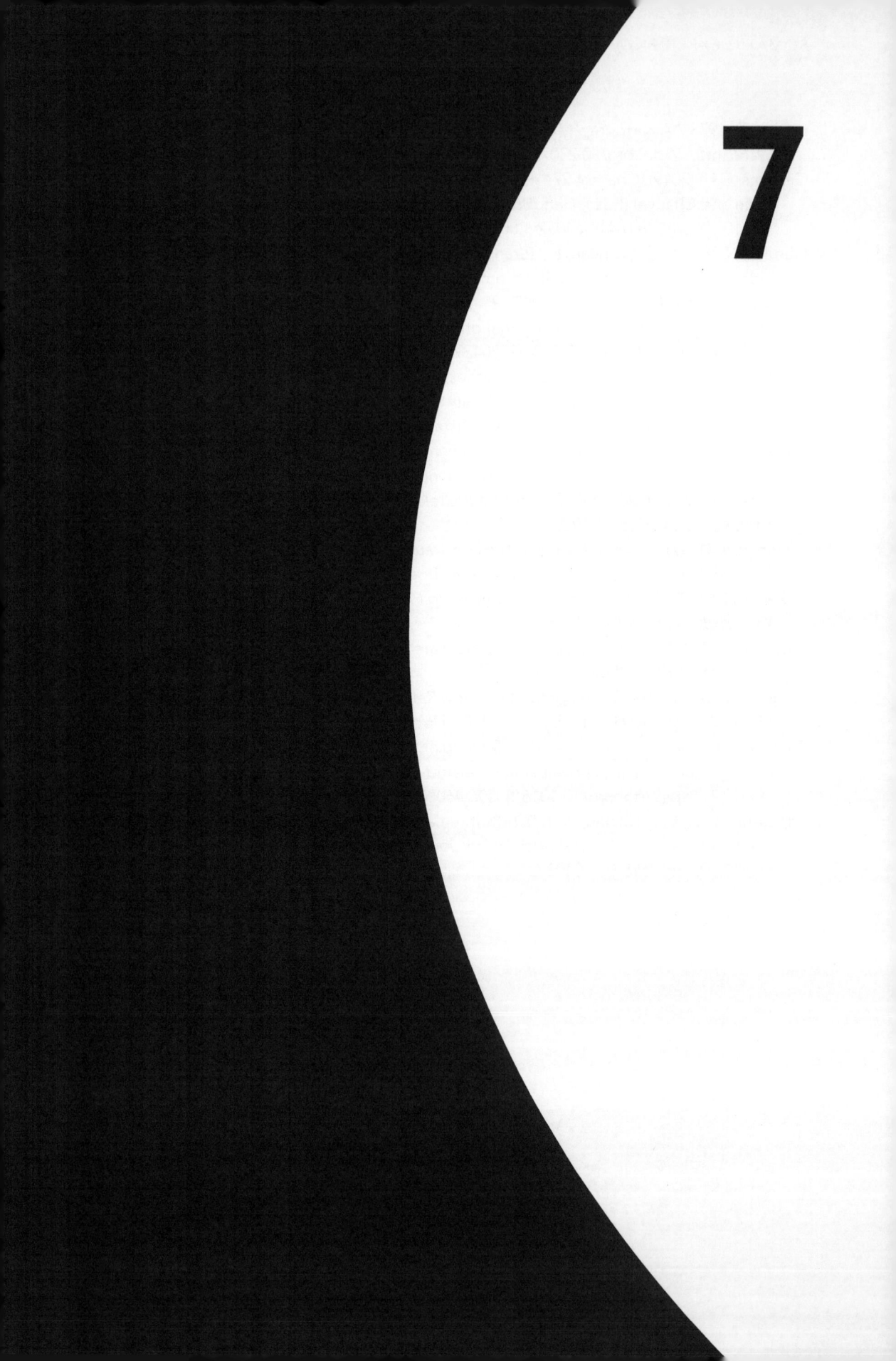

7

CHAPTER 7
HAKOMI MINDFULNESS-CENTERED SOMATIC PSYCHOTHERAPY

Benjamin Kagedan and Rebecca Stone

INTRODUCTION

Hakomi mindfulness–centered somatic psychotherapy (or the Hakomi method for short) is an experiential approach to psychotherapy that emerged out the work of Ron Kurtz and his students in the 1970s. Hakomi specializes in helping individuals gain insight into and transform the unconscious core beliefs and defensive character strategies that perpetuate emotional suffering and limit life satisfaction. It does so by inviting clients to pay mindful attention to body sensations and other nonverbal phenomena, helping them to study the ways they make meaning of and habitually respond to their experiences, moment to moment. Hakomi uniquely integrates Eastern principles of nonviolence and mindfulness, offering a gentle and holistic path toward reprocessing and integration of developmental and attachment trauma.

BRIEF HISTORY

Hakomi emerged in the mid-1970s out of the work of its pioneering founder, Ron Kurtz. Kurtz had a degree in experimental psychology and was versed in wide variety of spiritual and academic disciplines, including Buddhism, Taoism, physics and mathematics, Gestalt therapy, Reichian psychoanalysis, bioenergetics, Feldenkrais, and general systems theory. Dissatisfied with the popular clinical strategies of his time, Kurtz began to experiment with ways of facilitating spontaneous emergence of unconscious beliefs, emotions, and behavior patterns through gentle attention to the body and present moment experience. Over time, the techniques that Kurtz tested and developed in his many workshops were organized into a coherent and teachable system of experiential psychotherapy, which since the 1990s has been taught all over the world through multiple institutes. Hakomi distinguished itself from the field by incorporating mindfulness as a means of therapeutic exploration, by centering somatic and nonverbal experiencing over verbal exchange, and by maintaining a firm grounding in the Buddhist principle of nonviolence, such that transformation is achieved not by trying to challenge or modify the client's way of being, but by supporting and witnessing its natural unfolding. The name Hakomi comes from a dream had by one of Kurtz's students, and is a word in the Hopi Nation language meaning "Where do you stand in relation to these many realms," or more colloquially, "Who are you?", reflecting the method's emphasis on awareness and self-observation.

DOI: 10.4324/9781003455851-7

FUNDAMENTAL CLINICAL CONCEPTS

Hakomi possesses a unique conceptual structure, in which the practitioner's thought process and behavior are guided by two separate, co-equal, mutually reinforcing sets of ideas: The Principles and the Method (Johanson, 2015). The principles articulate the core tenets, ideals, and aspirations of the approach, and the method spells out a practical technique that flows from the principles and is constrained by them. We define the five principles.

MINDFULNESS

Hakomi was among the first approaches to incorporate mindful awareness directly into flow of the session, rather than as adjunct to therapy in the form of assigned meditation practice. In different moments throughout a session, the therapist invites and supports the client to turn inward, relax from analytic thinking, and bring receptive, non-judgmental attention to present experience. This slowing down of the nervous system and quieting of internal noise permits clients a more intimate and expansive apprehension of specific experiences in the moment, such as a given sensation, emotion, or memory. Simultaneously, the therapist themself maintains a state of mindfulness throughout the session, staying curious and attentive both to their client's experience and to their own responses to the client.

MIND-BODY HOLISM

Hakomi affirms a radically nondualistic account of the nature of mind and body. The human person is viewed as a complex and unified system, an embodied consciousness. Rather than favoring a physiological or psychological account of human nature, we assume that every state of being has physiological, emotional, and cognitive dimensions. Thus, any given dimension of experience – sensation, emotion, memory, image, or thought – when offered mindful attention, may serve as an access point for deepening and expanding self-awareness and facilitating the emergence and reprocessing of unconscious material.

ORGANICITY

The organicity principle arises from the belief that every person possesses what is now often referred to as an "inner healing intelligence," an intuitive, though not fully conscious, understanding of what is behind their suffering and how their healing ought to proceed. In practice, this means placing great trust in the natural movements of the client's consciousness to direct our joint attention and steer our inquiry into deepening layers of insight. We orient primarily toward the objects of their curiosity, privilege their sense of what is important, and give mindful focus to whatever is most salient in their awareness.

UNITY

The unity principle points to the fact that every person is a complex system, a whole comprised of many interdependent parts. It frames the work of therapy as the task of bringing disconnected parts of the system (e.g. unwanted emotions, repressed memories, parts that feel unacceptable or shameful) back into communication so that the system may function harmoniously. As therapists, we are asked to consider the way our clients' issues and experiences arise within a multiplicity of dimensions – physical, intra-psychic, inter-personal, familial, cultural and spiritual – all at once, and to bring this comprehensive view to our work.

NONVIOLENCE

The Hakomi practitioner strives to remain attentive to the safety of the client, and to avoid wielding their power in a way that undermines the client's autonomy. This is not to say the therapist never plays an active or leading role in the process. However, care is always taken to ensure that a client feels securely connected, resourced, and willing to follow the therapist's lead. When a client feels a "no" to any given inquiry or suggestion, the therapist does not attempt to push past it to achieve the desired outcome, but rather respects the boundary as an intelligent response and invites curiosity about it. As much as possible, we avoid bringing our own agenda to the therapeutic encounter.

LOVING PRESENCE

Though not strictly an original principle, a sixth foundational idea articulated by Hakomi's founder is that the therapist should work to cultivate an attitude of "loving presence" when sitting with clients (Kurtz, 2015). Simply put, this means sitting with an open-hearted and accepting demeanor, such that clients may feel genuinely seen and liked for who they are. Loving presence helps facilitate a strong rapport and secure attachment between client and therapist, which goes a long way toward softening defenses and allowing access to painful or shameful material.

THE METHOD: STUDYING THE ORGANIZATION OF EXPERIENCE

The Hakomi method consists of a variety of techniques to assist the client in studying their core unconscious organization. This approach is founded on the theory, put forward by Wilhelm Reich (1972) and elaborated by others, that children go through a series of developmental stages, each of which is characterized by a central developmental need and a central dilemma. As a child goes about seeking sufficient safety, nourishment, power, autonomy, and self-worth, they develop an internal "map" of how things work based on the physical, social, and cultural particulars of their early life. This map consists of unconscious beliefs about reality (the world is basically safe/unsafe; there is enough nourishment for me here/there is scarcity here; I can follow my own impulses/I must conform in order to belong; etc.), and adaptive strategies that arise as intelligent responses to that internalized reality. Thus, for example, a child whose spontaneous expressions of self are made to feel strange, unwanted, or transgressive in their family or cultural setting may well develop the belief that in this world, one must surrender self-expression in exchange for love and belonging. An adaptive strategy in such a world might then be to forego spontaneous movement and expression, becoming highly considered in speech and behavior while instinctively attuning to feelings and desires of others. What's more, the adaptive unconscious may well erect what Hakomi calls a "nourishment barrier" around the missing experience of autonomy and free expression, so as to prevent any re-experiencing of the pain of the original suppression. Thus, even when one's present-day environment does afford opportunities for autonomous expression, the individual will have great trouble identifying and making use of them.

As adults we are largely still using the maps we make as children, but with little insight into this state of affairs. Our core beliefs refract the information we receive from the world in highly particularized ways, which then appear to us as the simple truth of things. Our behavioral strategies can be so reflexive, or seem so necessary, as to severely limit our sense of choice around how we would like to respond to a given situation. Our beliefs and strategies are like the proverbial water in which the fish swims. The method therefore supports the cultivation of insight regarding the nature of our inner map, by facilitating access to core material – the unconscious memories, traumas, feelings, meanings, and body states that undergird our beliefs and strategies. Through insight and awareness, we open the possibility for corrective emotional experiences both in the therapy room and in life lived. This process will become clearer in the description of the method and case examples offered in the following. Ultimately, the method aims to cultivate more flexibility and choice in the ways a person interprets and responds to their inner and outer environments.

DESCRIPTION OF THE THERAPY PROCESS

EXPERIMENTAL ATTITUDE

Hakomi encourages therapists to bring an attitude of not-knowing to the therapeutic encounter. Rather than come in with a priori assumptions, we study the organization of client's consciousness through an iterative cycle of mindfully attuning to their experience, having hunches about the significance of that experience, checking out those hunches, gathering the feedback, and attuning once more. Illustratively, a favorite expression of many a Hakomi practitioner is "See what happens when …." We are not committed to being right, only to being curious.

TRACKING

Tracking is the bedrock of the Hakomi method, and simply means consistent mindful observation. In Hakomi, it is said that the therapist tracks the client while the client tracks themself. Tracking occurs on multiple levels simultaneously, as we attend to the narrative themes, level of autonomic activation, emotional quality (or lack thereof), somatic markers (e.g. leg shaking, eyes darting, breath quickening, volume or pace of speech changing, etc.), and interpersonal behaviors (e.g. a client looks down every time they speak about themselves, seems to reject every suggestion and invitation, laughs and jokes when speaking about their sadness, etc.). Through tracking, we begin to observe the patterns that will point us toward the core organization of experience.

CONTACT

At root, contact is the technique of maintaining presence and connection with one's client by demonstrating and verbalizing awareness, understanding and acceptance of who they are and what they are going through. It also functions to bring unconscious dimensions of the client's experience into shared awareness. Contact often takes the form of a small guesses about the client's present state (e.g. "Some sadness, huh?"; Seems like some anger comes in here") or observations of somatic phenomena (e.g. "Looks like your upper body is caving in a bit as we explore this").

ACCESSING AND DEEPENING

A guiding assumption in Hakomi is that that unconscious core material is always close at hand, like "flakes of gold in the ore of the present moment" (Gaskin, Cole & Eisman, 2015). Accessing is then the process of starting to pan for this gold, by immersing the client's awareness in a given experience, feeling, sensation, or theme in the present. We accomplish this through invitations to mindful attention ("See if it's okay to bring more attention to that sensation") and experientially oriented questions ("Where do you notice it? Is it moving or still? If it could speak, what would it be saying?"). By dwelling in one phenomenon at a time and remaining receptive rather than analytical, we open space for the emergence of important associations, meanings, and memories, thus "deepening" our inquiry toward the client's core unconscious organization. We further the deepening process by creating little experiments in mindfulness, as explained in the next paragraph.

EXPERIMENTS IN MINDFULNESS

The most unique element of the Hakomi method is a set of techniques that allow the client and therapist to gather insight and elicit unconscious material through little experiments undertaken in a state of mindfulness. Experiments are utilized to help elucidate a particular defense or adaptive strategy and the missing developmental experience that necessitated it, and can function in one of two ways: (1) The therapist offers a morsel of the missing experience, intended to evoke the defense or associated core material, or (2) the therapist lends support to a defense that is already engaged, "taking over" the protective action so that the client can more easily sense the painful material being repressed or avoided (Lavie, 2015).

Experiments are always done with informed consent of the client. The general structure is to (a) propose and explain the experiment, (b) invite or guide the client toward a state of mindful awareness or inner witnessing, (c) add a particular stimulus in the form of a verbalization, movement, image, action, interaction, or specific kinds of physical touch, and (d) study the client's automatic responses to the stimulus.

There are many types of experiments and plenty of room for creativity. But for purposes of this brief introduction, one example will suffice: In session, a client is describing feeling afraid of telling their partner that they don't want to come to the next big family event. The therapist hypothesizes that some core belief/adaptive strategy is standing in the way of the client speaking freely. After proposing the experiment and inviting the client into mindfulness, the therapist says, "Notice what happens when you hear me say – your feelings matter, too." The words are chosen specifically to elicit the opposing core belief and inhibiting strategy, which may show up as a tightening of musculature; autonomic arousal; an emotion like fear, anger, or sadness; a contradictory thought; an image or symbol of suppression or punishment; a memory of or memory fragment of a relevant developmental experience; or combination of these. The client tracks whatever arises and shares their observations with the therapist, who then collaborates in making meaning of the response and continuing the exploration from there.

WORKING AT THE CORE

The pathway toward the core always starts in the present but inexorably leads into early life, bringing us in touch with the young "mapmaker" whose traumas, impressions, and adaptive responses form the basis of today's limiting patterns. In Hakomi, we often invite clients to fully embody this child self, to step into their shoes and into their worlds, to feel deeply the fear, anger, disappointment, deprivation, loss, or powerlessness of the child's situation. The client's willingness to embody the "child state" permits a profound level of insight into the subjective and conditioned nature of the client's present-day perceptions and responses, which can in itself be transformative. For instance, one may become acutely aware that a recurring fear of requesting assistance from a coworker or boss is rooted in the repeated experience of incurring the wrath of an overworked and overstressed parent when needing help as a child. This kind of insight is not merely a conceptual connection between past and present, but an experiential shift in one's sense of truth and possibility, gained through a re-experiencing of the child's traumatic reality in the safety and warmth of the therapeutic situation. In some cases, this state does not include episodic content, but rather manifests as an intense bout of emotion, or an uncanny and total experience of being small, weak, alone, or depleted. As in many therapies, the opportunity for the client to experience such repressed emotion through to completion can be enough to release them from its neurotic hold on their interpersonal functioning.

Beyond the facilitation of insight, working with core or child states affords the therapist and client the opportunity to facilitate a missing developmental experience. Often this involves inviting a "magical stranger" into a painful memory, someone real or fictional who can help the missing experience happen. This can be the therapist themself, a grown version of the client, or any being the client identifies as a wise and safe presence. The magical stranger can intervene in various ways. Sometimes they will speak on behalf of the child to let a parent or caregiver know the kind of harmful impact they are having and help them find a better way of relating. Other times they might speak to the child, bringing in missing information that would have helped the child make better sense of the experience. For instance, the therapist might explain to the child in simple terms that the parent is totally overwhelmed by their job, and that the harshness of their response to the child has nothing to do with the child themself, nor does it mean that asking for needs to be met is wrong or bad. This allows the client to disidentify from the limiting belief formed through this and related experiences and make room for a new, more realistic belief to form. Much can happen somatically and emotionally in these moments, as archaic patterns of protection and self-reproach around these wounds start to relax. The effect is not always immediately easeful, as decades of unconscious grief and anger over what has been lost may rise to the surface. Yet, ultimately this kind of work can facilitate the long-sought freedom to feel, identify, express, and satisfy the full range of emotional and interpersonal needs.

INTEGRATION

The final step of the Hakomi method is helping clients integrate the insights and corrective experiences that arise in therapy into their lives in the world, encouraging new, adaptive beliefs patterns to take root neurologically and experientially. This is another place where options abound and the therapist can get creative. For the sake of this introduction, here are a few common integration techniques:

- The therapist leaves time at the end of the session to talk about and make meaning of intense or anomalous experiences that occurred in mindful and regressed states, and how they relate to current dilemmas.
- If, at the end of the session, a client is experiencing a new state of confidence, equanimity, freedom, or sensing the truth of a new adaptive belief, the therapist invites them to visualize handling stressful parts of life from within this new state.
- Client and therapist may role-play a difficult conversation, offering the client an opportunity to embody a new interpersonal strategy (e.g., clearly stating their needs or naming their boundaries).
- The therapist may inform the client about practices, communities, or resources outside of therapy that will support them in embodying and installing new beliefs and strategies (e.g., self-compassion practices, martial arts, ecstatic dance, assertiveness training, art-making, spiritual practices, community service, inspiring works of philosophy or poetry, etc.).

UTILIZATION OF THE MODALITY FOR THE TREATMENT OF TRAUMA

Generally speaking, Hakomi is very well suited to clinical presentations rooted in developmental trauma; in other words, trauma arising from life contexts that were not specifically life threatening or dangerously abusive, but which in some fashion suppressed, discouraged, or penalized the fulfillment of basic socio-emotional needs over a long span of time. However, Hakomi is contra-indicated for what is commonly called acute or shock trauma. The reason for this is that Hakomi's use of mindfulness, its frequent invitations to immerse oneself in difficult sensations and memories, and its embrace of regressed states all depend upon the client feeling a basic ground of safety. In cases of treating shock trauma, such a basic safety feeling cannot be presumed, given the high likelihood of hyper- and hypoarousal when accessing terrifying memories. Thus, contemporary somatic approaches to trauma (including sensorimotor psychotherapy, which grew out of the Hakomi method) emphasize abundant resourcing and stabilization of the client's nervous system and facilitate clients moving through, rather than dwelling in, the traumatic material. That being said, a course of therapy that draws heavily on the Hakomi method can easily be supplemented by complementary somatic modalities such as sensorimotor psychotherapy or somatic experiencing when working with shock trauma material.

This same rubric can be applied when dealing with trauma rooted in the experience of cultural oppression. When the traumatic material centers on racial or cultural violence, incarceration, starvation, or any kind of ongoing threat to physical safety, Hakomi is likely not the ideal choice of technique, for the reasons stated previously. However, in many cases, the trauma of cultural oppression does not involve experiences of concrete violence, but rather more subtle, chronic, and systemic forms of oppression like marginalization, economic disadvantage, micro-aggressions, lack of representation in media, or shame over difference or minority status. Simply existing in a cultural context that includes systemic oppression of these kinds can easily engender core beliefs and adaptive strategies that will set the stage for psychological suffering in adulthood. In such cases, the Hakomi method makes a fine choice of approach. However, it is crucial that the therapist working with individuals from oppressed communities exercise care not to invalidate or minimize the reality of the oppressive conditions that gave rise to the client's suffering, and especially the fact that those conditions are likely still true and ongoing in society. Extra attention must also be paid to class, race, gender, and sexuality differences in the therapeutic dyad and how they impact the client's sense of safety.

RESEARCH EVIDENCE

While a good deal has been published in the *Hakomi Forum*, the Hakomi Institute's own annual journal, illustrating the efficacy of the Hakomi method through case studies and the experience of practitioners, to date the method has not been studied by statistical means. Johanson (2013) attributes this to a conceptual discrepancy between the Hakomi method and the "gold standard" of modern psychotherapy research, the randomized control trial. Namely, whereas Hakomi training and practice sees the efficacy of the method as dependent equally upon the personhood and character of the therapist as proper performance of technique, the RCT model attempts to fully separate the technique from the person practicing it. The effectiveness of Hakomi can, however, be argued based upon empirical research demonstrating the validity of its component parts, specifically regarding mindfulness and interpersonal neurobiology (Hanson & Mendius, 2009; Siegel, D., 2007, 2010), psychodynamic psychotherapy (Shedler, 2010), and the "common factors" research showing the fundamental importance of the therapeutic rapport (Laska et al., 2014). Future research supporting the efficacy of the Hakomi Method, according to Johanson, while important, will depend both upon the availability of funding as well as the expansion of the scientific consensus around what constitutes empirical evidence. One immediate way forward may be for Hakomi practitioners to publish more accounts of their work using Fishman's (2013) model of the "pragmatic case study," which integrates aspects of qualitative and quantitative research design. The pragmatic case study method was used effectively by Kaplan and Schwartz (2005) to show how in detailed ways how body-centered psychotherapy was helpful for several individual clients undergoing short-term treatment.

CASE EXAMPLE

A client presents for treatment complaining of problems in her relationship with her husband. She finds herself taking on too much responsibility for the practical and emotional needs of their family, leaving her feeling resentful, lonely, and dissatisfied with their partnership. In learning about her history, the therapist discovers that the client struggled as a child with being compared to her high-achieving older sister. The client likely had undiagnosed attention deficit/hyperactivity disorder, and rather than getting the compassion and help she needed, was held accountable for whatever difficulties she experienced keeping up with life and deemed lacking in intelligence. As such, the client learned to stop expecting to be seen and supported, and turned to a strategy of being overly supportive of others in order to ensure her value and belonging. This strategy is still in effect today, and underlies the problematic cycle in her marriage. In session, the therapist and client are exploring the theme of deserving and receiving support:

T: How about we go into mindfulness to study this theme of support.

C: Okay.

T: Great, so close your eyes ... notice your breath ... feel your feet supported by the ground ... notice any current sensations. (Pause) I see you took a deeper breath there ... perfect .... So now, notice what happens all by itself when you hear me say ... I'm here for you.

C: I feel tightening in my chest, and I hear the word "no."

T: Great, let's stay with the tightening in your chest and the word "no," and see if we can make them even louder. What happens when you make the tightness even tighter? You can apply even more pressure to your chest with your hands and hear the "no" more intensely ... just notice what happens next.
        The client collapses in tears and can't stop crying. She repeats over and over again, "There is no support for me, there is no support for me." Therapist stays attuned and available, offering affirmations like "it's so painful" and "it's ok to really feel this" and waits for this wave of emotion to ease.

T: That was a big wave of grief, huh? Seems like those words may be coming from a young part of you who is really sad and confused, does that feel true?

C: Yes. She really is so sad and confused. (*More tears*).

T: I see, like she just can't understand why the support isn't available ... like, what did she do wrong?

C: Yes. (*more tears*)

T: As if she is the reason that she doesn't have what she needs. (*Here the therapists makes a guess about the core belief underlying this pain, that somehow she is at fault for the emotional deprivation.*)

C: Oh yes, she is. She's not smart enough, not interesting enough ... I have this picture in my head of being at the dinner table. My parents and sister are engaged in an intellectual debate for an hour – they are completely engrossed. I am silent and bored. And I share my opinion early on, but they don't hear me. An hour later, my sister arrives at the same conclusion I offered in the first

5 minutes, and my parents agree with awe and admiration for her intelligence. (*More tears*)

T: Sounds so painful, like you really felt invisible to them.

C: I was.

T: Yes, and so it sounds like that child started to believe something like: Don't expect much, no one will give you the love you need.

C: Yes. And so instead I give and give all the love I ever wanted and never got. Otherwise, (raising voice) NO ONE sees me.

T: Yes, what a recipe for disappointment and pain.

C: Yes, but there is no other way.

T: I wonder if we can work with this memory a little bit.

C: Sure. How?

T: Well, someone needs to get information to this little girl and her parents. Who can help the family see what they are doing to her and adjust? Her parents need help to understand her better ....

C: I always loved Mr. Rogers (the television personality).

T: Perfect, what do you imagine Mr. Rogers saying?

C: He says, "Hey, you are making your daughter feel like shit. You need to include her more and value what she says."

T: Great, what's it like for her little you to hear that from him?

C: It's good.

T: And how about if he also says to your parents: Just because she doesn't like to debate the way you do doesn't mean she has nothing valuable to add. She has a different kind of brain and so she learns differently, but she is just as intelligent as you and her sister. But she needs your help to feel valuable.

CLIENT TAKES A DEEP BREATH

T: Nice big breath, huh? Seems like the little you is feeling some relief.

C: Yes, it does feel nice. But they're still not warm. It's like, even if they value me more, I am still not going to get the love that I need.

T: Yes, that is important. So, what about having Mr. Rogers turn to you and speak to you directly now?

C: Sure.

T: Hmm, so how about he says: I know that you grew up in a family that isn't very warm. And it's not easy. But I want you to know something: Soon, you're going to leave this house and create relationships based on what people can give back. Your family might be cold, but they're just three people. The world has plenty of warm people for you to connect with. And this is just who your parents are. Their coldness has nothing to do with who you are.

CLIENT TAKES A DEEP BREATH AND SIGHS

T: Seems like that landed.

C: Yes, that felt good. I can see myself at the table but less upset. Like, I know I have value and I deserve warmth.

T: Great, stay with that.

C: It feels nice. I see my sister hogging all the attention, and I am reminding myself that soon I will find people who like being around me and hearing what I have to say.

T: Beautiful. And what happens when you want more from them emotionally than they can offer – like warmth?

C: It's painful but it's not about me.

T: Wow, how amazing.

C: Yes, it is.

          Therapist invites client to quietly stay with this new sensation and new belief about her deservingness of love and support for a couple minutes, "savoring" it mindfully. Then, therapist begins to offer integration of the new experience.

T: So what happens when you bring this new belief with you into your current relationship with your husband?

C: Hmm, that's hard, because I still feel so angry.

T: That's okay. Let yourself feel the anger alongside this new sense of what you deserve. See what happens.

C: Oh yes, that feels better. I am still angry because I deserve more. But I no longer collapse in self-pity and shame. I no longer feel like the reason I am emotionally deprived is because I am not enough. I see his limitations – I see how emotionally cut off he is. It's not about me ... I feel stronger!

This exchange is an example of how the Hakomi method charts a path from awareness of present-moment experience to deep re-experiencing and reprocessing of developmental wounds. By offering words of support in an experimental fashion, the therapist enables the client to directly perceive how much she unconsciously distrusts and rejects help from others, a consequence of not receiving enough help around her learning differences when it was needed as a child. (This is the protective "nourishment barrier" discussed earlier.) By supporting rather than confronting the defensive response, the therapist next enabled the client to touch into the sheer depth of the grief of that early deprivation. This willingness on the part of the client to fully experience a challenging emotion facilitates the emergence of a core traumatic memory into awareness, such that the client gains experiential insight into the formation of her negative beliefs about her value and deservingness. Having re-opened this developmental moment, the client can integrate new and important information about the meaning of the experience, and disidentify herself as the cause of her parents' misguided actions. Back in her present-day life, she may now approach her husband with a newly clear sense of her own value. Rather than stay in the cycle of overfunctioning and collapse, she now feels ready to risk naming her discontent and asking for more of what she needs.

STRENGTHS AND LIMITATIONS

The Hakomi method is well suited for a wide variety of clinical presentations, as well for clients experiencing troubling patterns or emotional cycles that lack the specificity of a formal diagnosis. This versatility is one of its great strengths. By orienting toward the unconscious conflicts and unintegrated developmental traumas that perpetuate symptom formation, Hakomi can be helpful in resolving a plethora of presenting problems. Another strength is how easily the method can be integrated in small or substantial ways into other therapeutic modalities. Whether one takes a psychodynamic, cognitive-behavioral, humanistic, or even coaching-style approach to the work, it is highly valuable to have a set of techniques at one's disposal for bringing the body more fully into the therapy process and making meaning of its signals. Hakomi makes an excellent choice for clients who prefer a good deal of spaciousness, freedom, and collaboration in therapy, and may struggle with therapies that are more systematic or goal oriented, as well as those who feel they have exhausted the benefits of verbally processing their issues in talk therapy.

In terms of limitations, owing to its consistent use of mindful self-awareness, Hakomi can be cumbersome for clients who have either no experience nor any positive feeling toward mindfulness practice. The same goes for clients who have great difficulty holding attention in one place, such as in cases of severe ADHD. Similarly, given its emphasis on tracking emotion and sensation in the body, Hakomi may be overly taxing for clients who are dissociated from the somatic layer of their experience, who are alexithymic, or for whom the body is the site of severe pain or trauma. At the same time, it is precisely the aforementioned types who are most in need of growing their capacity to slow down and safely connect with somatic experience. A skilled practitioner can offer such "somatic beginners" the patience and scaffolding required to take the first steps toward this new and rewarding possibility.

In addition, Hakomi is not well suited for individuals whose ego structures are highly fragmented or who cannot easily observe emotional and somatic states without being engulfed by them. Thus, the method is contraindicated for the treatment of personality disorders, especially borderline and narcissistic formations, as well psychotic, bipolar, and severe dissociative disorders.

RESOURCES FOR LEARNING

Body Centered Psychotherapy: The Hakomi Method by Ron Kurtz
Grace Unfolding: Psychotherapy in the Spirit of the Tao-te Ching by Greg Johanson and
    Ron Kurtz
Hakomi Mindfulness-Centered Somatic Psychotherapy: A Comprehensive Guide to
    Theory and Practice, by Halko Weiss, Lorena Monda, and Greg Johanson
The Hakomi Forum, the annual journal of the Hakomi Institute www.hakomi.com, featur-
    ing a library of videos featuring the work of Ron Kurtz, and other learning resources

REFERENCES

Fishman, D.B. (2013). The pragmatic case study method for creating rigorous and systematic, practitioner-friendly research. *Pragmatic Case Studies in Psychotherapy, 9*(4), 403–425.

Gaskin, C.L., Cole, D., Eisman, J. (2015). Accessing and Deepening. In Weiss, H., Johanson, G. J., & Monda, L. (2015). *Hakomi mindfulness-centered somaticpsychotherapy: A comprehensive guide to theory and practice* (pp. 41–57). W.W. Norton & Company.

Hanson, R., with Mendius, R. (2009). *Buddha's Brain: The Practical Neuroscience of Happiness, Love and Wisdom.* Oakland, CA: New Harbinger.

Johanson, G. (2013). Hakomi and the ambiguous nature of research. *Hakomi Forum, 26,* 11–26.

Johanson, G. (2015). Hakomi Principles and a Systems Approach to Psychotherapy. In Weiss, H., Johanson, G. J., & Monda, L. (2015). *Hakomi mindfulness-centered somaticpsychotherapy: A comprehensive guide to theory and practice* (pp. 41–57). W.W. Norton & Company.

Kaplan, A.H., & Schwartz, L.F. (2005). Listening to the body: Pragmatic case studies of body-centered psychotherapy. *Body Psychotherapy Journal, 4*(2), 33–67.

Kurtz, R. (2015). The Essential Method. In Weiss, H., Johanson, G.J., & Monda, L. (2015). *Hakomi mindfulness-centered somatic psychotherapy: A comprehensive guide to theory and practice* (pp. 19–32). W.W. Norton & Company.

Laska, K.M., Gurman, A.S., & Wampold, B.E. (2014). Expanding the lens of evidence-based practice in psychotherapy: a common factors perspective. *Psychotherapy, 51*(4), 467.

Lavie, S. (2015). Experiments in Mindfulness. In Weiss, H., Johanson, G.J., & Monda, L. *Hakomi mindfulness-centered somatic psychotherapy: A comprehensive guide to theory and practice* (pp. 178–193). W.W. Norton & Company.

Reich, W. (1972). *Character analysis.* Macmillan.

Shedler, J. (2010). The efficacy of psychodynamic psychotherapy. *American psychologist, 65*(2), 98.

Siegel, D.J. (2010). *The mindful therapist: A clinician's guide to mindsight and neuralintegration.*New York, NY: W. W. Norton.

Siegel, D.J. (2007). *The mindful brain in human development.* New York, NY: Norton.

8

CHAPTER 8
FOCUSING-ORIENTED THERAPY FOR THE TREATMENT OF TRAUMA

Jeffrey L. Morrison and Riley Paterson

INTRODUCTION

This chapter introduces focusing-oriented therapy (FOT), discusses how it emerged from research, and describes its relevance to the treatment of trauma. We begin with central clinical concepts including a philosophy of change, the felt sense, experiential listening, an approach to experiencing, and relational interactions that facilitate change. From there, we demonstrate how the central component of FOT – the *felt sense* – can be used in therapy broadly and trauma treatment specifically. The felt sense is a term coined by the founder of focusing, Eugene Gendlin, meant to describe a holistic, present, and embodied way of sensing complex situations. A felt sense is a type of embodied knowing from which steps of change emerge freshly in a *life-forward* direction. Further, we show how a felt sense can be used to access frozen and speechless aspects of trauma, and how to bring those aspects into explicit awareness (or focus) to facilitate symptom transformation. Finally, we will discuss the felt sense from an indigenous and noncolonized relational place of "knowing" and its ability to work with ancestral and systemic trauma.

HISTORY

Eugene Gendlin, Ph.D., discovered focusing through his research on what produces positive change in psychotherapy. As a philosophy student at the University of Chicago in the 1950s, Gendlin was curious about how a preconceptual, embodied experience becomes an idea framed in clear words and concepts. For Gendlin, there is a kind of experience from which a person speaks: The embodied, felt meaning that precedes the concepts and language we use to describe experience. So, as a graduate student Gendlin was faced with a puzzle: How does one study the process by which a person articulates his or her experience?

At that time, Carl Rogers, the founder of client-centered therapy, was the head of the University of Chicago Counseling Center and was continually engaged in relevant research on person-centered therapy. Gendlin joined Rogers's team of therapists and researchers to learn from and collaborate with them. They and others researched the question: Why is it that some people make progress in psychotherapy and others do not? They were interested in two key interdependent factors: (1) how the therapist relates to the client and (2) how the client relates to their own experiencing (Cornell, 2013).

DOI: 10.4324/9781003455851-8

They recorded hundreds of therapy sessions by many different therapists from different orientations. From the recordings, they were able to successfully predict which clients would make progress during a year of psychotherapy, as measured by the client's self-report, the therapist's report, and other specific outcome measures.

Gendlin and his colleagues found that improvements in therapy hinged on how clients paused to consult their feel of a situation before finding the words to express their sense of it. They had a recognizable pattern of slowing down, becoming less articulate, then finding unique words and phrases that matched what they were trying to say. This guiding touchstone of embodied knowing became known as a felt sense.

FUNDAMENTAL CLINICAL CONCEPTS

In this section we outline five concepts central to FOT. First is Gendlin's philosophy and psychology of change. Second is the felt sense, Gendlin's term for our embodied awareness of a situation. Third, we discuss experiential listening, the contact it creates with the client and how it facilitates felt sense formation. Fourth, we explore FOT's approach to experience, or the attitudes most appropriate to listening to someone's felt sense of a situation. Finally, we discuss "interaction first" and the central role of relationality in FOT.

A PHILOSOPHY AND PSYCHOLOGY OF CHANGE

All modalities for treating trauma evolve from assumptions about what a human being is, how trauma affects a person, and how change occurs. FOT emerged from the tradition of humanistic psychology and shares many of its key assumptions (Krycka, 2014). The central assumption of both humanistic psychology and FOT is that human beings, like all living organisms, are in an ongoing process of self-development and actualization. All living bodies, by their nature, are trying to develop themselves further.

An organism's further development is bodily implied; what is needed can be felt experientially and often seen externally. This means that, in some sense, the body *knows* what is needed for growth to occur. This kind of knowing can be sensed as a vague, yet intricate whole. It can be felt into as the unclear edge of an issue the client is trying to speak from and find words for. This holistic embodied knowing is what we refer to as *implicit experience*. It is not already formed but emerges as we bring awareness to it. FOT gives therapists a method for helping clients pause and speak from their implicit experience, allowing that to come into explicit *focus* with cognitive and conceptual clarity.

A child is born with a bodily implying of searching for its mother's breast and being cared for. A child living with abuse wants love and attention, but it is not there. Even worse, the child is confronted with ongoing abuse. The child's *life-forward implying* is interrupted and becomes trapped and frozen in what FOT refers to as a *stopped process*. A stopped process refers to a blockage of life-forward implying. The child grows up with both the abuse and the bodily implying of what would have been right from early on. The child grows into adulthood. Perhaps he or she has accepted what happened in childhood, but he or she may have lost touch with the younger self that held the implying of a different, more supportive life. *Trauma disconnects us from our ability to sense and trust our embodied (implicit) knowing of our needs and wants.* The child lives with a sense of something missing. The feel of the missing experience continues until a person can bodily access their implied needs and *carry forward* their next steps of living.

A FELT SENSE

There is a natural human process that can reestablish the lost connection to self, interrupted and stopped by trauma: A bodily felt sense. The forming of a felt sense contains both the feel of what's wrong (the problem) *and* the missing interaction that would feel right, that is needed to carry experience forward. The bad feeling and the knowing what would have been right come together, all at once, in a felt sense.

The felt sense sets FOT apart from other psychotherapeutic modalities. It is Gendlin's term for the embodied feeling of a situation in which we are living. At first there is a bodily felt, yet unclear or wordless sense of something. It is the "place" the client is trying to "get at" and speak from. This deeper place is found underneath explicit or surface thoughts and feelings; it is implicit in words and expression. The client can feel it stirring and may say, "I can sense it right here (their hand on their solar plexus), but I don't know what it is."

Ann Weiser Cornell (2013), a prominent focusing teacher and writer, defined it this way: "A felt sense is a fresh, immediate, here-and-now experience that is actually the organism (or body) forming its next step in the situation the person is living in" (p. xix). A felt sense forming is a new step of living beyond the stuck place the client was in a moment ago, it is the arrival of something new. The stopped process the client was up against begins to loosen as something new emerges. The client's "I" (or self) becomes stronger as he or she senses little steps in a life-forward direction. Looking back at this change, we can see how we got there but we could not have predicted its arrival.

A felt sense comes into focus once the right symbols are found and checked against our bodily feel. Symbolization is a process of finding words, vocalizations, gestures, and images that fit the feel of the intricate whole. Felt sense expression is often metaphorical and comes out in peculiar or funny phrases that capture a unique quality for the client. It may not suffice to simply call an interaction simply "unpleasant"; we may need a more precise phrase like "a comical interrogation." Once symbolized, the felt sense unfolds into greater cognitive detail with explicit fresh meaning. A client can *feel* when a word fits or resonates with a felt sense. There is often bodily relief, a deeper breath, and a new perspective on the situation. The client's experience comes into focus (focusing), integrating and carrying forward the experience.

EXPERIENTIAL LISTENING

Our third concept that is essential to FOT is *experiential listening*. All therapists listen. Doing it well is an art. Listening is a complex, multilayered process. It is the foundation of *contact* and *connection* between therapist and client. As Neil Friedman (2005) wrote: "Experiential listening is listening to the not yet fully articulated felt sense from which the speaker is talking. It comes out of a combination of Eugene Gendlin's philosophical work and Carl Rogers' reflection of feeling response" (p. 217). The client is encouraged to check the therapist's response. Do the therapist's words hit the mark? If not, the client checks inside, then shares what the therapist missed. This contact not only allows the client to feel heard, it also helps the therapeutic relationship develop.

A therapist's responses are meant both to check understanding and to point clients toward edges of awareness where a felt sense might form. A client may have a good deal to say about a situation with their family, for example, but then run into a less clear place, an edge in their understanding. An FOT therapist would support a client in finding a felt sense by reflecting *both* what is clear and what is unclear: "You can feel something in you that is angry at your parents, but you are still wondering what that anger is about. Take a moment and sense below the anger where it's not so clear." This is a reflection that both shows understanding (listening) and encourages a client to stay with their felt sense of things to see what comes next. This dialectic of listening and reflecting is essential to helping clients work with their felt senses.

AN APPROACH TO EXPERIENCING

Our fourth concept involves how an FOT therapist approaches inner life – a client's and our own – with reverence, presence, and a welcoming attitude that allows us to be with whatever experience is there. We want to befriend experience, to develop a relational and inner process of acknowledging, accepting, and welcoming the client's experience. FOT begins from a place of trust, meaning an FOT therapist presupposes that all experience comes for meaningful reasons. Therapist and client do not need to know what the bad feeling is or why it is there. It is something to be curious about, honored, and explored. Sensing unformed implicit experience requires a process of being tentative, gentle, and curious. We want to say "Hello" to what is emerging without pushing it away or trying to change it. We want to get to know it and listen to it, *just as it is.*

In the beginning of therapy, clients seldom approach their experience this way. When bad feelings come, the last thing they want to do is welcome them. They may believe the point of therapy is to find "tools" to get rid of those feelings. The therapist might then say, "The feeling you're trying to get rid of is your body's way of telling you, 'Something here needs help.' Our approach is to listen to what it has to say, so we can learn what it needs to heal." Being with something unwanted and letting it inwardly be, perhaps more than anything else, is the essence of how FOT approaches client experiencing.

Yet clients are often identified with reactive, emotional states. To say, "I am so angry," suggests I am identified with my anger. This does not leave any safe space from which to explore "anger." To facilitate a safe inner experiencing process, the therapist needs to be able to help a client be present with whatever experience comes in the session. *Presence* is our innate ability to hold our experience calmly with compassion and without judgment. A client might say, "I'm so angry at him." The therapist might reflect, "You're sensing something in you that is so angry at him." By making the anger a "something," clients can create a little space between themselves and the something in them that is angry. They can now relationally explore the something further. The development of what Cornell (2013, p 57) called *facilitative language* is particularly useful in helping clients be present and safely explore their experience.

In this way, FOT employs something like "parts work." Parts are seen as aspects of self that have a protective, critical, or vulnerable process designed to manage experience and keep the client safe. All parts are somethings we can be with. When we are present, we can welcome and be curious about each part. Parts bring some partial experience that needs listening and a reparative process. In FOT, unlike some other treatment modalities, parts are seen as temporary forms that will dissolve when given the attention they need.

INTERACTION FIRST: THE RELATIONAL HEART OF FOCUSING-ORIENTED THERAPY

"FOT is inherently relational and interactive," FOT therapist Lynn Preston writes:

> Gendlin's concept of *interaction first* is the cornerstone of his philosophy. It speaks to the nature of living as inherently interactive. If we look at an individual as a *process* rather than an *entity*, it changes everything we think about and do in our work. … For us as clinicians, the crucial question then is: What is the kind of interaction that makes the client better, and how can we be that?
>
> (2014, p. 99)

Focusing is often regarded solely as an inner process of self-responding. If we understand that a human being is process-in-interaction-with-everything, then we can see that we always focus within an interaction – we are always responding to our environment. FOT opens the door to a relational world with the client. A client's process is different with us, and we can respond differently to them. A different living process forms as the client says "the same old things" to the therapist, who can hear, see, and feel the old interaction, sense how it keeps the client stuck, and respond from their own felt sense to carry the client's process forward.

DESCRIPTION OF THE THERAPY PROCESS

As noted, FOT is not defined so much by a technique or protocol but by an orientation, a way of being with ourselves, our clients, and our experience together. More specifically, a FOT therapist is oriented to working in the present while recognizing that the past is always implied in the present. FOT therapists reflect a client's experience, welcoming what comes with curiosity, facilitating felt sensing moments, and being a *real other* to whom the client can relate. They maintain a dual focus of being present to their own experiencing while also tracking the client's process. They listen to stories while reflecting what the client is trying to convey. It is their job to be the kind of interaction (relationship) that leads to steps of change.

A session begins with helping the client speak from where they are in the present moment. Some FOT therapists offer a grounding attunement to help the client sense their embodiment, come into presence, and begin speaking from the edge of a situation that is puzzling or bothersome. It is common for clients to tell stories about their problems. The therapist engages in reflective listening, helping clients touch into what is just below the surface of familiar thoughts and emotions. The therapist is oriented to listening for what is underneath or implicit in the story. Their responses "point" to the emerging edge of what clients are trying to get at, an edge of an awareness where a felt sense might form.

For example, a client describes an issue he has with his partner. He gets to the edge of what he knows clearly about the situation and then becomes inarticulate. He has a hard time describing this complex mesh of thoughts, emotions, and something more that is difficult to put into words. In frustration he says, "Oh I don't know, it's just so confusing." The therapist might reply by saying, "You know a lot about the situation, and it seems like there is something more you are trying to say." The therapist gestures with her hand, bringing it to her chest and says, "Take a moment to sense what comes here and what more wants to be said." The therapist is pointing to a spot where something more might come if the client can pause and notice. The client may say something like, "This is odd, but this memory just came of me as a little boy with my mother."

At first neither client nor therapist knows how the memory relates to the current situation. The therapist may invite the client to sense the feel of the memory. The client says, "It's like a turning away." This response is not a thought or an emotion. It formed freshly from inwardly sensing the feel of the whole situation prompted by the memory. The therapist invites the client to explore this turning away in the memory and then with the current problem. The client says, "How I turn away from my partner is just like what I did with my mother when my parents were divorcing." The past turning away from an emotionally charged situation is implicitly functioning in the present with his partner. The client's experience has shifted from a narrow understanding of how he relates to his current partner to a wider bodily felt awareness of his own behavior and its deep roots in an old pattern of relating to significant others.

The client now has a new perspective on his current relationship that brings vulnerable feelings. Perhaps the client feels ashamed and begins to experience an inner criticizing process. "I always turn away. It's like I'm afraid to be seen as needing someone. Instead of reaching out, I turn away. I've done that my whole life." A new awareness is present, but it might be shut down by the client's self-criticism. The change step that emerged from this session brought more than just the experience of turning away. It brought a deeper context, the awareness that it's about turning away *when help is needed*. The therapist might say, "You needed your mother during the divorce, but you turned away, and are doing that now with your partner. Is that right?" The client, responds, "Yes, I do need her help. My turning away causes conflict between us."

The therapist can now guide the client into a listening relationship with his younger self. The therapist might say, "Let's listen to what he needs, or what he might show us." Together they listen to his experience speak from the memory. Once the client can sense the challenges he faced during the divorce, he might be able to feel empathy for his experience. What he could not do then, he might be able to do now.

The session might end with integrating the client's new experience of turning toward himself with inner empathy and how it feels to have done all that with his therapist. The experience of the past (the memory) can be explored relationally through a felt sense in the present (the partnership issue). Here, the essential missing experience was filled in and carried forward by a caring FOT therapist turning toward the client, and the client turning toward his own experiencing.

UTILIZATION OF FOCUSING-ORIENTED THERAPY FOR THE TREATMENT OF TRAUMA

Therapists work with trauma, which can be both acute and complex. With acute trauma, there is typically a singular event with immediate impact, like a car accident, assault, or natural disaster. Acute needs must be met before processing the event over time. Complex and developmental trauma, on the other hand, is caused by repeated and cumulative events that occur over time and within relationships. FOT can be adapted to work with all traumas if we understand the need to meet clients where they are and acknowledge what they face. This helps clients sense what is important for them and opens the doorway to change.

As we begin describing how FOT is used specifically in the treatment of trauma, let us first construct a basic frame for understanding what happens to a person who experiences trauma. Trauma overwhelms the organism and, consequently, memory becomes fragmented.

Some aspects of trauma are remembered while others remain out of awareness yet continue to function. What is absent from cognitive awareness is not forgotten by the body. The client might report a social situation that is not overtly threatening in which she "froze and couldn't speak up." She asks the therapist, "Why did I do that?" Her behavior does not make sense to her. This is what is meant by functioning implicitly or out-of-awareness. Something in the client holds the terror of what happened; she may be unaware of the trauma, lack a feel for what happened, or lack words for the experience … or all three. It is a mystery that haunts her.

The promise of experiential and embodied therapies is that they include our left hemisphere's clear, explicit, cognitive knowing and our right hemisphere's embodied, felt sensing, implicit knowing. Fragmented and dissociative experience is the speechless terror that is puzzling for both client and therapist. How do you work with experience that is fragmented, difficult to sense, and wordless?

FOT therapist Peter Afford has contributed significantly to the integration of contemporary neuroscience and FOT, reporting:

Neuroscience describes how emotionally overwhelming experiences are traumatic when the brain cannot integrate external sensory signals with internal bodily ones. This leaves what Allan Schore, a therapist who writes about neuroscience, calls 'dis-integration of the right brain'…. If right [hemisphere] doesn't marry external senses to internal senses, it may have no message at all to send to the left [hemisphere]—blank. The consequence is an ongoing dissociated state around the memory fragments of an experience and any reminders of it.

(Afford, 2014, p. 255)

The question becomes, what kind of process helps a client access right hemisphere experience and marry it to left hemisphere knowing? A felt sense arises from the right hemisphere's grasp of a whole situation in the present moment. This felt sensing ability is the key to accessing fragmented, traumatic experience. If a client can have a felt sense of a traumatic moment and find symbols (words, phrases, gestures, metaphors) that bring the experience into focus, right hemisphere sensing will marry with left, providing cognitive access to the whole experience.

We stated before the unique and essential use of felt sensing in working with trauma. But to do so requires clients to shift from experientially unsafe, dysregulated states to more consistently regulated, safe, present moment experiencing. Having a safe, grounded therapeutic relationship helps clients feel secure enough to explore the uncomfortable edges of trauma work. Here a therapist needs to help clients understand they *have* feelings, but they *are not* their feelings. They can learn to disidentify from merged experiencing using facilitative language or metaphors like stepping back and finding the right distance between you and your problem or being an observer of your experience. These are ways to help clients separate themselves from their trauma. Trauma is something that *happened* to our clients, it is *not who they are*. Once clients are able to step back, observe, and be with their experience, they can more easily contact their felt sense and listen to it.

In the remainder of this section, we will highlight the relational healing nature of this approach, and how a felt sense can be used to work with past trauma spots, regression, partial experience, and vicarious and intergenerational trauma, as well as address systemic and historical trauma.

WE HEAL RELATIONALLY

FOT does not offer a protocol for treating trauma. It does, however, offer what Preston (1985) referred to as "two miracles." The first is the miracle of felt sensing: A human capacity to know what is right from the inside. The second is the uniquely relational process of FOT itself. Human beings heal when they feel safe enough (within a relationship) to access and explore their inner world and share that with another person. In most cases, trauma has interrupted their innate ability to trust their felt knowing about situations and people.

FOT works with two kinds of responding: (1) the therapist responding to the client in a way that allows the client to relate to his or her experience compassionately and (2) the therapist using his or her own felt sense as a guide to form responses to the client, with the intention of building a secure connection. The metaphor of being in the same boat together applies here. Together, therapist and client sit through periods of not knowing, misunderstandings, and painful stories. As they work together, the relationship deepens, offering a concrete experience of a "new us" forming. *The relationship itself becomes a vehicle of change* as the therapist's responses support the client's felt sensing. The therapist models pausing, being present, sitting with the uncomfortable unknown, and working through relational troubles; the more this occurs, the more likely it is for the client to remain regulated when entering the unclear edges and shaky feelings of long-held trauma, with inner empathy, curiosity, and acceptance.

THE FELT SENSE: THE NEW "WAS"

A felt sense allows us to enter past experience frozen in trauma and bring it forward into the present moment. A felt sense requires a new understanding of what is meant by body and time. Gendlin (2007), put it this way:

> Your physically felt body is in fact part of a gigantic system of here and other places, now and other times, you and other people—in fact the whole universe. This sense of being bodily alive in a vast system is the body as it is felt from the inside.
>
> (p. 88)

If we are, "in fact, the whole universe," our felt sense allows us to enter the past in a consistent and reliable way to work with the past trauma that is frozen and speechless in our right hemisphere. *The new was* is Gendlin's concept for our ability to experience something new (explicitly) that was only implicit before in a past experience. A felt sense of a present situation holds the implying (what was needed but could not occur) and stopped process (what stopped it from occurring) from an earlier time. Almost all client issues are current iterations of past, unprocessed (traumatic) experience. The feel of a current situation can often easily be tracked back to an earlier age. It can be as simple as asking, "When do you first remember having that feeling?" or, "How long has that kind of experience been around?"

A felt sense of a present situation allows clients to access to their past. Some are intergenerational, some are from the womb, and others are from infancy and childhood. Most are moments in time when something significant happened that bring bits of memory and a feel of a situation. Here is where we find the trauma spots that can be opened, explored, and then closed within an hour session. We don't work with the past to resolve the past. We work with the living past because it wants to move forward for healing, resolution, and integration in the present.

WORKING WITH REGRESSION: OBSERVING THE BODY
AND WHAT IT SHOWS US

Her knees come up in front of her, forming a ball in the chair. Her voice and affect change to childlike tones. The therapist asks, "When do you first remember having that feeling? When did it start? What was happening then?" She replies, "Mother was in a car accident. She almost died. I was so scared. Where was my father? I had to care for my younger siblings."

Trauma is embodied; it occurs at a place in time and most often in relation to others. Regression is a return to an earlier state and occurs in micro-moments of interaction. There is often a childlike voice and expression that reveals a place in time (the age of the client when the trauma occurred). Clients will show you what happened if you watch and listen.

WORKING WITH "PARTS" OR PARTIAL EXPERIENCE

A part or partial self is an aspect of our experiencing that we are either identified with or that is functioning out of awareness, or both. When trauma occurs, experience becomes fragmented, resulting in partial experience or parts forming. Some parts are protective, some are traumatized, and others are critical. The first thing an organism does after experiencing trauma is try to get back control. Parts help to manage a kind of fragile and fragmented control while at the same time "freeze" a person's experience in time. Parts often need to be worked with before the deeper work of trauma can occur. Cornell (2013), has written well about parts work in FOT:

"Parts" are not the same as felt senses. The stopped process that results in the experience of parts can persist over many years, resulting in the experience that these inner states are nameable entities. A felt sense, however, is always freshly formed, arising in this moment and therefore not a nameable entity. One can, however, get a felt sense of a part.

(p. 109)

Partial selves may then need a kind of reparative process, which includes giving them acknowledgment, respect, compassion, and a kind of deep listening for what they have been trying to contribute to the person. Finding and listening to the "inner child" who went through the trauma can be very moving and healing for the client. When lost aspects of self are found and integrated, a client's deeper continuity can be restored.

WORKING WITH VICARIOUS AND INTERGENERATIONAL TRAUMA

Vicarious trauma refers to trauma that is held in a person's body and lived by him or her, but is not caused by their own life experiences. Intergenerational trauma refers to vicarious trauma that is picked up and passed along through generations. Emotions that were too much for one person may be picked up or taken on by another as a way of helping or coregulating another. Family survival sometimes depends on sharing the burden of trauma within and over generations.

FOT therapist Shirley Turcotte (2009) has written powerfully about intergenerational trauma:

I have met many a client who had swallowed their parent's depression, or rage, or family shame, so that the family could carry on. Many a child has absorbed and shared their mother's or father's depression to keep a parent from possible suicide, for the sake of the family.

(p. 13)

When a client's reaction to a current situation is out of proportion to the situation, it often points to a past trauma with vicarious aspects they are carrying from a family member or significant person in their life. Some trauma survivors vicariously adopt emotions of those who abused them. Helping a client distinguish between their own depression, shame, or anger and that of someone else can alleviate chronic symptoms rather quickly. Working with a felt sense helps in two ways. First, the felt sense can lead client and therapist to the trauma spot. Then felt sensing can be used to differentiate what was mine from what was someone else's experience. A depressed client may come to realize their depression was intertwined with their father's. Once the client can set down what was not theirs, they can more easily address their own.

ADDRESSING SYSTEMIC AND HISTORICAL TRAUMA

Turcotte is a Metis (of indigenous and European parents) woman from Canada who informs our experience of treating trauma. She practices Indigenous focusing-oriented therapy (IFOT; formerly referred to as Aboriginal FOT). Her understanding is that a felt sense offers access to ancestral knowing. A felt sense becomes the knowing of "all my relations." Turcotte & Schiffer (2014) explained it this way:

> A felt sense in AFOT [now IFOT] can be defined as a bodily experience of interconnected emotion, energy and sensations that are an expression of knowledge of collective experiences through time. This collection of traumatic experiences informs our minds, our bodies, our emotions, and our spirits. It is this implicit and ancestral memory knowledge, through the generations, that teaches us when to trust, how to trust and where to move ourselves forward for all life concerned.
>
> (p. 51)

IFOT centers on the ecology and interconnectedness of human existence. Human beings are not seen as separate from one another or from the land. Human beings are profoundly relational; we are embedded in and constituted by our relationships with the world, people, language, and landscape. IFOT offers a noncolonized understanding of the world that sits next to a Western, scientific understanding. Indigenous woman, author, and biologist, Robin Wall Kimmerer (2022) expressed this beautifully in a phrase from her book, *Braiding Sweet Grass*: "All flourishing is mutual" (p. 15).

To address and work through issues of systemic and historical trauma – such as the Indian residential schools in Canada and the United States – requires new thinking and experiencing. The body has not been colonized. Uncolonized knowing can be accessed through a felt sense. We believe FOT and a felt sense is a doorway to the mystery of life and all our relations.

ASSESSMENT OF RESEARCH EVIDENCE REGARDING EFFECTIVENESS IN TREATING TRAUMA

Focusing has been heavily researched as a therapeutic modality. Mary Hendricks (2002) chapter, "Focusing-Oriented/Experiential Psychotherapy," has surveyed and summarized the large body of research showing the general therapeutic effectiveness of focusing. Additionally, several studies have connected focusing and the treatment of trauma. For example, Klagsbrun and Lennox (2012) found that focusing can improve the quality of life for women who are dealing with the trauma of breast cancer. Through an exercise called "Clearing a Space," they demonstrated that focusing can help women feel safe and grounded during a time when their bodies have become unsafe.

Katonah (2012) has similarly shown how focusing exercises make it possible to move beyond the stuck patterns of traumatic experience. The fresh, embodied attention of focusing, Katonah claimed, creates "an experiential process that moves beyond the [stuck] patterning of the trauma," leading to "a significant reduction in trauma symptoms" (p. 149).

Additionally, Hudek (2007) has demonstrated how focusing can be used to treat vicarious traumatization, offering strategies for feeling safe and grounded in the face of overwhelming experiences. As Hudek argued, "The Focusing Attitude of curiosity (friendly interest), openness and acceptance ... is a healing attitude that can be helpful to anyone in attending to the effects of vicarious traumatization whether for themselves or for others" (p. 100).

FOT is difficult to fit into contemporary quantitative and evidence-based frameworks. There are no rules for sensing into your body's awareness of a situation, only approaches. FOT is not alone in this, as many other therapies have foregrounded the unpredictable, collaborative, and intersubjective nature of therapeutic change (Krycka, 2014).

CASE EXAMPLES REGARDING THE TREATMENT OF TRAUMA

Sarah is married with two daughters and is confident in her home and work life. As her oldest daughter enters high school, Sarah begins to have disturbing dreams in which she is trying to get away from something terrifying. She describes herself as someone who "pushes through and takes control" of situations, but recently she has struggled with a vague shakiness. What follows are two sessions with Sarah, to demonstrate different aspects of FOT trauma work.

Session 1 demonstrates how a vague bodily feeling can become a felt sense, which brings a memory of a past trauma and can then be addressed.

SARAH:	Usually, I can push ahead and take control, but recently that's not working. I can't seem to get control over this shaky feeling.
THERAPIST:	Usually, you can get control over unclear situations, but recently you have been experiencing something shaky. Perhaps you can describe the shaky feeling a little more. Take your time and allow a feel of it to form, that whole feel of shakiness.
SARAH:	My body shakes and I ... I want to run. There is also a kind of terror like something bad is about to happen.

She can be curious about something shaky and find words to describe it. She touches into her bodily felt yet unclear shakiness. A felt sense is forming.

THERAPIST:	Check and see if all that is about something happening now, or is it from an earlier time in life? How far back does the shaky feeling and wanting to run go?
SARAH:	There is a memory of being at a party during my freshman year of high school. I was kind of drunk. I can feel being pulled … pulled into a room.
THERAPIST:	Let's go slowly. Take time to notice the sensations in your body. You're here *now* with me remembering something that happened *then*. Let's help keep you present and safe while you visit that place in time. Sense your breathing and feel your feet on the floor. *The therapist helps her distinguish between then and now and be with her experience.*
SARAH:	I can't breathe, it's like my throat is closing. I feel a pressure on my chest. Something is happening to me I can't control. I want to scream but I can't. It feels like I'm going to … die. Why couldn't I do something? It's like I left my body. I wasn't there anymore.

Waves of emotion, bits of memory, and tears come.

THERAPIST:	Sarah, can you create a little space between you and your younger self who went through all of that? Let all that energy flow through you. *What was "frozen" needs to be felt, and the body needs a chance to sense "what would have been right" in terms of self-preserving actions.*
THERAPIST:	Notice what would have felt right back then, if you could have moved and used your voice. Allow your body to do what feels right now. *Energy comes into her limp body, and gestures of pushing away, kicking, and screaming come.*
SARAH:	Get off me! Get the f … off me! You have no right to me! *Her body is mobilizing to complete a process frozen by the trauma. It feels right.*

The rape was terrifying. She almost died, and perhaps something in her feels like it did die, but she survived. What was dissociated and unprocessed continued to live as a "shaky feeling." As her oldest daughter began high school, her trauma appeared in the form of shakiness and nightmares. This was her body's implying: An attempt to speak up and live beyond the stoppage. Now that she has the memory, her whole being can heal the wound.

Session 2 takes place later in therapy, reflecting the healing that has occurred. In this session, the therapist references a time prior to the trauma as a resource to use as Sarah is guided to find and integrate the "lost self" who endured the trauma and its aftermath.

SARAH   High school was awful. I felt lost and broken. I pretended to be what others wanted from me. I didn't feel seen. At home, it was even worse. My parents divorced, and I had no one to talk to. I was a mess. Somehow, I got into college and things began to change.

THERAPIST   Sarah, see if it would feel right to be with your younger self before all that happened. Go back to a place in time when things felt safe and good.

SARAH   I'm remembering my 14th birthday. I feel a lightness, a playfulness. I can see myself smiling and doing cartwheels on the front lawn. Oh, that feels good. I'd forgotten the good times and who I was then. I had big dreams and a carefree nature.

THERAPIST   Let yourself feel all those good qualities of you then, and let them be there now.

SARAH   I feel her sweetness and my body feels different, lighter. No shakiness.

THERAPIST   Keep those good feelings and bring them to the person you were shortly after the assault. Find a place in time that feels safe and right to be with now.
                The therapist encourages Sarah to connect to a time when she can experience her life-forward implying *and then bring it to a time when that implying had stopped and wasn't felt.*

SARAH   I can sense her sullenness. I'm maybe 16 here. Full of rage and shame. I hated myself then. I became a loner, cut on myself, and thought about ways to disappear.

THERAPIST   Notice how she would like you to be with her now.

SARAH   She is so angry with me. I see her folding her arms and looking away. That is painful. She's letting me know I betrayed her. I left her there alone in the aftermath of being assaulted and my parents' divorce. God, that was awful. She is so alone. It breaks my heart.

THERAPIST   Stay with her there. Give her some time to express what needs to be seen by you now. Maybe she can show you what she needs or wants from you going forward.

SARAH   I am approaching her slowly. She is sobbing. Now she is letting me touch her, hold her. She wants to know what she did to deserve this and why no one saw her suffering.

THERAPIST   She has suffered alone for a long time, but now you are with her, holding her. Notice if it would feel right to remind her of her 14th birthday. Let her see herself then and your strong adult self now. She made it through the dark night of the soul. Allow her to both remember her past and see the light in her future.

SARAH   That is so helpful. All of me is here now. There is a kind of through line, which is me, that I can feel in my heart. She feels seen by me and recognizes things have worked out. What happened then has made me who I am today. I see that now. I don't want to get rid of anything inside. When I feel shaky now, I will know it is her voice whispering from below, asking me to turn toward her and these big feelings. I can keep them company. I can do that now.

Sarah was able to integrate felt experience from the past into her present self. What was missing filled in and carried forward. Nothing changes what happened, but a client can change his or her bodily implying through felt sensing if the interaction makes it possible.

STRENGTHS AND LIMITATIONS OF THE MODALITY AS A TREATMENT FOR TRAUMA

At the heart of trauma treatment is the need for an approach that supports both the client and the therapist being in contact with emerging experience and being able to bring that into focus. FOT does this by (1) orienting toward the edge of how a situation is experienced bodily, spatially, and interactionally; and (2) using a felt sense to bring forth fragmented and dissociated experience for integration and healing. FOT is also inherently relational, as both therapist and client consult their felt sense to empathetically attune with each other, thus overcoming the many dead ends of talk therapy and past relational difficulties.

A limiting factor in FOT is that the process relies on the ability of the client to engage in felt sensing. Clients with rigid and structure-bound process often struggle to connect with inner experience, sometimes requiring a more didactic and cognitive process until the capacity for felt sensing emerges. Similarly, clients with complex trauma may require support with emotional regulation and building an experience of safety with the therapist before felt sensing occurs.

RESOURCES FOR LEARNING

WEBSITES

International Association of Focusing-Oriented Therapists. Focusing-oriented therapy. (n.d.). https://www.focusingtherapy.org/
Seattle Focusing Institute. Focusing-oriented therapy and complex trauma training program. (n.d.). https://seattlefocusing.org
International Focusing Institute's Gendlin Online Library. (n.d.). https://focusing.org/gendlin/

YOUTUBE

YouTube. (n.d.). Focusing-oriented therapies. https://www.youtube.com/c/FocusingOrientedTherapies

BOOKS

Cornell, A.W. (2013). *Focusing in clinical practice: The essence of change.* New York & London: W.W. Norton & Company.
Gendlin, E.T. (1996). *Focusing-oriented psychotherapy: A manual of the experiential method.* New York: Guilford.

Madison, G. (2014a). *The theory and practice of focusing-oriented psychotherapy: Beyond the talking cure.* London & Philadelphia: Jessica Kingsley.

Madison, G. (2014b). *Emerging practice in focusing-oriented psychotherapy: Innovative theory and applications.* London & Philadelphia: Jessica Kingsley.

REFERENCES

Afford, P. (2014). Neuroscience and psychological change in focusing. In G. Madison (Ed.), *The theory and practice of focusing-oriented psychotherapy: Beyond the talking cure* (pp. 245–258). London & Philadelphia: Jessica Kingsley.

Cornell, A. (2013). *Focusing in clinical practice: The essence of change.* New York & London: Norton.

Friedman, N. (2005). Experiential listening. *Journal of Humanistic Psychology, 45*(3), 217–238.

Gendlin, E.T. (2007). *Focusing.* New York: Bantam Books.

Hendricks, M.N. (2002). Focusing-oriented/experiential psychotherapy. In D.J. Cain (Ed.), *Humanistic psychotherapies: Handbook of research and practice* (pp. 221–251). Washington, DC: American Psychological Association. https://doi.org/10.1037/10439-007

Hudek, C. (2007). Dealing with vicarious traumatization in the context of global fear. *The Folio, 20*(1), 95–101.

Katonah, D.G. (2012). Research on clearing a space. *The Folio, 23*(1),138–154.

Kimmerer, R.W. (2022). *Braiding sweetgrass.* Minneapolis, MI: Milkweed Editions.

Klagsbrun, J., & Lennox, S.L. (2012). Clearing a space: An evidence-based approach for enhancing quality of life in women with breast cancer.*The Folio, 23*(1), 155–167.

Krycka, K. (2014). Thinking and practicing FOT in the twenty-first century: Challenges, critiques, and opportunities. In G. Madison (Ed.), *The theory and practice of focusing-oriented psychotherapy: Beyond the talking cure* (pp. 52–66). London & Philadelphia: Jessica Kingsley.

Preston, L. (1985). *Two interwoven miracles: The relational dimension of focusing-oriented psychotherapy* [Unpublished manuscript].

Preston, L. (2014) The relational heart of focusing-oriented psychotherapy. In G. Madison (Ed.), *Theory and practice of focusing-oriented psychotherapy: Beyond the talking cure* (pp. 98–112). London & Philadelphia: Jessica Kingsley.

Turcotte, S., (2009). *Focusing oriented therapy and relational consideration of unresolved trauma.* [Unpublished manuscript].

Turcotte, S., & Schiffer, J. (2014). Aboriginal-focusing oriented therapy (AFOT). In G. Madison (Ed.), *Emerging practice in focusing-oriented psychotherapy: Innovative theory and applications* (pp. 48–64). London & Philadelphia: Jessica Kingsley.

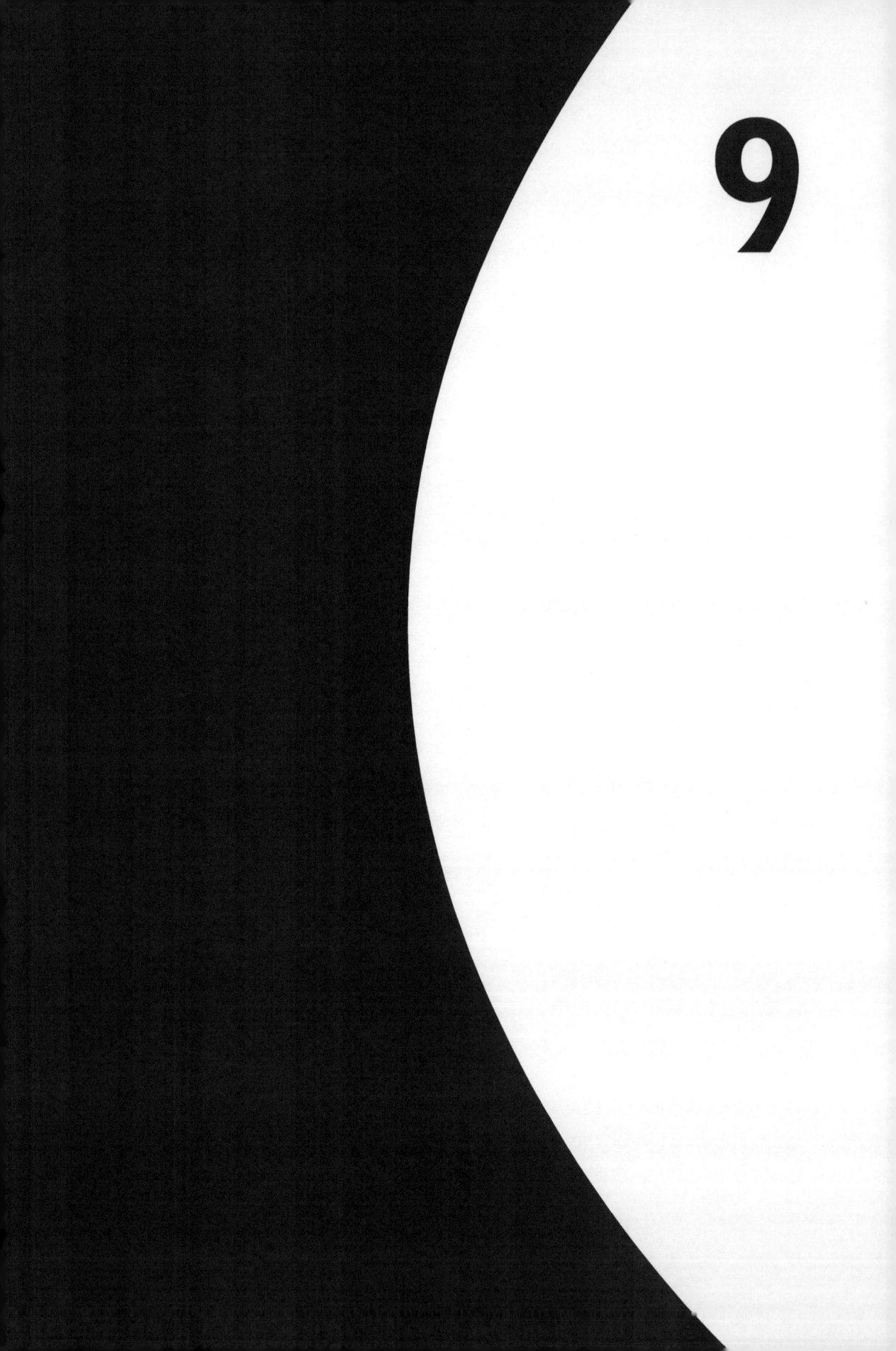

9

CHAPTER 9
EMOTION FOCUSED THERAPY FOR COMPLEX TRAUMA

An Overview of the Model

Anna Gartshore

INTRODUCTION

Emotion focused therapy for complex trauma (EFTT) is a short-term, evidenced-based, process-experiential therapy designed to address the specific symptoms stemming from the enduring impact of interpersonal trauma, including child abuse and neglect. This chapter covers a brief history of the general model of emotion focused therapy (EFT) and the underlying theory informing the eight key clinical constructs as a foundation for understanding the development of EFTT and its distinct features for practice. It offers an overview of the process and the intervention strategies tailored to the unique needs of trauma survivors. It describes how the therapist promotes emotional change through a corrective relational experience and a step-by-step process that fosters awareness, acceptance, expression, utilization, regulation and eventual transformation of the core maladaptive emotion schemes keeping survivors of child abuse and/or neglect stuck in their lives. It concludes with a case example to illustrate the principles and process in action.

BRIEF HISTORY

In the early 1970s, a young engineering student from South Africa became fascinated by an experience he had when he solved a difficult math equation without knowing how. He sensed that, beyond rationality or intellect, there was more at the source of human intelligence. His curiosity eventually led him to enroll in a PhD psychology program. which he completed in 1975. This young man was Dr. Les Greenberg, now an award-winning and Distinguished Research Professor Emeritus of York University in Toronto, Canada, and one of the main founders of emotion focused therapy (EFT) for individuals and couples.

While obtaining his PhD, Greenberg studied a variety of therapy methods and began to sense that emotion, or "gut feeling," was not only at the source of peoples struggles, but also acted as a kind of guiding wisdom (Bourne, 2022). He was deeply curious about the role of emotion in people's lives, how it influenced people's choices and, at times, the resolution of their suffering. He was mentored by Dr. Laura North Rice, who had worked with Dr. Carl Rogers at the University of Chicago in the 1950s. The EFT model has been richly influenced by the Humanistic traditions including Rogerian person-centered therapy and Fritz Perl's Gestalt therapy. In fact, EFT is well-known for its extensive research

DOI: 10.4324/9781003455851-9

on and refinement of the two-chair process originating from Gestalt therapy. In the early 1980s, Greenberg collaborated with Rice and Dr. Robert Elliott to develop and research an early model of EFT which combined Gestalt and person-centered therapy for depression and published one of the earliest studies on EFT for individuals (Greenberg, Rice & Elliott, 1993). By the mid-1980s, then–PhD candidate Sue Johnson collaborated with Greenberg on a model for the treatment of couples, publishing their first book in 1988 (Greenberg & Goldman, 2008). Sue Johnson continued to focus on couples becoming well known for her extensive work on the further development and promotion of EFT in this treatment area.

By 1995, Dr. Sandra Paivio was completing her PhD in Counselling Psychology at York University under Greenberg. She conducted research on the use of a standard EFT procedure for resolving *unfinished business* with another. *Unfinished business*, a concept derived from Gestalt therapy, is a process in which "primary emotional experience is inhibited or avoided … with the results that they [individuals] are apt to become psychologically and/or emotionally stuck (Greenberg & Malcolm, 2002, p. 406). Paivio became interested in a cohort of research participants who did not benefit from treatment. The common factor was complex and relational trauma stemming from child abuse and neglect (Paivio & Greenberg, 1995). This began her work, along with others such as Antonio Pascual-Leone, to adapt the EFT model to address the unique needs of this population.

The general model of EFT and emotion focused therapy for complex trauma (EFTT) have evolved as the evidence drawn from nearly 40 years of process-outcome research has shaped and refined the structure for practice. While EFT has its origins in humanistic, neo-Piagetian, constructivist, evolutionary and attachment theories, over time it has expanded to include newly emerging research on the neuroscience of emotional change and reconsolidation theory. EFTT is now a trans-theoretical and trans-diagnostic therapy that uses an experiential approach with a refined process for tracking in-session markers to initiate specific interventions and tasks to facilitate emotional transformation. To understand some of EFTT's distinctions, it is helpful to first look at the fundamental clinical concepts grounding emotion focused therapy.

FUNDAMENTAL CLINICAL CONCEPTS

EFT theory views emotion as an **adaptive orienting system** replete with valuable information organizing a person toward the fulfillment of basic needs. Being aware and accepting of our adaptive emotions helps us decipher what they are telling us and provides a reliable system for wisely guiding our choices, the way we relate to others and how we take action in the world. **Emotion schemes** take shape during our critical developmental years. They involve a network of cognitive, affective, motivational, somatic, behavioral and relational information consisting of neural networks that dynamically encode memory and provide automatic and efficient motivational responses (Greenberg, 2021).

All emotions can be regarded as relational signaling systems providing important information about needs for proximity and closeness or distance and boundary. Motivation springs from the emotion system and action tendencies mobilize the body towards the fulfillment of these needs. Emotion arises within the context of interrelated and co-occurring phenomena including external relational stimuli and internal stimuli such as thought, feelings, sensations and impulses or action tendencies.

> Emotion can be understood as a highly complex meaning system that is able to integrate all relevant facets of one's circumstances into an overall visceral experience. Thus, emotions provide information about the self and, at the same time, direct the self toward the fulfillment of needs.
>
> (Paivio & Pascual-Leone, 2023, p. 57)

While emotions are fundamentally adaptive, it is important to recognize what the symptoms showing up in the therapy office convey and how these relate to emotional processing problems arising in the context of current difficulties. Exposure to mis-attuned caregiving and adverse childhood experiences including abuse and neglect during our critical developmental years harms this system. This early learning shapes these emotional memory networks resulting in the development of our **maladaptive emotion schemes** as we become organized by the fear of lonely abandonment (attachment injuries) and core maladaptive shame (identity). Impairments to emotion regulation capacities, attachment style and the developing sense of self cause difficulties across a lifetime as we become cut off from our adaptive emotions and carry the burden of unmet childhood needs.

To understand the EFT treatment process, it is important to understand the unique way EFT describes and differentiates emotion. EFT theory distinguishes between different types of emotions including **primary adaptive** and **primary maladaptive** emotion (the feelings that come first), **secondary** emotion (the emotion about emotion such as fear of anger or shame about vulnerable sadness) and **instrumental** emotion (manipulative qualities such as anger used to over-power or dominate). Understanding their differences is a critical skill for the emotion focused therapist. The ability to recognize the markers for specific types of emotion as they arise in session signals the implementation of the associated EFT tasks and interventions. These moment-to-moment emotion cues present therapeutic opportunities that are harnessed to facilitate emotional transformation (Greenberg, 2021; Auszra et al., 2013)

INTERVENTION PRINCIPLES

"Feel it to heal it" is a key principle guiding the EFT process. It is by evoking and directly experiencing painful, stuck emotion in the safety of an empathically attuned relationship that we have access to the maladaptive emotion schemes that leave us caught in repetitive and reflexive responses. EFT theory counters the behaviorists by emphasizing that, while cognition does play a role in making sense of what we feel, it is not cognition that comes first. We cannot change a core, amygdala-based emotion by modifying thoughts and behaviors. Rather, it is by working through an experiential and co-regulatory relational process directly through the emotional system that the possibility for new meaning emerges.

Greenberg is often quoted as saying we have to "arrive at a place before we can leave it" and emotion focused therapies offer a precise process for the well-trained, empathically adept and attuned therapist to guide clients toward experiencing and regulating that which has been previously avoided or resisted in the service of an emotional change process. (Auszra et al., 2013)

EMOTIONAL CHANGE PROCESS

EFT theory and research indicates that emotions change not by venting, releasing, or talking about them but rather in relationship to newly emerging and contrasting emotion. For example, core maladaptive shame rooted in the sense of "I am bad" is transformed when clients have access to healthy, adaptive anger expressed directly in session to the imagined other who caused them harm in the past. The action tendencies held in the experience of shame lead the body to withdraw, collapse and hide. The action tendencies held in adaptive anger lead the body to grow tall, aligned, with an impulse toward boundary assertion. The EFT therapist tracks markers for emerging adaptive anger and helps the client by guiding their awareness of and acceptance toward the experiencing and expression of the adaptive anger through specific tasks and interventions designed to elicit this. In this example, the adaptive anger can be thought of as the antidote to the maladaptive shame. By following the full impulse and expression of this anger toward the imagined other, in the safety of the relationship with the therapist, the client's sense of self begins to shift. The belief "I am bad" dissolves and the understanding "what happened to me was wrong" revises the narrative.

In contrast to other models, rather than simply expressing or reflecting on emotions through cognitive processes, EFT offers a precise process for evoking specific adaptive emotions to change other (maladaptive) emotions (Greenberg, 2021). In doing so, the therapy moves beyond behavioral coping skills and strategies. As clients gain access to the underlying adaptive emotions through a process of increasing awareness and acceptance, they are connected to an essential source of healthy information about what they need to make wise choices.

EIGHT KEY CONSTRUCTS

EFT has developed eight key constructs guided by the process outcome research that has shown how to work productively with emotions in psychotherapy to help facilitate an enduring change process. The first construct is focused on helping clients to increase **awareness** of their emotions as they arise in session. This leads to further **acceptance** of emotion, which is the second key construct. The third key construct focuses on facilitating **expression**. As a more accepting relationship develops with internal states, clients are assisted to recognize, find words, metaphors and symbols to describe and express their emotions. This is essential to make sense of the information they hold and to discern maladaptive from adaptive emotion. **Utilization of emotion** is the fourth key construct: With the resolution of maladaptive emotions, clients can harness and make use of the information arising from adaptive emotions and use this to take action toward the fulfillment of the needs associated with them.

People seeking therapy present on a spectrum of emotional experiencing ranging from emotional flooding and feeling overwhelmed at one end and over-control, numbing or alexithymia at the other end. The therapist's warmth and skillful use of self enhances further safety and trust in support of the fifth key construct: **Emotion regulation and co-regulation**. By providing attuned presence expressed through prosody, pace, posture, tone and a vast repertoire of appropriately engaged empathic responses, the therapist fulfills a co-regulatory function. In addition, at times the therapist teaches skills and provides emotion coaching to enhance capacities for self-regulation. Gradually, acceptance and expression of internal experience is practiced and new ways of relating to and regulating distress are internalized.

The sixth key construct involves **reflecting on emotion**. Insight continues to grow over the course of therapy and an increasing perspective provides clarity as past recurring patterns are recognized and changed and a new narrative understanding emerges.

Emotional transformation is a hallmark principle of EFT as therapists help clients change maladaptive emotions by accessing and expressing contrasting adaptive emotions. The EFT perspective is that maladaptive emotion schemes are restructured in relationship to newly experienced adaptive emotion and hence the view that transformation occurs by changing emotion with emotion.

The eighth key principle of EFT emphasizes the importance of the therapist's role in providing an ongoing **corrective emotional experience**. Since emotions are regarded as relational signaling systems giving important information about our needs for closeness and connection or fairness, respect, understanding and boundary, the adaptive responses provided by the therapist begin to elicit newly experienced and corrective feelings. If a client has come to expect to be judged, blamed and shamed when vulnerable and honest and instead is attended to with a consistency of presence, validation and warmth, the corrective experience begins to reshape old schemes. Gradually, the newly experienced emotions emerging from feeling respected, appreciated, believed and valued begin to change old, stuck emotion. By looking at how change happens in specific sessions and over the course of a psychotherapeutic process, the process-outcome research methodologies have informed the evolution of EFT practice and reinforced its major position that emotional suffering changes in relationship to newly arising adaptive emotions made available in the context of the empathically attuned relationship. In the safety of the therapy office, painful, stuck and avoided emotion can be accessed, tolerated and changed as previously blocked adaptive emotion is experienced and expressed.

EFT posits that emotional suffering and emotion regulation difficulties are at the root of most mental health diagnoses. Helping clients to increase their awareness and acceptance of emotional experiencing in session leads to more capacity for expression, utilization, regulation and reflection. This leads to newly emerging adaptive emotion states that change and transform the old structures. In effect, the therapeutic relationship provides the corrective experience necessary to access and experientially relate to the core maladaptive emotion schemes to address and resolve the unmet needs (Greenberg, 2021).

UTILIZATION OF THE MODALITY FOR THE TREATMENT OF TRAUMA

Emotion focused therapy for complex trauma is founded on the theory and key constructs of the general model. In addition, it has some special features tailored to the specific symptoms and needs of survivors of child abuse and neglect, chronic interpersonal trauma and complex PTSD. It offers compassionately attuned interventions to address mental health symptoms such as emotion dysregulation, chronic avoidance, low emotional awareness, alexithymia and gaps in narrative memory so prevalent with this population. The model is also equipped to address the often comorbid symptoms of depression and anxiety (Paivio & Pascual-Leone, 2023).

EFTT offers a carefully scaffolded, step-by-step approach with consistent attunement to the client's capacity to tolerate and regulate their feelings. Unlike the general model, EFTT also includes principles of gradual trauma exposure as further research in EFTT has led to precise steps for working directly with traumatic memories in the middle phase of therapy. It is also one of the few therapies that has a specific process for working through grief and sadness during the resolution stages of the therapy as clients come to terms with the impact of all that was lost because of the traumas they survived.

Compared to the general model, EFTT uses a more directive approach and therapists are trained in an advanced set of skills to sustain accurate attunement using a vast repertoire of empathic responses to help evoke and upregulate or downregulate emotion as needed. It places a greater emphasis on fostering a secure attachment bond and offers a broader range of interventions to address emotion regulation challenges including emotion coaching, psychoeducation and guided skills practice such as breathing and trauma-sensitive yoga (Paivio & Pascual-Leone, 2023).

EFTT also places a greater **emphasis on client strengths and areas of resilience** wherever possible. This helps to nurture awareness of and increase access to adaptive emotion, which strengthens the sense of self as opportunities are harnessed to resolve core maladaptive shame, powerlessness, self-blame and worthlessness so prevalent among childhood abuse survivors. EFTT employs the **use of imagery and enactments** including evocative empathy, experiential focusing and Gestalt therapy–based procedures to evoke core maladaptive emotion and trauma content encoded in experiential memory (Paivio & Pascual-Leone, 2023).

Earlier we defined EFT's general view of emotion schemes. In EFTT, empathic exploration elicits further articulation of the problems that keep survivors of childhood abuse trauma stuck as client and therapist **collaboratively build a case conceptualization** to identify the core maladaptive emotion scheme across four dimensions: 1. The primary maladaptive emotion (e.g. core shame, lonely abandonment, fear); 2. Sense of self/negative self-evaluation; 3. Perception of others (e.g. as threatening, dangerous, untrustworthy); and 4. Core unmet needs (e.g. for respect, safety, love).

Primary maladaptive emotion related to child abuse trauma such as fear and shame are a result of exposure to unsafe, threatening and repeated interactions that include humiliation, harm and neglect. Children growing up in environments that included abandonment or where their emotional needs were denied or ignored may have a core maladaptive emotion scheme organized around the feelings of chronic sadness, loneliness and fear of abandonment. "Accurate intervention involves determining which core emotional experience is most dominant for the client – overall and at any given time" (Paivio & Pascual-Leone, 2023, p. 91). A clearly articulated case conceptualization built in collaboration with the client will determine the focus of the work, including a specific intention to work directly with a traumatic memory during the middle phase of therapy.

A key finding that emerged from the early research on the classic two-chair EFT intervention to resolve unfinished business with another person in the patient's life indicated that this procedure was not suitable for many survivors of relational trauma. It involves imagining the other in the empty chair (also referred to as **imaginal confrontation (IC)**. For some trauma survivors, visualizing their perpetrators in the empty chair proved to be too overwhelming and they therefore refused to engage at all (Paivio & Pascual-Leone, 2023). While EFTT does move toward resolution procedures with perpetrators of abuse, it has been adapted to include the **evocative empathy procedure (EE)** as a less threatening alternative. It applies the exact same intervention principles as IC. However, the other person is imagined through visualization and feelings that are evoked and expressed directly to the therapist rather than to the imagined other in the empty chair. It is often the case that once clients have gained some practice with EE they become more comfortable engaging in imaginal confrontation.

DESCRIPTION OF THE THERAPY PROCESS

EFTT is a short-term, semi-structured approach that typically consists of 16–20 weekly one-hour sessions. The duration will vary depending on the client's particular needs and response to the process. As with the general EFT model, EFTT places a special focus on the formation of a strong therapeutic alliance before proceeding to the deeper work of emotional experiencing, processing and resolution.

There are four distinct phases in EFTT. In the **initial phase**, the focus is on forming the alliance, promoting emotional experiencing and introducing the first experiential tasks. In the **middle phase**, the focus shifts toward memory work while reducing maladaptive fear, anxiety and avoidance, as well as shame, guilt and self-blame. The **late phase** of EFTT shifts to resolution work through interventions designed to support the expression of adaptive anger, sadness and grief. The **final phase** focuses on preparation for ending and termination (Paivio & Pascual-Leone, 2023).

INITIAL PHASE

The first three sessions are devoted to alliance formation. The therapist leads from compassion by providing appropriate empathic responses, validating experiences and feelings that are shared, offering reassurance, encouragement and hope while also eliciting the trauma story by asking directly about it. Trust is also nurtured through transparency by clarifying therapist and client roles, fostering realistic expectations for the therapy and working collaboratively to build a case conceptualization. Client and therapist work together to identify and clarify the client's core maladaptive emotion scheme in order to establish goals. A secure base founded on trust and safety offers a corrective experience to early attachment injuries, neglect and mis-attuned caregiving. In addition, it provides the stability needed for a client to accept the therapist's guidance toward a gradual process of ever-deepening emotional experiencing as awareness of different types of emotions (e.g. maladaptive vs. adaptive, primary, secondary or instrumental) are identified, accepted and resolved.

The EFTT therapist assesses client readiness using a process–diagnostic approach as they attend to client markers for emotion regulation and experiencing capacities as well as the ability to focus on the trauma (s) that have been identified as the focus of therapy. They refrain from emotional deepening and re-experiencing at this early stage and track the quality of the alliance using the Horvath & Greenberg (1989) Working Alliance Inventory (Paivio & Pascual-Leone, 2023).

HOW EFTT PROMOTES EXPERIENCING

EFTT offer a step-by-step process for deepening emotional experiencing with every step informed by the process-diagnostic approach (Paivio & Pascual-Leone, 2023). From the very first session the EFTT therapist is assessing the client's capacity for experiential deepening and tracking their responses to interventions that are used to support this. Resistances to deepening exploration and factors that may affect this such as difficulty regulating high states of arousal, scattered narratives, fear of experiencing, avoidance and low emotional awareness will contribute to the case conceptualization as well as the pace and guidance provided. Grounded in the EFT research on optimal arousal for productive experiencing, the EFTT therapist will either be eliciting or reducing arousal to help the client relate to their subjective internal reality within their window of tolerance (Auszra et al., 2013).

An important experiential task first introduced in the initial phase and frequently used throughout EFT and EFTT is the **Structured Focusing Procedure** originally developed by Eugene Gendlin. EFT research indicates that focusing is most effective for clients who present with a vague and unclear sense of their feelings or when they are confused about their feelings. It provides a gently scaffolded structure for deepening emotional experiencing and processing (Paivio & Pascual-Leone, 2023).

By the end of the third session, the EFTT therapist and client will have established a clearly defined contract based on collaboratively articulated goals and agreements to engage processes to support emotional deepening. The client should have a clear rationale and an emerging felt sense for how engaging in all further procedures will lead them toward the resolution of the trauma they have come to therapy to work on. All of this contributes to a strong therapeutic alliance and sets the stage for the first **Imaginal Confrontation Procedure** usually introduced in session 4. Foundational research conducted by Paivio and Nieuwenhuis (2001) indicated that, along with the quality of the therapeutic alliance, the placement of the IC intervention at this point of the therapy strengthened change outcomes.

Imaginal confrontation involves imagining the perpetrator of the abuse in the empty chair to communicate and express the painful truth regarding the impact of abuse and/or neglect and to hold perpetrators accountable for the damage they caused. The technique has features of exposure-based approaches but is distinct in its emphasis on the resolution of harm caused in the context of interpersonal relationships (Paivio & Pascual-Leone, 2023). When clients find this step too threatening, then **evocative empathy** can be introduced as an alternative.

Imaginal confrontation has the power to evoke core emotional processes, making maladaptive schemes available to explore and articulate. Therapists need to gauge the pace while guiding clients toward an awareness of their internal experience in order to facilitate the expression of this directly to the imagined other. The eight key constructs of EFT are the foundation as clients are supported to find the words to describe their feelings so that they can be directly expressed to the perpetrator of their abuse in the session. "Resolving interpersonal injuries related to childhood maltreatment is the primary task of therapy and IC is the procedure most frequently used to accomplish this" (Paivio & Pascual-Leone, 2023, p. 45).

For some clients, assistance with emotion regulation will be necessary. The EFTT therapist will offer support through their use of self in addition to practices to help ground the client such as guided breath practices, trauma-sensitive yoga practices and behavioral skills drawn from other approaches including CBT and DBT. In other instances, the therapist may need to elicit more for clients who are disconnected from their internal experiences. The EFTT therapist is always tracking tendencies toward over-control or feelings of being overwhelmed and rely on the EFT evidence to gauge and guide just enough emotional experiencing for the therapy to be productive (Auszra et al., 2013).

MIDDLE PHASE

The focus of the middle phase of EFTT therapy focuses on memory work. Based on the neuroscience of emotional change, traumatic memory is malleable once it is activated. Middle phase interventions are designed to evoke the experiential memories held in emotions, sounds, smells, images and bodily experience. An ongoing collaborative process-diagnosis approach helps the therapist and client attend to and distinguish between different types of maladaptive emotions such as fear and anxiety to help reduce avoidance of internal experience as memories are approached.

The client is supported to access and allow primary emotional experience to be felt and articulated as associated unmet needs begin to be addressed. The middle phase also addresses shame, guilt and self-blame and offers associated interventions that have been identified through the EFTT research to help distinguish between and resolve adaptive and maladaptive shame. As vulnerable sadness and grief is also explored, the therapist can initiate interventions that focus on compassionate self-soothing (Paivio & Pascual-Leone, 2023).

LATE PHASE

The late phase of therapy moves toward the resolution of interpersonal trauma as clients have more access to adaptive anger – a key EFTT process. Here again the process-diagnosis approach helps to identify and distinguish maladaptive from adaptive anger and to facilitate clinical choice points to engage interventions that further expression. Consistent with EFT's principle of changing emotion with emotion, having access to and expression of adaptive anger is the key to transforming core maladaptive shame and self-blame. Lastly, EFTT supports the resolution of grief and sadness that emerges in the later stages of therapy. It is one of the few trauma therapies that offers a specific process to attend to the natural and adaptive grief that arises as clients come to terms with the profound losses stemming from childhood trauma and neglect.

To summarize, EFTT is a short-term therapy that typically consists of 16–20 sessions. An empathic and collaborative alliance is essential for the success of further trauma work as clients are guided through the eight key constructs described earlier. The process helps to transform maladaptive emotion schemes by reducing fear, anxiety and avoidance of internal experience as well as guilt, shame and self-blame as direct work with traumatic memory is approached. The late phase supports an ever-deepening process toward the resolution of interpersonal trauma by resolving maladaptive anger and promoting primary adaptive anger and eventually toward the resolution of traumatic grief.

ASSESSMENT OF RESEARCH EVIDENCE REGARDING EFFECTIVENESS IN TREATING TRAUMA

EFT founder, Les Greenberg, made an impressive contribution to the field of counseling psychology and to the expansion of its research methodologies. He is considered to be a pioneer in the development of process–outcome research methodologies and has challenged the view that the randomized control trial be upheld as the gold standard in psychology research methodologies. He has proposed innovative strategies for research design focused on the in-session specificity regarding linking particular markers to specific tasks with a focus on what leads to enduring change in psychotherapy. The EFT theory and research canon has significantly influenced the field's overall understanding of the important role emotion plays in change processes in psychotherapy and Greenberg's contributions have been widely recognized.

As the research on EFTT has grown since the late 1990s, it stands out as one of the few psychotherapies for complex/developmental and relational trauma that has a body of evidence supporting the rationale for emotional experiencing to therapeutically provide enduring change, filling a much-needed research gap regarding addressing the needs of child abuse survivors. It is exciting to see EFTT being applied in broader contexts, including refugee trauma, transgender populations, human trafficking and domestic violence for example (Paivio & Pascual-Leone, 2023). While there is a growing body of evidence supporting the effectiveness of EFTT there is a need for further meta-analyses and longitudinal studies with a broader spectrum of participants from diverse backgrounds. Further comparative effectiveness studies that compare EFT with other evidence-based treatments for trauma would contribute valuable insights.

CASE EXAMPLE REGARDING THE TREATMENT OF TRAUMA

Louisa, a 37-year-old married, lesbian, cis-gendered mother of two, diagnosed with complex PTSD, was referred for EFTT therapy by her psychiatrist. She had recently completed a shorter program of DBT therapy but continued to struggle with marital issues and feelings of disconnection. She also expressed her readiness to "get to the root" of her issues when exploring next steps with her psychiatrist. Louisa completed 24 sessions of EFTT with a focus on resolving a key traumatic memory that she described as "the worst" part of her past.

At her initial session, Louisa stated that she had prepared by doing a Google search to learn more about EFT. She admitted that she almost cancelled because she did not want to be "forced" to participate in chair work or go digging into painful memories from her past. She explained, that until very recently, she'd been able to keep the memories "locked up in a box on the shelf." The therapist acknowledged that starting EFTT was a brave step. She reassured Louisa that she was in the driver's seat, that she and the therapist could set the pace together and that it was perfectly fine if she did not want to engage in chair work by reassuring her that "EFT for trauma offered a less stressful alternative." She briefly offered further psychoeducation about the process, mentioning that

> EFTT does indeed focus on the resolution of past trauma through memory work, but we can go slowly. The first three sessions are focused on getting to know each other. From there we can decide what seems right to do next.

Once Louisa had a chance to catch her breath and get comfortably settled in her chair, the therapist began by asking her to share more about her decision to begin therapy to gain further clarity about her current struggles, identify goals and discuss how EFTT might help with this.

THERAPIST: So, Louisa, I'm curious to learn more about you and especially today to hear more about how you came to the decision to begin EFTT therapy. I get that it was difficult to come today and yet, here you are. Can you tell me more about what helped you decide to come?

By joining with her hopes and motivations, the therapist begins to form a good collaboration with Louisa by clarifying her goals. By exploring her hopes and fears about starting therapy, realistic expectations are fostered for what can be accomplished in 16–20 sessions.

LOUISA: Well, I'm not exactly sure, to tell you the truth. I'm really not into the touchy-feely stuff. I met with my psychiatrist, and she suggested I try something different. I did learn some good skills in the DBT program,

	I guess. But I still feel like I'm circling around the "same old, same old." My wife is fed up with me … I'm afraid she's going to leave me if I don't get to the root of this.
THERAPIST:	Right. So, you've invested quite a lot already. You've learned some good coping skills and I imagine that took some effort and I hear the frustration in your voice as you mention feeling stuck in the "same old, same old." I also hear the concern – the fear that your wife might leave you. There's a lot at stake here.
LOUISA:	Ya. She's off on a trip right now. Says she needed to get a break from me.
THERAPIST:	Ok. So, I'm getting how important it is that we find a way to help. EFTT does offer some ways that we can "get to the root" as you say. Can you tell me a little more about what you believe is lying at the root of this? [beginning to elicit the trauma story]
LOUISA:	It's like … sometimes I just feel like I'm that ten-year-old kid again. It's so stupid. I just shut down. She said she was fed up with my walls. She says I ice her out. It's hot/cold, you know?
THERAPIST:	Yes, "hot/cold" … so difficult. Feels like that little girl again, just ten. I have some sense of how bad things were for you as a child. [empathic affirmation] Can you tell me a bit about what happened? [directly eliciting the trauma story]

Over the course of the next three sessions Louisa and her EFTT therapist are developing a secure attachment bond as the therapist nurtures trust and safety by responding with interest, reassurance, compassion for her suffering, validation of the fears she raises and by offering hope. By providing further education about how the EFTT process can help her, Louisa begins to see the value in feeling her feelings and preparing to work with a painful memory from her past.

By the end of session three, they have established an agreement to focus on the traumatic memory that has been most intrusive for Louisa with the understanding that the therapist will support her to go at a pace that will both help her feel her feelings and also regulate her distress before memories are approached.

THERAPIST:	This is difficult, getting in touch with such painful feelings. I'm here to help you feel these here where it's safe so they can change and heal. We'll do this together but your job is to let me know when it's feeling like it's too much.

The therapist has also been listening for Louisa's strengths and resilience and harnessing opportunities to highlight the adaptive emotions. The second major task in the initial phase is to begin to promote awareness and exploration of internal feelings and meanings such as thoughts, images and bodily sensations. It is "essential to treat experiencing as a capacity that can be improved with practice - collaboration on the goal to improve this capacity is the first step" (Paivio & Pascual-Leone, 2023, p. 119).

Louisa reported feeling disturbed by an intrusive memory that had been plaguing her most recently – an image of her ten-year-old self standing at the bottom of a staircase, feeling frozen but about to ascend the stairs. The coercive perpetrator who sexually abused her was waiting for her there. As she described the image, the felt sense of her feelings was vague and unclear – a marker for the structured focusing procedure – which was introduced by session three.

The procedure begins with helping the client to relax by guiding basic breathing or progressive muscle relaxation practices as clients are encouraged to place a gentle focus on their inner experience. This may be enough for some clients – especially if they are prone to emotional flooding or high states of mental distraction. However, since Louisa tolerated this first step well, she was guided to attend to her bodily felt experience, to allow more of the sensation into her experience.

THERAPIST: Now that you are noticing your breath just a little more, see if you can clear your mind of any distractions, just bringing a gentle focus inward – noticing just to notice.
[*Louisa's* body gradually begins to appear more relaxed as her shoulders soften and her breathing steadies]

THERAPIST: Just being with that place in your body where you notice the whole of that frozen feeling ....

The therapist patiently supports Louisa to follow the sensation and attend to her experience without pushing and to allow the experience to naturally evolve. Gradually, Louisa is supported to find the words to describe the quality of that experience.

THERAPIST: Say a little more about the quality of that sensation there, of feeling frozen. Is there a phrase, maybe a word or image that seems to fit?

LOUISA: Like, I'm just a robot. My body is walking up the stairs but I feel frozen in ice.

THERAPIST: Yes. Like a robot, moving but somehow feeling frozen. So scared. Can you say more about that. Like, something bad is coming? [evocative empathy]

LOUISA: Yes! A part of me is just so angry at her: "You're such a fool! Why did you walk up those stairs!" [marker for self-blame]

THERAPIST: So scary. Such a scared little girl knowing what's about to happen but feeling so caught without a choice with no one there to protect her.

Here the therapist made use of empathic responses that pointed toward the needs held in previously unexpressed feelings and aligned closely with Louisa's own language. Hearing her own words reflected helped nurture an increasing clarity of awareness and expression. Further deepening was fostered through evocative empathy, empathic conjecture and exploration by sensitively asking questions building on the leading edge of Louisa's own processing.

By the fourth session we are moving into the middle phase of therapy where earlier markers of shame, self-blame, fear and avoidance will begin to be addressed and resolved and set the groundwork to further explore episodic memory and activate the maladaptive sense of self as blame-worthy and shameful, while simultaneously drawing on her adaptive adult strengths and inner resources.

For Louisa, the process began in session four by using evocative empathy, but she was eventually ready to try the imaginal confrontation (IC) procedure as her sessions progressed with more trust and safety established. Two-chair dialogue between her self-critic and the ten-year-old caught in the traumatic memory at the stairs helped her access her adaptive adult capacities where she was eventually able to have compassion for the little girl and adaptive anger towards the perpetrator. During the late phase of Louisa's therapy, she was further supported to access and express her anger by holding her perpetrator accountable using the IC intervention. This eventually led to the resolution of her traumatic memory and the final stages of allowing and expressing her unprocessed grief and sadness stemming from all that was lost. By the end of her 20 sessions, Louisa's wife noticed that she was no longer shutting down and icing her out. Louisa noticed a sense of confidence in her body and, although she still remembered her experience, it did not arise intrusively or with the prior symptoms of feeling frozen. By gaining further awareness and acceptance, she was better able to identify, regulate and express her feelings and access the important qualities held in her adaptive emotions.

STRENGTHS AND LIMITATIONS OF THE MODALITY AS A TREATMENT FOR TRAUMA

EFTT is designed to help those who have experienced severe and chronic interpersonal trauma with a particular focus on childhood maltreatment. While EFTT has shown great promise as an evidenced-based therapy at the leading edge of trauma approaches, like any model, it holds both strengths and limitations. For example, EFTT is not appropriate for clients presenting with anxiety as the principal symptom resulting from single-incident or shock trauma. Here the APA best-practice guidelines continue to emphasize treatments such as exposure-based CBT or EMDR.

A key strength of EFTT is its emphasis on helping individuals transform the maladaptive emotion schemes that keep them caught in repetitive and reflexive cycles of pain. It aims for enduring change and offers a finely attuned and compassionate process built on a 30-year program of process-outcome research. EFTT has filled a major gap in the trauma canon, providing great relief for many who have not benefited from other approaches. By fostering a deeper understanding and integration of traumatic experiences, clients who respond well to EFTT often experience the resolution of their symptoms, thereby freeing them from having to perpetually manage with coping skills alone. EFTT also recognizes the importance of secure attachments and interpersonal relationships in the healing process. The therapist works to create a safe and supportive therapeutic relationship that offers a corrective experience for individuals with a history of relational trauma. The comprehensive and holistic approach of EFTT helps to address the multifaceted aspects of complex trauma including cognitive, emotional, somatic and behavioral elements.

A major limitation of the model is that the success of the treatment hinges entirely on the quality of the therapeutic relationship. If there are challenges in establishing trust or if the therapeutic alliance is compromised, progress may be hindered. It also requires a high level of skill in combination with a consistency of heart–centered presence from the therapist. EFTT may not be suitable for all survivors of complex trauma and not all therapists are suitable to use EFTT. Some individuals may require more structured or directive approaches, and therapists need to carefully assess the appropriateness of EFTT for each case.

RESOURCES FOR LEARNING

READING

Sandra Paivio and Pascual-Leone: Paivio, S.C., & Pascual-Leone, A. (2023). *Emotion-Focused Therapy for Complex Trauma: An Integrative Approach*. International Society for Emotion Focused Therapy. https://www.iseft.org/eftresources

VIDEOS

Greenberg, Les: Working with current and historical trauma. http://www.counsellingchannel.tv/ or https://www.cpcab.co.uk/shop/les-greenberg-wwcht-video
American Psychological Association. (2014). *Series II – Specific Treatments for Specific Populations, Sandra C. Paivio, PhD, CPsych – Emotion Focused Therapy for Trauma* [DVD]. USA; APA Psychotherapy Videos.

FURTHER TRAINING

Workshops at York-Emotion-Focused Therapy Clinic: https://www.yorku.ca/health/eft/training-institutes-york/
Greenberg Institute of Emotion Focused Therapy: https://www.cpeh.ca/copy-of-about
International Society for Emotion Focused Therapy: https://www.iseft.org/
Cyprus Institute for Emotion Focused Therapy: https://www.eft.cy/team/leslie-les-greenberg/

REFERENCES

Auszra, L., Greenberg, L.S., Herrmann I. (2013). Client emotional productivity-optimal client in-session emotional processing in experiential therapy. *Psychotherapy Research* 23(6): 732–746. https://doi.org/10.1080/10503307.2013.816882. Epub 2013 Jul 15. PMID: 23848974.

Bourne, D.T. (Host). (2022, May 6). Dr. Leslie Greenberg's Journey, Thoughts on CBT, and-Development of Emotion Focused Therapy [Video Podcast Episode]. In *DTB*. Apple-Podcasts. Retrieved June 6, 2023, from https://podcasts.apple.com/ca/podcast/dr-leslie-greenbergs-journey-thoughts-on-cbt-and/id1576127599?i=1000559837685

Greenberg, L.S. (2021). *Changing emotion with emotion: A practitioner's guide*. Washington, DC: American Psychological Association. https://doi.org/10.1037/0000248-000

Greenberg, L.S., &Goldman, R.N. (2008). *Emotion-Focused Couples Therapy: The Dynamics of Emotion, Love, and Power*. https://doi.org/10.1604/9781433803161

Greenberg, L.S., &Malcolm, W. (2002). Resolving unfinished business: Relating process tooutcome. *Journal of Consulting and Clinical Psychology, 70*(2), 406–416.

Greenberg, L. S., Rice, L. N. & Elliott, R. (1993) *Facilitating Emotional Change: The Moment-by-Moment Process*. Guildford Press.

Horvath, A. O., & Greenberg, L. S. (1989). Development and validation of the Working Alliance Inventory. *Journal of Counseling Psychology, 36*(2), 223–233. https://doi.org/10.1037/0022-0167.36.2.223

Paivio, S.C., & Greenberg, L.S. (1995). Resolving "unfinished business": Efficacy of experiential therapy using empty-chair dialogue. *Journal of Consulting and Clinical Psychology, 63*(3), 419–425. https://doi.org/10.1037/0022-006X.63.3.419

Paivio, S.C., & Nieuwenhuis, J.A. (2001). Efficacy of emotion focused therapy for adultsur-vivors of child abuse: A preliminary study. *Journal of Traumatic Stress, 14*(1), 115–133. https://doi.org/10.1023/A:1007891716593

Paivio, S.C., & Pascual-Leone, A. (2023). *Emotion-Focused Therapy for Complex Trauma: AnIntegrative Approach*. American Psychological Association.

10

CHAPTER 10
EYE MOVEMENT DESENSITIZATION AND REPROCESSING (EMDR) IN THE 21ST CENTURY

Noora Niskanen

INTRODUCTION

In 35 years, eye movement desensitization and reprocessing (EMDR) therapy has evolved from Francine Shapiro's chance personal discovery to becoming one of the leading psychotherapy treatments for post-traumatic stress disorder (PTSD) worldwide. EMDR treats the whole person – their cognitions, their emotions, their body, and their stored traumatic memories. Grounded in Shapiro's adaptive information processing (AIP) model, EMDR proposes that traumatic memories are incorrectly stored and need to be reprocessed for symptoms to resolve and learning to occur. The EMDR therapist activates the patient's innate self-healing process. It also uses dual attention awareness, one foot in the present and one foot in the past, in the form of bilateral stimulation of the brain to help keep patients in the window of tolerance. New research shows that overloading working memory while reprocessing traumatic memory could lead to even greater speed, efficiency, and cost savings. While EMDR is currently recommended by the World Health Organization and the Institute of Traumatic Stress Studies for the treatment of PTSD, the new ICD-11 diagnosis of complex post-traumatic stress (C-PTSD), which includes "disorders of the self," presents new clinical challenges. Continued research needs to be conducted in the form of randomized control trials (RCTs) in PTSD treatment while also developing new protocols and techniques for C-PTSD.

BRIEF HISTORY

Eye movement desensitization and reprocessing (EMDR) was initially developed in 1987 by psychologist Francine Shapiro. As she recalls in her book, *Eye Movement Desensitization and Reprocessing Therapy* (2018), while working on her doctoral dissertation on Thomas Hardy she was diagnosed with cancer. She decided to quit her English PhD program and enroll in a doctoral program in psychology to research the connection between stress and disease. In the spring of 1987, Shapiro (2018) writes:

> While walking one day, I noticed that some disturbing thoughts I was having suddenly disappeared. I also noticed that when I brought these thoughts back to mind, they were not as upsetting or valid as before …. Fascinated, I started paying very close

DOI: 10.4324/9781003455851-10

attention to what was going on. I noticed that when disturbing thoughts came into my mind, my eyes spontaneously started moving very rapidly back and forth in an upward diagonal. Again, the thoughts disappeared, and when I brought them back to mind, their negative charge was greatly reduced.

(p. 7)

Shapiro began experimenting on friends, colleagues, and patients. After having them bring up disturbing memories, beliefs, and present-day stresses, she found that the easiest method for them to replicate the way she moved her eyes in the park was to move her fingers across their field of vision and have them follow her hand. After working with 70 people for six months, Shapiro (2018) began developing a standard protocol, "Eye Movement Desensitization" (EMD), that produced a reduction in their anxiety symptoms. At that time, she found that it worked best with clients' distant memories rather than recent ones.

Shapiro believed that this technique would also be effective with people affected by trauma. To test that hypothesis, she first worked with a Vietnam veteran, "Doug," who was haunted by a disturbing memory of unloading dead bodies from a helicopter. Shapiro asked him to hold that memory in his mind while following her hand. After two or three "sets" of eye movements, he reported that the auditory part of the memory was gone. After several more sets, he reported that the memory was like "a paint chip under water" (Shapiro, 2018, p. 9) and that he felt calm. Then he said, "I can finally say the war is over, and I can tell everyone to go home" (Shapiro, 2018, p. 9). Later when he was asked to think about Vietnam, some positive images of the beauty of the countryside emerged. Six months later, he said the memory still looked like a "paint chip." Giving the staying power of the EMD technique, Shapiro moved on to a study with patients who suffered from PTSD.

Following her positive experience with "Doug" in 1989, Shapiro set up a controlled pilot study of EMD with 22 victims of rape, molestation, or Vietnam combat who fit the PTSD criteria as defined by the *Diagnostic and Statistical Manual of Mental Disorders* (DSM-III, American Psychiatric Association, 1980). She utilized a treatment and control group. All group members described their traumatic memories in detail and identified a disturbing image of their traumatic memory and a negative thought or belief about themselves in that situation. She called these negative beliefs, "negative cognitions" and used the 11-point Subjective Units of Disturbance scale (SUD) to rate their anxiety (Shapiro, 2018, p. 10). She also asked each research subject for a positive cognition of what they would like to believe about themselves and rated these for how true it felt using a 7-point scale called Validity of Cognition (VOC). Shapiro's treatment group showed two changes: A decrease in anxiety and an increase in the VOC of positive cognitions. In the control group, anxiety increased, and sense of self-efficacy decreased. While the pilot study lacked standardized measures and blind evaluations, it was one of the first published controlled studies assessing a reduction in PTSD symptoms using EMD (Shapiro, 1989).

In 1991, the name EMD was changed to EMDR (eye movement desensitization and reprocessing) to reflect the change from mere desensitization of anxiety to an information processing model (Shapiro, 1991; 2018). Based on case reports from hundreds of clinicians, in addition to decreasing anxiety, EMD also resulted in the cognitive restructuring of memories, the elicitation of spontaneous insights, and an increase in self-efficacy, "… all of which appeared to be the by-products of the adaptive information processing of disturbing memories. This realization led to my renaming the technique Eye Movement Desensitization and Reprocessing (EMDR)" (Shapiro, 2018, p. 12). Thus, over a span of 20 years, EMDR progressed from a technique to a protocol to a comprehensive psychotherapy (Laliotis et al., 2021).

FUNDAMENTAL CLINICAL CONCEPTS

In 1995, Shapiro developed a theoretical framework to explain treatment outcomes and to help guide future EMDR clinicians. Initially calling it A.I.P, the accelerated information processing model (Shapiro, 1995), she later revised it to stand for the adaptive information processing model (AIP) (Shapiro, 2001). Shapiro (2018) developed this model as a "working hypothesis only and is subject to modification based on further laboratory and clinical observation" (p. 26) and utilized neurophysiology terminology and research introduced by Bower (1981) and Lang (1979). In particular, Shapiro (2018) used the term "neural network" to refer to the "neurobiological configuration of an individual memory" (p. 28), which accounts for the cognitive reprocessing that is a hallmark of EMDR. Although the AIP model has not yet been validated by neuroscience, it has served as the primary guide for EMDR therapists.

As Shapiro (2018) states, "Adaptive Information Processing (Shapiro, 1995) represents the general model that provides the theoretical framework and principles for treatment and an explanation of the basis of pathology and personality development" (p. 26). She built upon Freud's (1955) and Pavlov (1927) ideas about how humans process information. Believing that information is processed to an "adaptive resolution," that is, "… a resolution in which the connections to appropriate associations are made and the experience is integrated into a positive emotional and cognitive schema" (Shapiro, 2018, p. 26). In other words, a person learns what is helpful from the experience and stores this information with the appropriate affect for use in the future. For example, if you forgot to do the reading for a class and are called upon by the professor, you register a certain amount of embarrassment and do the reading for the following class. The AIP model is a learning model about how we adaptively process our life experiences and learn from them.

When a traumatic event occurs, it creates physiological changes including cortisol release, spikes in adrenaline, and fluctuations in neurotransmitters, resulting in neural disequilibrium (Griffin, Charron, & Al-Daccak, 2014; Rodrigues et al., 2009, Weiss, 2007). Shapiro hypothesized that in traumatic moments the adaptive information processing system is overwhelmed, and the information retrieved at that moment, including images, sounds, emotions, and physical sensations, is stored in this hyperaroused state rather than being adaptively processed into our existing schema. According to Shapiro (2018), trauma is a result of "insufficiently processed memories inappropriately stored in the brain" (p. 38). Therefore, traumatic memories are not just remembered, but relived with all the accompanying emotions, physical sensations, and images present at the moment of occurrence. It is this hyperarousal state that makes trauma reprocessing so intense and difficult.

In EMDR treatment, when you pair bilateral stimulation with the traumatic memory, a physiological state is created that allows reprocessing of the trauma that could not be metabolized during the traumatic incident. Bilateral stimulation (BLS) began with eye movements where the patient followed the therapist's fingers back and forth. Since then, other forms of BLS have emerged, including adding tactile and auditory options. According to Shapiro (2018), "bilateral stimulation during EMDR processing sessions (1) taxes (overloads) the working memory, (2) stimulates the orienting reflex and an associated parasympathetic response, and (3) elicits the same or similar processes that characterize rapid eye movement (REM) sleep" (p. 27). According to Laliotis et al., 2021, "It is generally agreed that dual attention, that simultaneously maintaining two distinct focuses, allows for the client to process their experience in a more detached manner" (p. 191). While the exact mechanism of action is still not completely understood, it is generally accepted that the inadequately processed memory is "reprocessed" by feeling the accompanying emotions and physical sensations and moving from a "negative cognition" like "I am powerless" to a "positive cognition" such as "I did the best that I could in those circumstances." In other words, instead of "reliving" the traumatic memory with the original emotional, cognitive, and physical sensations, the memory is "remembered" without the accompanying "charge" or hyperarousal symptoms of PTSD.

A key component of the AIP model is that all patients have an innate self-healing mechanism and that the goal of EMDR treatment is to create the clinical conditions to facilitate this operation. Shapiro (2018) used this analogy: When you cut your hand, your body knows how to heal the wound. In the EMDR process, a person's "stuck" self-healing mechanism is able to resume operation, enabling the traumatic experience to be metabolized at last and viewed in a healthy, self-affirming way. Another important aspect of the AIP model is the concept of memory or neural networks, "… where related memories, thoughts, images, emotions, and sensations are stored and linked to one another" (p. 30). In EMDR reprocessing, clinicians ask a patient to focus on a specific "target" memory, part of a "node" that has physiologically associated material. For instance, a client may have intense anxiety in relation to the changing light in September, which would be considered a node because of its associated material. The fall light might be related to a back-to-school trauma from childhood or other past experiences that happened at that time of year. The goal of EMDR therapy would be for the patient to react calmly to the target by reprocessing the dysfunctionally stored material (Shapiro, 2018).

Since a memory or neural network is linked associatively, multiple traumatic memories can be worked on simultaneously. Unlike traditional talk therapy that relies exclusively on verbal cues or insights, EMDR therapy can reprocess groups or channels of traumatic memories along with the associated images, beliefs, and bodily sensations. "According to our model, psychological dysfunction, with all its complex elements of lack of self-esteem and self-efficacy is caused by the information stored in the brain. By means of EMDR therapy, this information is accessed, processed, and adaptively resolved" (Shapiro, 2018, p. 43). This process affects shifts in emotion and self-assessment with new thoughts and beliefs changing how the experience is now stored and remembered. One can shift from the belief, "It was my fault" to "I did the best that I could."

There are times during EMDR trauma reprocessing when things grind to a halt and the patient is stuck in an abreaction or in a negative belief about themselves. Generally, this is when the patient lacks sufficient information to bring the processing to a positive outcome. Shapiro (2018) called it "blocked processing" or "abreactive looping" and suggested using a "cognitive interweave" to get the processing back on track. For example, when an adult patient is looping in fear of a childhood abuser who is dead, the therapist can ask, "Can he hurt you now?" (p. 273). A popular trainer, Laurel Parnell (2013), used the broader term "interweave," noting that in addition to cognitions, one can invoke attachment figures (nurturing, protective, and wise) to imagine a more desirable outcome to the event ("If you could redo the scene, what would you do now?"), to sort information with a "split screen," and to employ acquired knowledge ("As an adult, what do you understand now?"). Another technique that Shapiro endorsed to get to the root cause of a present-day trigger is the floatback technique. Here, the therapist asks the client to bring up a recent disturbing event along with the physical sensations and the negative cognition it generates, then asks her/him to float back to an earlier time so that the earliest version of a specific upset is available as a target for reprocessing. Parnell (2013) refined this technique calling it "bridging" or "tracing" back. Shapiro and Parnell's hypothesis is that reprocessing the earliest memory creates a more generalized effect so that fewer targets are needed to provide greater relief.

DESCRIPTION OF THE THERAPY PROCESS

Shapiro (2018) developed an eight-phase treatment protocol along with a temporal three-pronged approach that focuses on the past, present, and future aspects of a target memory. In EMDR protocols, according to Laliotis (2021), "The goal is partial or complete reprocessing of memories that contribute to the client's presenting problems. Protocols can be used as a stand-alone approach, or as part of a more comprehensive psychotherapy" (p. 190). All certified EMDR practitioners learn Shapiro's eight phase, three-pronged protocol, yet there is an art to applying them successfully. There is some confusion even among EMDR clinicians about the difference between utilizing the EMDR protocols and EMDR psychotherapy. As defined by Laliotis et al., 2021:

> EMDR psychotherapy is the comprehensive application of EMDR therapy that treats the whole person, addressing the full clinical picture to include individual, relational and behavioral domains … It regards the therapeutic alliance as an integral part of the therapy…treats presenting symptoms, low self-esteem, attachment issues, developmental deficits, and/or other personal characteristics that are mutually elaborated as goals for treatment across different diagnostic categories.
>
> (p. 190)

In practice, EMDR protocols work extremely well for a single incident trauma while more extensive EMDR psychotherapy is necessary for working with clients with complex post-traumatic stress disorder (C-PTSD) which includes disorders of the self, such as low self-esteem, difficulties with emotional regulation, and struggles in interpersonal relationships.

The eight phases in the standard EMDR treatment process (Shapiro, 2018) are: 1) Client history-taking to determine appropriateness and eligibility for EMDR, treatment planning, and the identification of potential targets to be reprocessed; 2) Preparation, in which the client is introduced to EMDR procedures, theory, and informed consent about the intensity of EMDR reprocessing; 3) Assessment to determine a target and baseline response using the SUD scale and VOC scale; 4) Desensitization to address physiological and emotional activation of the memories and the elicitation of "insights and appropriate associations" (Shapiro, 2018, p. 65) or positive cognitions; 5) Installation that focuses on working with the positive cognition and integrating it into the patient's cognitive schema or beliefs about the self; 6) Body scan to see if there is any physical activation left in body when bringing up the target memory; 7) Debriefing with the client about the session and bringing them to equilibrium following the reprocessing; and 8) Re-evaluation of the target to make sure that it has been fully processed and to determine if it is associatively linked to another neural network.

In Phase 1, the clinician obtains a detailed client history to gauge readiness for EMDR treatment and the need for psychological supports between sessions. EMDR reprocessing may activate intense emotions and physical sensations that were experienced during the event. This is described as an "abreaction" or re-experiencing the memory with a high level of disturbance as indicated by a SUD of 5 or higher. The target may also link to dissociated information that is connected to the traumatic memory, but outside of the patient's conscious awareness. As Shapiro (2018) said, "There is no way to predict exactly how a client will process a particular event" (p. 86). Part of informed consent with EMDR is alerting patients about the possible abreactions, the unpredictability and intensity of this type of psychotherapy.

In Phases 2 and 3, the clinician sets the stage for reprocessing.

> Client preparation involves establishing a safe therapeutic relationship, explaining in detail the process and its effects, and addressing the client's concerns and potential emotional needs. Assessment determines the components of a target memory and baseline measures of the client's reactions to the process.
>
> (Shapiro, 2018, p. 113)

EMDR therapists employ different strategies during the preparation phase, but resource development or ego strengthening is an important step. This includes the establishment of a peaceful place and positive attachment figures, both of which serve to assist with trauma reprocessing, especially when it is "stuck," and with emotional regulation that may be necessary between sessions. Another key part of the process is the identification of potential targets for reprocessing utilizing the three-pronged approach. Clinicians look for dysfunctional stored information as evidenced by high emotional activation, avoidance, and negative beliefs about oneself. They draw parallels between the past, the present, and the future in order to find the locus of the disturbance. The three-pronged approach helps guide the overall treatment plan of the client and consists of "(1) the past experiences that have set the foundation for the pathology, (2) the present situations or triggers that currently stimulate the disturbance, and (3) the positive templates necessary for appropriate future action" (Shapiro, 2018, p. 71).

As in most psychotherapy modalities, the EMDR therapist needs to form a strong thera-peutic alliance in which she guides the process. Given the common characteristic of help-lessness among people who have experienced trauma, EMDR is meant to empower the client in their own healing process. One way the EMDR therapist demonstrates this form of client-centeredness is by letting the client choose which form of bilateral stimulation to use – the classic eye movements following a therapist's hand, a lightbox, tactile stimulation either self-tapping or with pulsers, or auditory stimulation. Shapiro (2018) recommends developing a safe/calm place and adding slow, short sets of bilateral stimulation that pro-vides a place to return to when the reprocessing is too intense or the client needs a break.

In Phase 3, the client "determines the components of the target memory and establishes baseline measures for the client's reactions" (Shapiro, 2018, p. 124). The clinician does not need to know all the details of the trauma, but rather the way the client is experienc-ing the trauma in the present. In the standard protocol, the target consists of: 1) An image of the worst part of the memory; 2) The negative self-cognition as it relates to the event, for example, "I am a loser," "I am powerless"; 3) The positive cognition that the client would like to believe about themselves, such as, "I did the best I could," and how true it feels using the VOC scale before the reprocessing of it; 4) The emotion that goes with the memory as felt in the present when paired with the negative cognition; 5) The disturbance level of the overall target using the SUD scale of that emotion in the present; and 6) The physical sensations accompanying it.

The reprocessing of the traumatic memory occurs in Phases 4–7. Phase 4 is the desen-sitization phase which, ideally, removes the disturbing aspect of the target memory and brings it to an SUD of zero. Since there are associative channels for each target/node, new images, sounds, sensations, emotions, tastes, or smells may emerge in successive sets of bilateral stimulation. If change is happening, the therapist continues.

> Clinicians can assume a channel has been cleared out when the client has become progressively less disturbed, when the associations appear to have reached a reason-able stopping point, and when nothing new or significant emerges after two sets of eye movements.
>
> (Shapiro, 2018, p. 150)

Once the SUD reaches zero, the target is considered desensitized, and Phase 5, the instal-lation phase, begins. Here the therapist asks if the positive cognition that was developed before reprocessing still feels appropriate, or if there is another statement that feels truer. The client is asked to bring up the original image with the positive cognition, which is then strengthened or "installed" with another round of bilateral stimulation. Phase 6 is the body scan, which checks for any remaining physical "residue" of the trauma. "The importance of the body scan in complete reprocessing of the targeted event and associated material cannot be overemphasized" (Shapiro, 2018, p. 184). When the client can hold the event and the positive cognition in their mind with no physical disturbance, this phase is considered complete. Phase 7 involves closure. Shapiro (2018) recommends 90 minutes for an EMDR therapy session to ensure that the clinician has time to prevent the client from leaving in an abreactive state when the reprocessing is over. The opening of a new mem-ory channel toward the end of a session is also discouraged. The Safe/Calm place can be used to bring the client out of the target memory. If reprocessing is incomplete, the target is reassessed at the next session.

Phase 8, the reevaluation phase, is characterized by the three-pronged review of past, current, and future issues to create a road map for further EMDR treatment. This phase consists of "… targeting past and current issues, and preparing the client for alternative, more adaptive ways of dealing with whatever future issues may arise both personally and relationally" (Shapiro, 2018, p. 191). In focusing on past events, the goal is to clear out the dysfunctional material so the client can live fully in the present. Focusing on present triggers targets current life conditions that have a negative impact on the client. Both the past and present are sources of targets for reprocessing. Adaptive future functioning is important in helping the client make different choices going forward. "This is done by identifying and processing anticipatory fears, as well as targeting a positive "future template" that incorporates behaviors appropriate for the future" (Shapiro, 2018, p. 203). An extension of the installation phase, it helps the client integrate the positive cognition and envision how this thought could impact future relationships and life challenges. For example, with a target of performance anxiety at work, once the past event or "feeder memory" is reprocessed, the client is asked to imagine how giving a presentation will be different.

UTILIZATION OF THE MODALITY FOR THE TREATMENT OF TRAUMA

Trauma is generally characterized as an event that feels or is perceived as life threatening and makes one feel helpless. It can be a single incident like a rape, a physical fight, or natural disaster or it can be multiple, repeated incidents over time such as physical or sexual abuse by a family member, childhood neglect, genocide campaigns, or a tour of duty in a war zone. Post-Ttraumatic stress disorder (PTSD) is one of the most common psychological conditions and affects nearly 4% of the world's population (Koenen et al., 2017, p. 2260). Given ongoing wars and conflicts, climate unpredictability, and poverty in so much of the world, trauma is an ongoing part of many people's lives. When a person experiences a single incident of trauma, the risk of developing PTSD is between 9–14% (Nijdam et al., 2012, p. 224). Patients who come for EMDR treatment rarely have one incident of trauma. Resick (2012) states that in relation to trauma exposure, "complexity is the norm, not the exception" (p. 242). In the National Comorbidity Study (Kessler, Sonnega, Bromet, Hughes, & Nelson, 1995), 61% of males and 51% of females have been exposed to one trauma and 20% of males and 11% of females were exposed to three or more traumatic events (Resick et al., 2012, p. 242).

Although complex post-traumatic stress disorder (C-PTSD) was first proposed by Herman (1992) to describe the symptoms following trauma that is repeated, prolonged, and inescapable as a trauma of "captivity," it is still not included in the DSM-5-TR. According to the ICD-11 criteria for C-PTSD, patients not only have the three symptoms of PTSD (re-experiencing, avoidance, and hyperarousal), but also disturbances in self-organization

(DSO), which include difficulties regulating their emotions (excessive reactivity, anger outbursts, feeling disassociated), a negative concept of their self (worthless, low self-esteem, persistent feelings of shame and guilt), and ongoing, persistent difficulties in relationships (WHO, 2018).

EMDR is widely accepted as a PTSD treatment method in all national and international guidelines, including those of the World Health Organization (2013) and the International Society of Traumatic Stress Studies (ISTSS Guidelines Committee, 2018). An important question is whether the standard protocol developed by Shapiro is as effective with complex PTSD. De Jongh and Hafkemeijer (2023) states that "case conceptualization and treatment planning for people with C-PTSD do not need to differ much from the procedure used to treat PTSD" (p. 3). There is still debate among EMDR specialists about the amount of preparation time needed for complex PTSD symptoms – extensive preparation can feel like avoidance, which is a trauma symptom, but strong abreactions to reprocessing the emotion fully can lead to early termination of treatment.

RESEARCH EVIDENCE REGARDING EMDR THERAPY

Since the founding of EMDR therapy, "Currently, there are more than 30 randomized controlled trials (RCT) demonstrating the effectiveness in patients with this debilitating mental health condition, thus providing a robust evidence base for EMDR therapy as a first-choice treatment for PTSD" (De Jongh et al., 2019, p. 261). These studies show significant decreases in PTSD symptoms with symptom reductions ranging from 36% (Devilly & Spence, 1999) to 94–95% (Capezzani et al., 2013; Nijdam et al., 2012). EMDR is also being explored as a treatment for severe psychiatric disorders in which psychosis co-occurs with PTSD (Van den Berg et al., 2015). More research studies need to be conducted into the efficacy of EMDR to treat comorbidity of PTSD with severe psychiatric disorders and with the new ICD-11 diagnosis of complex PTSD. In addition, high-quality randomized controlled trials measuring the efficacy of EMDR in patients with PTSD are needed to ensure that EMDR remains a "first-line therapy for PTSD" (De Jongh et al., 2019, p. 267).

In 2013, the World Health Organization (WHO) recommended both EMDR and trauma-focused CBT as first-line treatments for PTSD. In 2018, the International Society of Traumatic Stress Studies (ISTSS) recommended EMDR along with variants of CBT therapy, particularly prolonged exposure, as treatments for PTSD in adults and children. However, in 2017, the American Psychological Association (APA) gave EMDR a "suggested" rating, but not the "recommended" rating given to CBT. Furthermore, the National Institute for Health Care and Care Excellence (NICE, 2018) recommended EMDR for youth only if they did not respond to trauma-focused CBT and for adults with noncombat-related trauma. However, EMDR and CBT variants continue to be the two dominant modalities included in the international guidelines for the treatment of PTSD.

CASE EXAMPLE TREATING TRAUMA WITH EMDR

Deborah, a high-functioning, overachieving cisgendered, heterosexual, Caucasian, 39-year-old woman, has sexual difficulties and periods of disassociation and low self-esteem. She is highly intelligent and a corporate lawyer in a large metropolitan area. She is wiry, athletic, and experiences difficulties resting, sleeping, and slowing down. She has a mild eating disorder where she binges, then restricts. Deborah is in a long-term relationship, but often thinks about ending it. She reports struggling with sexual intimacy, sharing that she is either highly sexually active or shut down, and sometimes uses alcohol to be able to have sexual intercourse. She remembers being sexually abused by her coach in adolescence. She has cheated on her current partner and reports having guilty feelings about that. Her treatment goals include wanting to feel more connected to her body, her emotions, and her partner.

Following the three-pronged assessment, in the present, her workplace is causing her the most anxiety. She also struggles with disassociation in her long-term relationship and feels a lack of safety in her body even when there is no present danger. In her past, the coach sexually abused her during middle school after which her severe disassociation and anxiety began. However, she states that the anxiety might have had its origins earlier in childhood, despite the lack of clear memories of an earlier trauma. Deborah wants to begin by working on her work stressors, then move on to the sexual abuse with the coach.

During the preparation and resource development phase, disassociation was clearly present. Deborah had racing thoughts and difficulties reporting physical sensations in her body. In addition, during the installation of her attachment figures, she was unable to imagine being inside her own body and had a bird's eye view of the peaceful place she chose (a quiet beach), rather than seeing it through her own eyes. When the EMDR therapist added her previous therapist and her nanny to the peaceful place, Deborah was able to feel the warm sand of the beach between her toes. The therapist began with working on smaller present-day targets and was able to help Deborah prepare for an upcoming presentation by helping her feel the anxiety in her body associated with the negative cognition "I'm not good enough." Deborah was pleased and felt empowered by the experience.

In the next session, she reported being triggered during a disagreement with her partner. When he raised his voice at her, she shut down and disassociated rather than speaking up. She felt disconnected from him and wondered about the future of the relationship. Deborah felt embarrassed about shutting down. Jim Knipe (2019), a seasoned EMDR therapist, has developed a way to target shame by asking the question, "What is the good thing about not …?" In this case, the therapist asked, "What is the good thing about not arguing with your husband?" She listed many reasons about avoiding conflict, keeping the peace, and not wasting time on this when she has a lot of work to do. The shame dissipated and then she felt fear. The therapist set up the target of her husband raising his voice, the fear in her stomach, and the negative belief, "I am powerless." Deborah said this was an old familiar feeling, so the therapist bridged back to an earlier memory of her swim coach yelling at her as she stood with her teammates unable to speak. She processed her fear of "getting into trouble," then she "looped" in her anger – the processing was stuck. The therapist used an imaginative interweave, in which her nanny was standing next her for support and gave her a baseball bat. She imagined smashing the coach's car and telling him to stop yelling at her. After processing her anger, she felt exhausted and imagined a close-up image of the coaches' forearm that was stuck in her head since she was a young teenager, a trailhead target for the next session.

Deborah was nervous about the forearm target, not knowing what it contained. It was a highly charged memory fragment but was missing the context of the incident. The therapist did a couple of short sets of bilateral stimulation to desensitize the target because it was accompanied by extreme tightness in her chest and thinking about it made it difficult for her to breathe. Once the physical sensation subsided, she felt tremendous fear. With her nanny brought in as a resource, she was able to feel this fear and felt ready to process the forearm target, using the image of the forearm, the sensation of anxiety in her chest, and her negative cognition, "I'm dirty." It brought her back to a memory beginning with massaging the coach's forearm in a hotel room and ended with her performing oral sex on him. First, she felt the shame, then processed the disgust, anger, and sadness. Employing another imaginative interweave, her current partner helped rescue her teenage self to get her out of the hotel room. The negative emotional "charge," SUD, or disturbance level, decreased to a 3, but wasn't totally gone. The therapist did a body scan that found that she felt nausea in her stomach. After a couple more sets, the nausea went away. The therapist returned to the original forearm target and installed her new positive cognition, "I was just a child. He's the disgusting one." Deborah was exhausted but had a SUD of 0 by the end of the session.

In the next session, Deborah reported feeling more physically and emotionally connected with her partner. She had spoken to him about the last session and, while difficult, she found that her shame about the sexual abuse had decreased dramatically. She was physically more relaxed in the session, saying that talking to her partner about the sexual abuse had made her trust him more and feel more connected to him, which surprised her. The work on her complex PTSD therefore occurred both in the EMDR session and with her partner outside the sessions. The therapist suggested that she attend a group for survivors of childhood sexual abuse, knowing how telling one's story to others who have gone through similar traumas can be helpful. Deborah said that she would consider that and given the improvement in her relationship would like to take a break from treatment and come back if necessary to work on additional targets.

STRENGTHS AND LIMITATIONS OF EMDR AS A TREATMENT FOR TRAUMA

EMDR has demonstrated effectiveness as a first-line treatment for PTSD, is multidisciplinary, and it integrates and continues to evolve by including elements of CBT, somatic therapies, relational psychotherapies, and scientific advances in neuroscience. According to the AIP model, healing in EMDR originates in the patient with the therapist facilitating and accelerating the healing process. Unlike traditional talk therapy, the therapist is not the locus of knowledge. The answers come from within the patient as the EMDR therapist uses the AIP model to access and reprocess the trauma, bringing the patient's system back into emotional regulation and homeostasis in the present. EMDR is client-centered and relies on a strong therapeutic alliance, which helps the patient tolerate potential abreactions. It builds resilience and confidence in a client, enabling the confrontation of PTSD symptoms, so he or she can live life in a body that is calm, in the present, and no longer haunted by dangers from the past.

EMDR also has limitations. If a patient cannot stay in the window of affect tolerance or completely dissociates, EMDR may not be suitable. More severe forms of trauma lead to dissociation, even dissociative identity disorder and/or an inability to recall memories. In these more extreme cases, somatic experiencing or dialectical behavioral therapy may help build the capacity for the body to tolerate highly charged emotions and recall the traumatic memories. For certain clients, the high level of activation is not tolerable, and they discontinue treatment abruptly. For other clients, the avoidance symptoms are so intense that they cannot begin treatment or also terminate treatment early.

In addition, the new ICD-11 diagnosis of complex PTSD presents a new set of challenges and complexity for EMDR. Prolonged trauma exposure in childhood has a developmental component where the same trauma can have a different effect at different ages. In these cases, internal family systems may be a more suitable treatment modality with its emphasis on a person's "parts" at different developmental stages. Early childhood defenses help a patient survive, but keep them isolated and alone in adulthood. Due to the lack of trust in others, clients can struggle to be vulnerable with a therapist or to do an intensive treatment like EMDR, when they have no social supports. When people have poor affect regulation, their ability to tolerate an intensive treatment like EMDR is low. Some studies have shown Chen et al., 2015)) that EMDR was more effective when delivered by more experienced therapists, so more inexperienced therapists may not be able to tackle these challenges. Complex PTSD requires a multilayered approach, which is why many current EMDR practitioners employ complementary techniques to assist, complement, modify, or add to the three-pronged, eight-phase standard protocol to meet these challenges.

CONCLUSION

EMDR has evolved from Shapiro's walk in the park into a cutting-edge trauma treatment through a spirit of innovation, curiosity, and caring about a world where trauma is a daily ongoing reality for many. Shapiro built a flexibility into the treatment so that EMDR can continue to evolve to meet the ever-changing and growing complexity of our 21st-century world and can include the latest research so EMDR therapists can play their part in reducing the suffering in our world.

RESOURCES FOR LEARNING

https://www.emdr.com/francine-shapiro-library/
https://emdrfoundation.org/emdr-info/for-professionals/
https://www.emdrhap.org/
https://www.nyctrn.org/
https://www.emdria.org/find-an-emdr-therapist/
https://emdrfoundation.org/toolkit/rtep-manual.pdf
https://emdrfoundation.org/toolkit/gtep.pdf
https://parnellemdr.com/
https://flashtechnique.com/wp/
https://brainspotting.com/
https://emdradvancedtrainings.com/product/simplifying-complex-ptsd-new-
    treatmenapproaches-and-emdr-2-0-an-enhanced-version-of-emdr-therapy-day-2-de-
    jongh-and-matthijssen/

REFERENCES

American Psychiatric Association. (1980). *Diagnostic and Statistical Manual of Mental* .

Bower, G.H. (1981). Mood and memory. *American Psychologist*, 36, 129–148.

Capezzani, L., Ostacoli, L., Cavallo, M., Carletto, S., Fernandez, I., Solomon, R., & Can-
    telmi, T. (2013). EMDR and cbt for cancer patients: Comparative study of effects on
    ptsd, anxiety, and depression. *Journal of EMDR Practice and Research*, 7(3), 134–143.

Chen, L., Zhang, G., Hu, M., & Liang, X. (2015) Eye movement desensitization and repro-
    cessingversus cognitive-behavioral therapy for adult posttraumatic stress disorder:
    Systematic review and meta-analysis. *The Journal of Nervous and Mental Disease*,
    203(6): 443–451.

De Jongh, A., Amann, B.L., Hofmann, A., Farrell, D., & Lee, C.W. (2019). The status of
    EMDR therapy in the treatment of posttraumatic stress disorder 30 years after its
    introduction. *Journal of EMDR Practice and Research*, 13(4), 261–269.

De Jongh, A., & Hafkemeijer, L.C.S. (2023). Trauma-focused treatment of a client with
    Complex PTSD and comorbid pathology using EMDR therapy. *Journal of Clinical
    Psychology*, 80, 1–12.

Devilly, G.J., & Spence, S.H. (1999). The relative efficacy and treatment distress of EMDR
    and a cognitive-behavior trauma treatment protocol in the amelioration of posttrau-
    matic stress disorder, *Journal of Anxiety Disorders*, 13 (1–2), 131–157.

Freud, S. (1955). Introduction to psychoanalysis and the war neuroses. In J. Strachey (Ed.,
    & Trans.), *The standard edition of the complete psychological works of Sigmund
    Freud* (Vol. 17). London: Hogarth Press. (Original work published 1919).

Griffin, G.D., Charron, D., & Al-Daccak, R. (2014). Post-traumatic stress disorder revisiting
    adrenergic, glucocorticoids, immune system effects and homeostasis. *Clinical and
    Translational Immunology*, 3(11), e27.

Herman, J. (1992) Complex PTSD: a syndrome in survivors of prolonged and repeated
    trauma. *Journal of Traumatic Stress 5*, 377–391.

ISTSS Guidelines Committee. (2018). Posttraumatic stress disorder prevention and treatment guidelines methodology and recommendations. http://www.istss.org/treating-trauma/new-istss-prevention-and-treatment-guidelines.aspx

Kessler, R.C., Sonnega, A., Bromet, E., Hughes, M., & Nelson, C.B. (1995). *Postraumatic stress disorder in the National Comorbidity Survey. Archives of General Psychiatry*, *52*, 1048–1106.

Knipe, J. (2019). *EMDR Toolbox* (2nd ed.). Springer Publishing Company.

Koenen, K., Ratanatharathorn, A., Ng, L., McLaughlin, K., Bromet, E., Stein, D., … Kessler, R. (2017). Posttraumatic stress disorder in the World Mental Health Surveys. *Psychological Medicine*, *47*(13), 2260–2274.

Laliotis, D., Luber, M., Oren, U., Shapiro, E., Ichii, M., Hase, M., La Rosa, L., Alter-Reid, K., & Jammes, J.T.S. (2021). What is EMDR therapy? Past, present, and future directions. *Journal of EMDR Practice & Research*, *15* (4), 186–201.

Lang, P.J. (1979) A bioinformational theory of emotional imagery. *Psychophysiology*, 16, 495–512.

National Institute for Health and Care Excellence (NICE). (2018). Post-traumatic stress disorder. NG116. 2018. https://www.nice.org.uk/guidance/ng116

Nijdam, M., Gersons, B., Reitsma, J., De Jongh, A., & Olff, M. (2012). Brief eclectic psychotherapy v. eye movement desensitisation and reprocessing therapy for post-traumatic stress disorder: Randomised controlled trial. *The British Journal of Psychiatry*, *200*(3), 224–231.

Parnell, L. (2013). *Attachment-focused EMDR: Healing relational trauma.* WW Norton & Company.

Pavlov, I.P. (1927). *Conditioned reflexes: An investigation of the physiological activity of the cerebral cortex.* Oxford University Press.

Resick, P.A., Bovin, M.J., Calloway, A.L., Dick, A.M., King, M.W., Mitchell, K. S., … & Wolf, E. J. (2012). A critical evaluation of the complex PTSD literature: Implications for DSM-5. *Journal of Traumatic Stress*, *25*(3), 241–251.

Rodrigues, S.M., LeDoux, J.E., & Sapolsky, R.M. (2009). The influence of stress hormones on fear circuitry. *Annual Review of Neuroscience*, 32, 289–313.

Shapiro, F. (1989). *Efficacy of the eye movement desensitization procedure in the treatment of traumatic memories. Journal of EMDR Practice and Research*, 9, 17–27.

Shapiro, F. (1991). Eye movement desensitization and reprocessing procedure: From EMD to EMDR: A new treatment model for anxiety and related traumata. *The Behavior Therapist*, *14*, 133–135.

Shapiro, F. (1995). *Eye movement desensitization and reprocessing: Basic principles, protocols and procedures.* Guilford Press.

Shapiro, F. (2001). The challenges of treatment evolution and integration. *American Journal of Clinical Hypnosis*, 43, 183–186.

Shapiro, F. (2018). *Eye movement desensitization and reprocessing (EMDR) therapy: Basic principles, protocols, and procedures* (3rd ed.). The Guilford Press).

van den Berg, D.P., de Bont, P.A., van der Vleugel, B.M., de Roos, C., de Jongh, A., Van Minnen, A., & van der Gaag, M. (2015). Prolonged exposure vs eye movement desensitization and reprocessing vs waiting list for posttraumatic stress disorder in patients with a psychotic disorder: A randomized clinical trial. *JAMA Psychiatry*, *72*(3), 259–267.

Weiss, S.J. (2007). Neurobiological alterations associated with traumatic stress. *Perspectives in Psychiatric Care*, 43(3), 114–122.

WHO (World Health Organization). (2013). Guidelines for the management of conditions that are specifically related to stress. Retrieved from https://iris.who.int/bitstream/handle/10665/85119/9789241505406_eng.pdf

CHAPTER 11
SENSORIMOTOR PSYCHOTHERAPY
A Body-Centered Approach for the Treatment of Trauma

Amy Gladstone

INTRODUCTION

This chapter provides an overview of sensorimotor psychotherapy, a method for treating trauma that addresses both the physiological and psychological impact of traumatic experience. Advances in neurobiology have revealed the impact of trauma on the nervous system, underscoring the importance of incorporating the body in therapeutic interventions. In essence, regulating the nervous system is crucial for cultivating a life free of trauma triggers and painful relational patterns. This approach places significant emphasis on the somatic dimension, recognizing its vital role in accessing memories encoded as sensory fragments or enduring physical patterns, often emerging as responses to traumatic events and attachment experiences. By discerning these embodied expressions, therapeutic interventions can be thoughtfully devised to foster the emergence of new adaptive behaviors, emotions, and cognitions. These transformations in a client's bodily responses not only enhance affect regulation but also facilitate the integration of past experiences, thereby diminishing the negative impact of trauma and problematic attachment patterns on present-day realities. This chapter includes a discussion of the history of sensorimotor psychotherapy, key clinical concepts, an explanation of the therapeutic process, and a case example.

BRIEF HISTORY

In the 1970s, Pat Ogden, the founder of sensorimotor psychotherapy, was mentored by Ron Kurtz in an experiential method of psychotherapy called the Hakomi method. In 1981, Ogden developed a Hakomi offshoot, Hakomi bodywork. Subsequently, the method's name changed, first, to Hakomi integrative somatics and finally, in 2002, to sensorimotor psychotherapy (SP). These name changes reflected Ogden's evolving vision, wherein the body was seen not merely as an expression of psychological issues, but as a means of transformation in its own right.

The establishment of SP coincided with developments in traumatology and attachment theory. This allowed for the refinement of therapeutic techniques that integrated advances in neurobiology, while preserving the original humanistic principles. Currently, SP can be

DOI: 10.4324/9781003455851-11

described as a somatic talking therapy – a method that combines sensorimotor processing with emotional and cognitive processing.

DEFINITION OF TRAUMA

Ogden and Fisher (2015) describe trauma as "any threatening, overwhelming experiences that we cannot integrate" (p. 66). Trauma can manifest as a single event, such as a car accident, or a chronic occurrence, like homelessness. It may involve other people as perpetrators, such as in cases of sexual assault, or be attributable to natural or political forces, such as earthquakes or wars. Trauma occurs when events are perceived as threatening and trigger instinctive, somatically based defenses unmediated by cortical processes. This definition of trauma suggests that regulating the nervous system is crucial in trauma treatment, regardless of the specific precipitating event or circumstances.

Early trauma experienced within caregiving relationships has profound developmental implications. Traumatic attachment experiences involve overwhelming affect that surpasses the child's developmental capacity for integration, potentially laying the neurobiological groundwork for chronic dysregulation and dissociation. According to Allan Schore (2003), in cases of structured insecure attachment, biases in the autonomic nervous system develop to manage dysregulating patterns of interaction with caregivers.

In SP, healing involves expanding clients' capacity to manage dysregulated arousal and developing flexible and integrated responses to trauma triggers and maladaptive attachment patterns, regardless of the type or origin of the trauma.

FUNDAMENTAL CLINICAL CONCEPTS

SP is characterized by a foundational belief in the body's innate wisdom and its organic drive toward health and healing within a facilitative environment. The following are four of the clinical concepts that guide the SP method.

THE LANGUAGE OF THE BODY

Everyone's story and history are told by wise bodies – bodies that freeze amidst overwhelming fear, stiffen at unrecognizable sounds, and retract from disapproving facial expressions. These bodily responses reflect learned patterns, ingrained through lived experience and shaped by past traumas. While traditional therapy primarily relies on clients' spoken narrative to inform clinical practice, autobiographical memory and verbal expression have inherent limitations. Unlike declarative memories, trauma memories are often stored in a nonverbal, sensory, or emotional form, making them inaccessible through conscious recollection or explicit awareness.

In SP, we recognize that clients' bodies convey implicit stories of their past through procedural somatic and affective patterns. Attachment styles are often expressed through bodily expressions; for instance, clients with dismissive attachment may lean away or restrict hand movements, while those with preoccupied attachment may lean forward and gesticulate broadly. These bodily actions communicate aspects of childhood trauma that may not be readily recalled or expressed verbally.

Understanding the language of the body is crucial for healing in SP. We invite clients to notice their bodies' flow of experience, including breathing patterns, muscle constriction, or subtle movements. As our clients describe their moment-to-moment internal somatic experience, and we observe their body communications, we utilize these present-moment expressions of their traumatic history to facilitate the transformation of deep-seated patterns.

MINDFULNESS OF THE PRESENT MOMENT

While mindfulness is a widely used technique in psychotherapy, in SP it serves a distinct function: Directing the clients' attention to elements of internal experience as related to moment-to-moment flow; Ogden (2021) refers to this as embedded relational mindfulness. SP practitioners utilize mindfulness to track the implicit manifestations of trauma, including physiological responses (such as increased heart rate or sweating), somatic sensations (such as tingling or tension), emotional reactions (such as fear or anxiety), and thought patterns (such as self-blame or learned helplessness).

In SP, the elements we ask clients to observe are called the five building blocks of experience: (a) body sensation, (b) movement, (c) sense perception, (d) emotions, and (e) cognition. Body sensation refers to the physical feelings that result from shifts in electrical, chemical, and muscular activity. Movement refers to the actions our bodies take automatically in the service of activity or preparation for activity. Sense perception encompasses sensory experiences of sight, sound, touch, taste, and smell, while emotions include feelings and nuanced aspects of emotional tone and mood. The last building block, cognition, is particularly relevant for the interpretations and meanings clients attribute to themselves and the events in their lives.

Mindful awareness of these building blocks serves as the foundation for discovering new response patterns. For example, a sexual assault survivor might exhibit a freeze response characterized by electric sensations throughout her body, constricted movement in her arms and legs, a narrowing of her visual field, feelings of fear and foreboding, and the thought, "I'm not safe." By guiding the client's attention to these distinct elements of experience, we can work to manage her internal activation and shift her awareness to the safety of the present moment.

WINDOW OF TOLERANCE AS AN ASSESSMENT TOOL

Conceived by Siegel (1999), the window of tolerance represents an optimal zone of activation in where "various intensities of emotional and physiological arousal can be processed without disrupting the functioning of the system" (p. 253). Within this zone, arousal is appropriately modulated to meet the demands of the moment, whether internal or environmental, enabling us to think, speak, remember, sleep, experience our emotions, and engage with our surroundings as needed. Regulation is facilitated by maintaining a manageable level of autonomic arousal in our bodies – not too high nor too low to assimilate new information – thus ensuring a state of equilibrium.

Hill (2017) wrote, "When affect is regulated the bodymind is integrated. When affect is dysregulated, the bodymind is dissociated" (p.40). In traumatized dissociative states, autonomic arousal exceeds the window of tolerance, hindering clients' ability to manage their emotions and reactions effectively. When triggered, the perception of danger and life threat evokes either hyperarousal (i.e., panic, rage) or hypoarousal (i.e., immobilization, numbness) – too much or too little arousal to process effectively. As a result of past experiences and/or sensitivities in the nervous system, trauma survivors often develop a pervasive perception of danger, frequently resulting in enduring states of hyperarousal, hypoarousal, or cycling between these extremes.

In SP, therapists discern where clients are in their window of tolerance through tracking (Ogden, 2021), observing subtle signs of shifts such as widened eyes or sudden changes in posture. For instance, Suzy described discomfort at being approached in a bar; her voice grew louder and higher, and her prosody faster as her arousal escalated. Conversely, Ralph, exhibited signs of hypoarousal, bowing his head and trailing off as he described his apprehension about confronting his ex-wife.

The window of tolerance serves as a foundational framework for understanding and addressing clients' affective states during therapy sessions in SP. Therapists carefully assess where clients are within this window through tracking and adapt their interventions accordingly. For instance, if clients exhibit hyperarousal or hypoarousal, therapists prioritize regulation to bring them back into their window of tolerance. In contrast, when clients are within this optimal range, it allows for the exploration and processing of challenging or compartmentalized material.

TOP OF FORM

THREE-PHASE MODEL OF TRAUMA RESOLUTION

Traumatized clients frequently begin therapy in extreme distress marked by feelings of rage, panic, hopelessness, or despair. They often perceive threat in ordinary daily life occurrences, such as the sound of a car door slamming, or a friend's expression of surprise. They may even find themselves frightened by their own spontaneous thoughts or unexpected bodily sensations. Developing and expanding the capacity to regulate affective responses to both external and internal stimuli is a cornerstone of successful therapy. As Schore (2012) wrote,

> Effective work at the regulatory boundaries of right brain low and high arousal states ultimately broadens the windows of affect tolerance, facilitating the acceptance of a wider variety of more intense and enduring emotions.
>
> (p. 104)

In pursuit of this goal, SP aims to gradually widen the window of tolerance for our clients, empowering them to navigate a broader spectrum of experiences. To accomplish this objective, we employ a three-phase model as a structured approach to expanding their window of tolerance. Phase-oriented treatment, a common approach for trauma treatment, originated with 19th-century psychologist Pierre Janet (1898), whose groundbreaking work significantly advanced our understanding of trauma and dissociation.

In the initial phase, the focus is on managing trauma symptoms that directly impact clients' daily functioning and overall quality of life. This involves addressing dysregulated arousal and helping them cultivate mindfulness skills and resources for stabilization in the face of trauma triggers.

In the second phase of treatment, with increased capacity to manage traumatic reactivity, we address the habitual immobilizing impact of traumatic events – patterns of freeze, collapse, or numbing – by reinstating active defenses. Utilizing sensation and movement primarily, we work on traumatized body states to help clients achieve an embodied sense of agency and empowerment. Additionally, we work through traumatic memories and affect at the boundaries of the window of tolerance by managing overwhelming arousal as clients recall activating aspects of traumatic experiences.

In the third phase, with greater resourcefulness and reorganization of trauma patterns from the previous two phases, clients can address the developmental and relational deficits created by trauma and attachment experiences. We focus on "adaptive strategies" reflected in somatic patterns, habits of relating, affective expression, and core beliefs related to the self and the world. Clients often confront their difficulties with expansive feelings like joy or pride, or vulnerable feelings like love or dependency. A wider window of tolerance allows clients to process emotions without fragmentation, enabling experiential exploration of new relational patterns.

Of course, therapy is not a linear process, and how humans organize their experience is complex and fluid within a therapeutic hour and across time. Therefore, as SP therapists in collaboration with each client, we notice the activation in the nervous system and what needs processing – that is, implicit trauma-related memory or adaptive patterns or attachment styles – and then select the relevant maps and interventions from the corresponding phase of treatment.

THE SENSORIMOTOR PSYCHOTHERAPY THERAPY PROCESS

This section outlines the overall method for SP sessions, the clinical application of the three phases of treatment, along with case examples.

In practice, an SP session might begin like any other therapy session. Clients describe the week's events and related feelings, raise burning issues, react to previous sessions, or share concerns or dilemmas. As clients speak, SP clinicians engage in a process of attunement that includes both affective engagement and body reading. We look for implicit cues in the narrative, paying close attention to the body's communication and we verbalize our impressions to help clients recognize the language of their bodies. For example, we might say, "I notice your body pulls back as you tell me what your girlfriend said to you." In addition, we assess whether they are within their window of tolerance, indicating regulation, or outside of it, suggesting dysregulation. This assessment guides the direction and pace of the session.

After attuning to clients and assessing their arousal levels, we ask if they would like to work on a specific aspect of their experience. If consent is given, we help clients mindfully explore their experience vis-à-vis their narrative, asking about the different building blocks in relation to the specific focus we've established.

For instance, a client with a history of child abuse might initiate the session by recounting a recent argument with an overbearing boss. As she shares her experience, we might notice her face flush. Bringing this observation to her attention, we shift focus from a description of a troubling event in the past to present-moment reactions. She may describe the sensation of flushing as heat, prompting us ask if she would like to explore further the physical sensation in her face when recalling her boss' harsh tone of voice. We might then ask, "As you notice the heat in your face, is there something your body wants to do?" This question refers to the building block of movement. If the client responds, "I want to hang my head," we would then explore an additional building block such as emotion: "As you feel the heat in your face and the inclination to hang your head, is there an accompanying emotion?" A child abuse survivor is likely to associate this body state with feelings of shame, in which case our next question might target the building block, cognition: "As you sense the heat in your face, the inclination to hang your head, and feel a sense of shame, are there any thoughts that arise?" She might respond, "I'm bad if I ask for what I need." In this way, we flesh out a mind/body state that involves all the building blocks – sensation, movement, sense perception, emotions, and cognition – related to the clients' presenting narrative. At this point in the session, we introduce targeted interventions, known as experiments, that advance the session by fostering therapeutic shifts.

THE USE OF EXPERIMENTS

When considering therapeutic action, we identify interventions that effectively create change– an important tool in SP is the use of experiments. As Ogden (2006) noted, "An experiment is a trial of change: a change in words used, a change in posture, a movement or a stilling of movement, a change in orientation, a change in sensory modality" (p. 197). Experiments are designed to bring the client's attention to the present moment, fostering a heightened awareness of the building blocks of experience. They are introduced with the question, "What happens when …."

In a typical verbal experiment, the therapist may make a statement such as "What happens when you hear me say, your needs matter?" The use of the phrase, "What happens when," prompts the client to notice any changes experientially by directing their attention to any spontaneous reactions.

We utilize experiments to uncover procedural tendencies and facilitate their transformation by eliciting new experiences within a mindful state. Experiments often catalyze shifts in clients' perception of themselves, their environment, or their sense of safety. In the previous clinical example, we could conduct experiments related to the client's feelings of shame regarding her needs by studying her body's participation in this shame-based state and exploring whether adjusting her posture could promote acceptance of her needs. For instance, we might ask the client to assume the shame-based posture and then notice the effects of lifting her head and making eye contact. This experiment might reveal that assuming an upright posture and engaging in eye contact grounds the client in the present moment within the therapeutic relationship, in which the therapist's responsiveness to her needs could foster a new belief, such as "It's okay to ask for what I need."

This is one of many experiments we might conduct. Others could utilize trials of experience involving movement, words, or gestures. Additionally, we might conduct the experiment ourselves, such as reaching a hand out to the client or turning away. The possibilities for experiments are endless and arise based on what we are processing in any given session.

The structure of a typical SP session – attuning to clients, framing a focus, fleshing out the elements of experience and introducing experiments – applies to each of the three phases of treatment.

PHASE 1: DEVELOPING RESOURCES – OUTSIDE THE WINDOW OF TOLERANCE

In SP, the initial treatment goal is to help clients develop the capacity to self-regulate in response to trauma triggers. Resourcing is a primary method we employ to stabilize trauma symptoms, utilizing clients' capabilities, competencies, and skills to create a toolbox of techniques for managing triggers. Mindfulness serves as the foundation for increasing awareness of triggers, followed by collaborative exploration and embodiment of stabilization techniques. Examples of resources include placing a hand on the heart, visualizing a supportive relative, or assuming a grounding posture.

In sessions addressing dysregulation, we may invite clients to focus on developing and practicing a resource. If they agree, we study how their system is organized across the building blocks of experience in the triggered state. We then suggest experiments to discover what resources will promote increased regulation and integration. For example, we might ask a client about the effects of imagining a boundary around themselves. As we work with resources and clients perceive a shift – such as deeper breaths, relaxation in the facial muscles, or a heightened sense of aliveness in the chest – we invite them to "stay with" these shifts mindfully. Following any experiment, we ask clients to connect these shifts to additional building blocks of experience deepening the transformation and enabling clients to embody the resource fully. We can ask, "As you notice your breath deepen, is there an image, an emotion, or a sense of yourself that comes?"

An example of resource development in Phase I involves Cindy, who endured abuse and intimidation from an older brother. He would frequently take her to unfamiliar places, abandon her, and she would be left feeling lost and fearful as she tried to find her way home. For Cindy, encountering unfamiliar surroundings became a trauma trigger. Several months into therapy, she missed an appointment when construction workers temporarily removed a street sign at the corner, leaving her disoriented. Following this incident, we started to explore her tendency to dissociate in unfamiliar environments. Cindy learned to identify somatic markers of what she referred to as "spacing out," such as a fuzzy sensation in her head and altered sound perception. Together, we developed and practiced grounding techniques, which included focusing on feeling her feet, observing colors, and utilizing breathing patterns. Equipped with these tools, Cindy gained the ability to recognize her trigger, effectively utilize resources, and return to a state of regulation, empowering her to confidently navigate unfamiliar environments.

PHASE 2: ADDRESSING MEMORIES – AT THE EDGE OF THE WINDOW OF TOLERANCE

In SP, memory processing involves addressing dysregulated arousal and procedural action patterns organized around survival strategies. While narrative memory reports are often utilized to access implicit trauma memories, explicitly recounting the traumatic event may not be necessary, particularly benefitting clients who experienced dissociation during the trauma.

During this phase, we intentionally evoke traumatic responses for reprocessing. Clients who habitually enter a freeze-or-collapse response are given the opportunity to discover truncated impulses for mobilizing defensive actions and to complete them. This intervention is also applied to clients triggered into dysregulated mobilizing responses (e.g., fight, flight, cry for help). By mindfully completing these truncated mobilizing actions, clients' systems can re- organize, leading to a sense of satisfaction or even triumph.

In this phase, we also use *Sensorimotor Sequencing* (Ogden et al., 2006). This intervention involves clients tracking internal sensations of hyperarousal related to traumatic activation, such as tingling, shaking, or quivering, and allowing the natural flow of sensations, movements, and impulses to progress through the body until the activation dissipates.

By mindfully sequencing activation, allowing patterns to complete, and/or reinstating active mobilizing defenses, the system can integrate and reorganize. Through their recently discovered or rediscovered embodiment, clients find new ways of experiencing themselves and the world, as demonstrated by the following case.

Jane was haunted by memories of a sexual assault, as they pervaded her dream life and interfered with her concentration. During a session, as Jane recalled the sound of glass breaking and the sight of a strange man coming through her window, she felt panicky. I asked Jane if she could set aside the memory and simply experience the panic as a bodily sensation without the associated fear. Encouraging her to become mindful of any micro-movements in her body, she reported a sensation of trembling in her face and upper body. I urged Jane to stay with the trembling, observing its progression. Mindfully noting the escalation of trembling, she eventually felt it subside as warmth filled her face and chest. Using resources we had developed, Jane reminded herself that she is safe now, in the present. As she returned to her window of tolerance, she could feel her resilience and capacity.

In another session, we revisited the same memory. Instead of going into panic, Jane was able to track the sensations in her body, leading to an inclination to make a fist. Exploring the words accompanying this action, she expressed, "Get off." Experimenting with repetition of these words, Jane noticed a newfound belief about herself emerging from her embodied experience – that she was a strong person capable of defending herself.

As illustrated by this case example, the process of sequencing arousal and reinstating active defenses often releases clients from habituated disempowerment as they recognize their body's agency in the face of life-threatening situations.

PHASE 3: MOVING FORWARD – INSIDE THE WINDOW OF TOLERANCE

In Phase 3, our focus shifts to the processing of emotional pain and the meanings our clients ascribe to themselves and the world around them. The goal is to evoke compartmentalized emotions and self-perceptions. Through experiential present-moment experiments, we invite new somatic, affective, and cognitive experiences of self and others.

Before Phase 3, our approach predominantly centers on physical sensation and movement as we address dysregulation and immobilizing defenses. However, during Phase 3, while the body remains our starting point, we primarily direct our attention toward the emotional and cognitive elements of experience, related to developmental and attachment issues.

The following case example illustrates Phase 3 work addressing the core belief, "I am alone." During a session, Anita discussed an interaction with her boyfriend that left her feeling hurt. She recounted a conversation with him about a work event in which her boss criticized and devalued her. While Anita was sharing her painful feelings, her boyfriend received a text message and glanced at his phone.

I asked Anita to recall the moment he reached for his phone and describe her present moment experience. She reported feeling the urge to withdraw and turn her head to the side. I encouraged her to execute those movements slowly and to notice what words might express and represent those actions. Anita said, "I must pull away and not rely on you."

When asked about associated emotions she began to cry and expressed feeling sad and alone. Tearfully she revealed the belief, "I'm alone with my pain." I proposed an experiment in which I make a gesture: Reaching out to her by extending my hand. As I reached out, Anita exhaled and described a sensation of relaxation in her core, an inclination to reach back, and feelings of surprise and joy. In this state, she identified a different belief: "I can be sad, and people will care." Through such interventions, we can help clients process painful affect and support them in cultivating new beliefs about themselves and others derived from embodied experience.

What follows is a detailed case example illustrating a session from Phase 2, during which a client works with a trauma memory involving fear and humiliation.

CASE EXAMPLE OF THE TREATMENT OF TRAUMA

Having witnessed domestic violence as a child, Steven, a 42-year-old gay white man, struggled with pervasive anxiety. As a boy, he often intervened to protect his mother from the violence inflicted by his alcoholic father. As a result, he became the target of his father's rage, often enduring forceful shoves and cutting verbal taunts. When Steven was 19, his father slapped him across the face for defending his mother. In that moment, Steven froze, later overwhelmed by a profound sense of shame as he couldn't forgive himself for not fighting back.

In his late 20s, Steven's father passed away, and among all the abusive memories, this one haunted him the most – the recollection of being slapped by his father. During the 20th session of a year-and-a-half-long treatment, the therapist helped Steven process this distressing memory.

This session started with Steven letting the therapist know that the past weekend was the anniversary of his father's death. He said he had felt both anxious and numb all weekend. Steven added that he kept thinking about the incident when he was 19 and felt ashamed and anxious, but also frozen. His voice was shaky, and he clasped his hands together stiffly in his lap.

The following dialogue illustrates the progression from a freeze response to the mobilization of a defensive action. The interventions are aimed at (a) bringing Steven's awareness to the body reactivity triggered by recall of traumatic events; then (b) helping him maintain focus on body sensations until he might perceive an impulse toward mobilized action; then (c) mindfully executing the action; and (d) connecting verbal expression, emotion, and cognition with the somatic changes that result from the action. This dialogue takes place about 10 minutes into the session:

STEVEN:	I wish that I had fought back, but instead, I just froze.
THERAPIST:	Yeah, that is a painful memory for you.
STEVEN:	Yes, when it happened, I felt numb. My mother was on the sofa crying after he laid into her about a question she asked, calling her names like moron and idiot. I yelled, "Stop." I can remember the look on his face. It was pure hatred. It looked like he wanted to kill me. When he slapped me, he shouted, "How dare you," and said it over and over again. At first, the slap stung, but then I couldn't feel anything, like I had died, and I was just a stiff corpse (he lowers his head).
THERAPIST:	Like you had died already, and you went numb.
STEVEN:	Yes, like I didn't survive it. It was the worst feeling.
THERAPIST:	Sounds very distressing. What's it like inside as you talk about this?
STEVEN:	I feel it again. (His posture is upright and leaning forward; a stiffness takes over his body as he says this. His voice gets higher.)

THERAPIST:	Oh, you feel it again. Can we notice what happens in your body when you remember this?
STEVEN:	Yes, it's here, like all in my throat. I feel like I'm going to throw up.
THERAPIST:	It's intense, huh? Maybe we could work with the body experience you're having as you remember the incident. Your body doesn't know that you survived. Would that be okay?
STEVEN:	Yes, I would like to feel better about how I reacted.
THERAPIST:	You feel really bad about it right now. I wonder if you could drop the actual memory for a moment and focus on your body; what it's like inside of your throat?
STEVEN:	Yes, my throat is very uncomfortable. Like an explosion is going to happen.
THERAPIST:	It's a lot of sensation, huh? Can you stay with the experience in your throat? What tells you that it's like an explosion is going to happen?
STEVEN:	It feels like a lot of pressure and like a buzzing in my throat.
THERAPIST:	I know it's probably a bit uncomfortable, but can you stay with that sense of pressure and buzzing? And just notice it as sensation. Is it throughout your throat or more in the center of your throat?
STEVEN:	It's throughout my throat, but it's starting to move towards my face. I can feel my jaw starting to clench.
THERAPIST:	Stay with the sensation moving towards your face and with the jaw clenching. Sense into that clenching, Steven, and see: Is there any movement that wants to happen?
STEVEN:	I can feel myself wanting to grit my teeth and my eyes want to nar-row (Steven is starting to move his forearms a bit as they rest in his lap).
THERAPIST:	As you feel the impulse to grit your teeth and narrow your eyes, is there anything happening in any other part of your body?
STEVEN:	I can feel some tingling in my arms.
THERAPIST:	So, stay with that tingling in your arms. Is there any impulse to move?
STEVEN:	They want to come up.
THERAPIST:	Up, huh? So, stay with that impulse. Sense how they want to come up.
STEVEN:	Like I want to raise my forearms and flex my hands.
THERAPIST:	Stay with that impulse to raise your forearms and flex your hands. Let's try that slowly but letting your arms move as you feel the impulse from inside. (Steven slowly lifts his forearms from his lap so they are parallel to his sides, leaving his hands extended upwards and flexed in a "stop" gesture.)
THERAPIST:	And let's see from this place, is there a movement that wants to happen?
STEVEN:	Yeah, a shove. I can feel myself wanting to shove.
THERAPIST:	Can we try an experiment? Let's see what it would be like to use the wall and maybe try a few shoves against the wall. How does that sound? Shall I join you?

(Steven nods and goes over to the wall and pushes against the wall. I position myself a few feet away and push as well.)

THERAPIST: What's that like?

STEVEN: It feels really good. I feel really alive.

THERAPIST: What tells you that you feel alive?

STEVEN: There is an energy running through my whole body.

THERAPIST: Sense that energy running through your whole body. And as you feel your body executing the shove, are there words that come with that?

STEVEN: Yeah, the words are STOP.

THERAPIST: Can we see what happens when you say that? Should we say it together?

STEVEN: Sure. (At the count of three, Steven and I say the word STOP loudly and repeat it a few times.)

THERAPIST: How was that? What's happening inside now?

STEVEN: I feel grounded and calm. I can feel it in my feet. And I can feel it in my core, there is an energized calmness.

THERAPIST: So, feel into that energized calmness in your core, and if it had a message for you about yourself or the world, what is it telling you? And see if you can let it come from the energized calmness.

STEVEN: It says, "I can defend myself" and "I can live."

THERAPIST: Ah, you can defend yourself and you can live. And is there an emotion that goes with that?

STEVEN: Relief and hope. I can see that when my dad slapped me, I was like a deer in headlights and I couldn't move, just like the way that I felt over the weekend. But now I know that I can defend myself and I can live! (broad smile and eyes gleaming) I feel so strong and so alive.

REFLECTION ON THE SESSION

At the beginning of this session, the therapist tracked Steven's level of activation and noted his hyperaroused state. Directing his focus to the sensations in his throat, the therapist encouraged him to let go of the visual and narrative memories exacerbating his arousal. The objective was to lower his arousal to a managing level by homing in solely on the physical sensations.

Once Steven was more regulated, the therapist guided him in observing the flow of the sensations throughout his body while also tracking for any signs of mobilized activity, such as muscle constriction or small motor movements. With Steven's permission, the therapist joined him in both the shove and vocalization to alleviate any self-consciousness. Completing the truncated somatic response brought Steven relief and renewed hope and he expressed optimism as he left the session. As the therapist and Steven consistently worked through similar memories, he no longer grappled with pervasive anxiety as his feeling of empowerment steadily grew.

SP THROUGH AN ANTI-OPPRESSION LENS

In *Sensorimotor Psychotherapy in Context*, Ogden et al. (2021) explore the impact of culture, racism, and biases on clients' psyches and bodies. They suggest that oppression can lead to chronic hypoarousal or hyperarousal because historical trauma, institutionalized racism, and intersectional oppression are ongoing assaults on the nervous system.

Practicing SP in context requires therapists to recognize that our clients do not necessarily experience us as inherently safe or neutral. The personal histories of both the client and the therapist influence their moment-to-moment embodied experience. Complex intersections of different aspects of identity related to power, privilege, or disempowerment and oppression impact the therapy and the relationship between therapist and client. Ogden et al. (2021) urge practitioners to solicit honest feedback with sensitivity and frequency, as power dynamics based on social location can foster clients' too-ready agreement with interventions. Additionally, they caution practitioners about the impact of implicit bias and privilege on body reading – an essential technique in SP; for example, interpreting a client's rapid and spacious gesticulation as hyperarousal when it might, in fact, be culturally determined. To this point, Ogden et al. (2021) wrote:

> … the meaning we make from posture and movement is…a result of idiosyncratic and family influences embedded in a community specific culture. At the most fundamental level, what we feel, see, and recognize in others' nonverbal communication is filtered through what we have personally experienced…. Our sense of safety and familiarity affects the way we read other people's movements and somatic expressions which can lead to misinterpretation when working with people from diverse backgrounds and locations.
>
> (p. 32)

Ogden et al. point out that Black, Indigenous, and People of Color (BIPOC) may elicit fear, judgment, or disdain from white practitioners. They suggest that practitioners track their somatic responses to catch implicit bias and bodily manifestations of disowned negative emotions such as constriction, impulses to move away, and freeze responses. Ogden et al. are not calling for "perfect practice," but for therapeutic intervention "grounded in mindful awareness of the effects of many histories of privilege/oppression and resilience present in both the client and the therapist" (2021, p. 36).

EVIDENCE REGARDING EFFECTIVENESS IN TREATING TRAUMA

At present, SP lacks the research base to be regarded as an evidence-based treatment. Nevertheless, there are two published outcome studies of a time-limited group therapy approach grounded in SP principles. Langmuir et al. (2012) conducted a study on a group of 10 participants receiving weekly group therapy sessions to stabilize PTSD symptoms in an outpatient hospital program. The results indicated improvements in dissociative symptoms, internal awareness, and receptivity to soothing, both at the conclusion of the group therapy and during a follow-up assessment six months later. Similarly, Gene-Cos et al. (2016) implemented a 12-week structured group protocol with 20 subjects incorporating psychoeducation, body awareness, and strategies for managing autonomic arousal. Upon completion, participants reported decreases in depressive and PTSD symptoms as well as improvements in overall health and social and vocational capacities. It is important to note that both studies have limitations, including small sample sizes and the absence of a control or comparison group.

While SP interventions have been refined based on clinical experience and client feedback, additional formal studies are needed to provide scientific support for SP's effectiveness as a general method and specifically as a treatment for trauma.

STRENGTHS AND LIMITATIONS OF THE MODALITY AS A TREATMENT FOR TRAUMA

In light of advances in neuroscience, clinical theorists have advocated for experiential models of practice that target the right brain. However, until now, clinical techniques have lagged behind. Previous experiential models either lack safeguards against re-traumatization because they fail to address the physiological basis of trauma sequalae as distinct from emotional and psychological processes, or the opposite – they focus almost exclusively on traumatic expression in the body, overlooking the range of emotional and psychic experiences that our clients bring.

The strength of SP lies in its systematic experiential method, which addresses both traumatic activation and attachment wounding utilizing specific techniques for each. As such, SP can address the oscillation of affect that commonly occurs during therapy sessions. One of Ogden's most important contributions to psychotherapy is the recognition that regulated and dysregulated affect necessitate distinct interventions.

SP offers much to both clients and clinicians as a holistic model of psychotherapy. Some clients become frustrated with traditional psychotherapy methods that privilege insight and find that active engagement with present-moment somatic and emotional experiences deepens therapy and provides access to previously inaccessible material. The method's reliance on spontaneity not only enlivens the therapeutic process for clients but also for clinicians. It facilitates creativity and fosters deep connections with clients. Additionally, SP's systematic method of dealing with dysregulated arousal guards against vicarious traumatization, a possible byproduct of less gentle methods such as exposure therapy.

However, like all models of practice, SP has its limitations. New clinicians may find it challenging to remain attuned to their clients while implementing the method without proper training in broader psychotherapeutic processes. SP is not a manualized treatment, and its founder emphasizes the organic unfolding of techniques and interventions within the specific therapeutic dyad. Yet, without grounding in general psychotherapy principles, new clinicians might be tempted to privilege technique over attunement. While clinicians seek expedient ways to ease the suffering of their clients, it is essential to avoid the temptation to implement SP interventions prematurely or with too much personal investment in the outcome. This could lead to enactments in which the client feels pressured or compelled to please the therapist rather than respond authentically. This danger exists with all models of practice, not just SP, and underscores the necessity of ongoing supervision and consultation for therapists.

CONCLUSION

This chapter explored the multifaceted landscape of sensorimotor psychotherapy, highlighting its clinical technique and distinct contributions to trauma treatment. Through its systematic method of expanding the window of tolerance, emphasis on present-moment awareness, three-phase treatment model, and distinct interventions for trauma and attachment, SP advances our understanding of how therapy can improve affect regulation and facilitate the healing of trauma and attachment wounds. Central to this approach is a profound recognition of the body's role in reliving and processing past traumatic and attachment experiences. This recognition challenges the traditional focus solely on emotional and cognitive processes, contributing to a broader understanding of how the body can serve as a valuable resource in the therapeutic journey.

RESOURCES FOR LEARNING

BOOKS

Ogden, P., & Fisher, J. (2015). *Sensorimotor psychotherapy: Interventions for trauma and attachment.* W. W. Norton.

Ogden, P. (2021). *The pocket guide to sensorimotor psychotherapy in context.* W. W. Norton.

VIDEOS

Ogden, P. (n.d.). Introductions to sensorimotor psychotherapy [YouTube channel]. Retrieved February 17, 2024, from https://www.youtube.com/playlist?list=PLPu4s3_ihY_b6-uJWxh1Z3DYzn87t_cmX

Sensorimotor Psychotherapy Institute (n.d.). Sensorimotor psychotherapy [YouTube channel]. Retrieved February 17, 2024, from https://www.youtube.com/c/sensorimotorpsychotherapyinstitute

REFERENCES

Gene-Cos, N., Fisher, J., Ogden, P. & Cantrell, A. (2016). Sensorimotor group therapy in the context of complex PTSD. *Annals of psychiatry and mental health, 4*(6), 1080. https://doi.org/10.47739/2374-0124/1080

Hill, D. (2017). *Affect regulation theory. A clinical model*. New York: W.W. Norton.

Janet, P. (1898). *Nevroses et idees fixes*. Paris: Felix Alcan.

Langmuir, J., Kirsh, S., & Classen, C. (2012). A pilot study of group oriented group psychotherapy: Adapting sensorimotor psychotherapy for the group treatment of trauma. *Psychological Trauma: Theory, Research, Practice and Policy, 4*(2), 145–151. https://doi.org/10.1037/a0025588

Ogden, P. (2021). *The pocket guide to sensorimotor psychotherapy in context*. New York: W. W. Norton.

Ogden, P., & Fisher, J. (2015). *Sensorimotor psychotherapy: Interventions for trauma and attachment*. New York: W. W. Norton.

Ogden, P., Minton, K., & Pain, C. (2006). *Trauma and the body: A sensorimotor approach to psychotherapy*. New York: W. W. Norton.

Ogden, P., Taylor, S., Jorba, L., Rodriguez, R., & Choi, M. (2021). Sensorimotor psychotherapy in context: Sociocultural perspectives. In P. Ogden (Ed.), *The pocket guide to sensorimotor psychotherapy in context* (pp. 1–73). New York: W. W. Norton.

Schore, A. (2003). *Affect dysregulation and disorders of the self*. New York: W. W. Norton.

Schore, A. (2012). *The science and the art of psychotherapy*. New York: W.W. Norton.

Siegel, D. J. (1999). *The developing mind: How relationships and the brain interact to shape who we are*. New York: Guilford Press.

12

CHAPTER 12
USING INTERNAL FAMILY SYSTEMS IN THE TREATMENT OF TRAUMA

Lia Avellino and Benjamin Seaman

INTRODUCTION

Internal family systems (IFS) is a non-pathologizing, trauma-informed, evidence-based psychotherapy modality developed over the last 30 years by family therapist Dr. Richard C. Schwartz and colleagues. IFS posits that the human psyche is composed of a system of subpersonalities Schwartz calls "Parts" that serve and protect the "Self," an observing level of the psyche that possesses the capacity for leadership and self-healing. When people have experiences that overwhelm the psyche, unbearable feelings become "Exile" Parts. Protector Parts, known as Managers and Firefighters, attempt to protect the Self from recurrences of the original distress. While all Parts have positive intentions, more extreme Parts can inhibit the ability of the Self to lead the system, causing mental health symptoms commensurate with the level of trauma. IFS treats trauma by softening defensive patterns enacted by Managers and Firefighters and by facilitating "unburdenings," a corrective emotional process that allows a client to reevaluate and relinquish maladaptive negative cognitions that stem from the trauma.

BRIEF HISTORY OF THE INTERNAL FAMILY SYSTEMS MODEL

The internal family systems (IFS) model of psychotherapy was developed by Richard C. Schwartz, PhD, in the 1980s. Schwartz, a trained family therapist, had been working with adolescent clients presenting with eating disorders and found they often referred to different aspects of themselves as having distinct thoughts, feelings, wishes, and behaviors, which Schwartz called "Parts." By treating Parts with curiosity, instead of trying to "fix" or eliminate them, Schwartz found these Parts "softened" and desisted from symptomatic behaviors (Schwartz & Sweezy 2021). Schwartz also found that many patients identified a place in their psyche, distinct in nature from Parts, that held a reservoir of positive leadership qualities such as compassion, courage, and curiosity, which he called the "Self" (Schwartz, 2020). Schwartz was aware that multiplicity of mind had been present since Freud's identification of the id, ego, and superego. Schwartz also found that early 20th-century psychoanalysts Roberto Assagioli and Carl Jung also saw the mind as multiple, and in addition, they had identified a Self in their clients. Numerous practitioners recognized

DOI: 10.4324/9781003455851-12

subpersonalities, most notably Fritz Perls (Gestalt Therapy), and developed techniques for dialoguing with Parts (Schwartz, 95). Schwartz expanded the focus on individual Parts to include the systemic and collaborative work of Salvador Minuchin, Jay Haley, Michael White, and Virginia Satir (Schwartz, 1995). In addition, Schwartz identified a phenomenon he called "legacy burdens," or beliefs and interactional patterns that are inherited from a person's family of origin and culture, accounting for the role of oppressive forces such as patriarchy and racism in trauma.

FUNDAMENTAL CLINICAL CONCEPTS OF IFS

IFS centers multiplicity, asserting from the beginning of treatment that all individuals possess subpersonalities, known as Parts, that make up an internal system; in addition to Parts, individuals have a place within them referred to as the Self, the seat of consciousness from which individuals view themselves, their Parts and their environment. Psychological symptoms are the result of Parts taking extreme positions in response to equally extreme experiences. Parts can be viewed and acted upon with the same systems theory we bring to family therapy; they can change and impact one another, often rapidly, with small changes leading to systemic changes.

UNDERSTANDING PARTS

Parts have their own beliefs, behaviors, ego states, physiology, and affect and interact internally with one another. All Parts have the positive intention to serve and protect the Self, even those that criticize the Self or engage in other harmful behaviors. No Part needs to be "fixed" or eliminated; if a Part has taken on an extreme role and is having a negative impact, it is because of the adverse experiences it has navigated. Parts correspond roughly to "psychological defenses" but without the pathologizing connotations.

TYPES OF PARTS

Parts are known as either *Protector* Parts, which include Managers and Firefighters, or *Vulnerable* Parts, known as Exiles.

Exiles: These are vulnerable Parts of the internal system that contain feelings that once overwhelmed one's system. These Parts hold memories, sensations, and emotions related to past events and carry "burdens" or maladaptive self-beliefs.

Managers: These Parts run day-to-day operations and, in extreme situations, protect the Self from the unbearable feelings contained by Exiles by adopting such roles as people-pleaser, caretaker, or inner critic. Managers' behaviors are often adaptive and socially sanctioned. Their motto is "never again," and they are *proactive* in nature.

Firefighters: These Parts come to the rescue when exiles are activated and aim to douse emotional pain quickly. They are *reactive* in nature, and their behaviors are often maladaptive. Common firefighter strategies include drug or alcohol use, cutting, suicidal ideation, violence, and binging.

Parts in relationship to each other. A young, male-identified child is bullied for displaying "effeminate" behaviors. The resulting hurt feelings are unbearable, and are thus dissociated, or "Exiled." The boy develops a Manager Part that adopts "masculine" attire and behaviors to protect himself from future bullying. As with many Manager behaviors, this strategy is socially sanctioned and, in a sense, adaptive. One day, the boy cries while watching a movie with friends and is teased; a Firefighter part may be activated to douse his humiliation by starting a fistfight. Like many Firefighters, their protective behavior can be maladaptive or have unwanted consequences.

UNDERSTANDING THE SELF

Each person has a governing Self (Schwartz & Sweezy 2021), an inborn entity of a higher level than Parts. The Self is distinguished by numerous leadership qualities: Compassion, curiosity, clarity, creativity, calm, confidence, courage, and connectedness, known as the "Eight C's." Emotional and psychological difficulties are not seen as evidence of gaps in development, nor damage to the Self, but rather arising from Parts that have obscured or blocked the Self. Crucially, IFS sees the Self as the agent of healing, rather than the clinician.

KEY CONCEPTS

Self Energy: This is the degree to which the qualities of the Self are accessible by the individual in a given moment. It corresponds to a state of emotional regulation and objectivity about one's emotions. A person with high Self-Energy feels capable of facing life's challenges and has greater leadership over their Parts. Such a person often states, "I feel like myself."

Blending: This occurs when a Part is undifferentiated from the Self. Consciousness narrows to the views and concerns of a particular Part. In psychodynamic terms, we are "overidentified" with the Part. Example: "I'm furious with you!" is the statement of a person blended with an angry Part, versus, "I want to let you know I have a Part that is angry with you," which is known as "speaking for a part."

Polarization: Refers to having Parts that have equal and opposing positions on a particular issue and corresponds to "inner conflict" in psychodynamic work. Example: "I am so sick of this job, but I could never quit in the current economy; I need the money." Most complaints of "stuckness" by a client are evidence of polarizations.

Legacy Burdens: These are beliefs, emotional patterns, and mental behaviors we inherit from family, social circles, and greater society regarding ourselves and others. The cultural legacy burdens of racism, patriarchy, materialism, and individualism combined with current structural oppression are overwhelming, and therefore traumatic (Gutierrez, 2022).

Backlash: Sometimes, the IFS process of helping protectors "skips over," or neglects a Part that has concerns about accessing an Exile. Example: A client reports feeling embarrassed to share vulnerable feelings. A well-intended therapist might encourage sharing, but the Part concerned with being exposed has not consented and may criticize the therapy process, leaving the client with mixed feelings about further exploration.

GOALS OF IFS

The goals of IFS treatment are fourfold: 1) help Parts release limiting beliefs and give up rigid protective behaviors through Unburdening; 2) help restore the Self to a position of sovereignty over Parts; 3) restore balance to the system as Parts give up extreme positions; and 4) bring the enhanced qualities of the Self to other people and society at large (Adapted from Schwartz & Sweezy, 2021).

UNDERSTANDING THE FLOW OF IFS

OVERVIEW

The IFS model offers a simple yet powerful protocol for conducting therapy sessions. The therapist begins by first working with a client's defenses, or protector Parts, and then working with vulnerable feelings, or Exile Parts, facilitating a release of constraining and obsolete beliefs. This process is repeated as necessary over the course of treatment, until symptoms are resolved.

ASSESSING READINESS AND APPROPRIATENESS FOR TREATMENT

As with any type of treatment, we recommend assuring that a client is not currently in an unsafe situation, and taking proper actions, for example, referral to a domestic violence shelter, before beginning IFS treatment (Anderson, 2017). Additionally, IFS is contraindicated for persons with traumatic brain injury (Hodgdon et al., 2022). Because IFS requires the individual to be able to reflect and tune into the internal world, if there is either an external or internal constraint, IFS is not recommended.

GOING INSIDE: BEGINNING THE IFS JOURNEY

An IFS session begins with inviting the client to "go inside" and notice their internal experience. Even this can activate the first layer of protective Parts; common concerns about going inside include fear of an unfamiliar process, a desire to recount the narrative directly to the therapist, fear of "doing it wrong," and others. The therapist develops trust by addressing these fears respectfully.

WORKING WITH PROTECTORS — THE SIX FS

Once a client has turned their attention inward, the therapist can begin work in the next protective layer of the client's system. A mnemonic known as the "Six Fs" is employed: Find, Focus, Feel Towards, Flesh Out, beFriend, and Fear (Pastor & Gauvain, 2021). Each step in working with protector Parts has the potential to activate other protector Parts with concerns that need to be addressed before they allow the process to move forward.

Find: The IFS process begins with identifying a "target" Part to work with by noticing internal images, feelings, and bodily sensations. The goal is to encourage openness toward one's internal experience and allow Parts to reveal themselves. Clients often have to be invited to choose the one they feel will most benefit from attention.

Focus: Once the Part is identified, the goal is to heighten the client's awareness of and focus on the Part. In this step, a client may benefit from help in "unblending" from the Part – that is, establishing compassionate objectivity and separation from the feelings held by the Part.

Feel toward: Once one Part reveals itself, it is essential to see what other Parts in the system may be influencing it. People often have Parts that hold frustration, sadness, or shame related to a Part that acts like an "inner critic," which persists in communicating negative messages toward the Self of the client. These Parts often have concerns that contacting the inner critic could amplify its harsh judgments. A client may also have Parts who appreciate or agree with the target Part's feelings, opinions, concerns, and behaviors. Many people have a Part that attributes their success in life to a tough inner critic they feel has pushed them to achieve great things. Positive or negative, strong feelings toward a target Part inhibit the client's ability to connect usefully with the target Part. The therapist must help the client validate these reactions and invite them to "step back," until the client reports a significant amount of compassion, curiosity, or other qualities of the Self to allow a supportive connection with the target Part.

Flesh out: In this step, the goal is to allow the Part to become vivid by asking the client to notice as much as possible about it. It's common to ask what the Part's emotional age is, how it makes itself known, whether the Part has a visual manifestation, and other ways the Parts attempts to communicate with the Self of the client.

beFriend: Once reactions to the target Part have stepped back, the therapist supports the client in connecting with the target part with a friendly "getting to know you" tone, free of agenda, presuming positive underlying function for the Part.

Fear: This step aims to identify the core fear or concern that keeps this Part in place. For instance, an inner critic may reveal, "I have to criticize you to keep you accountable."

WORKING WITH THE EXILE (UNBURDENING)

With a safe and secure connection established between the Self of the client and the target Part, the therapist can begin the unburdening process. When someone experiences a difficult or traumatic event, they adopt a particular belief about oneself or the world as a way of organizing the experience. For instance, a client may have learned while growing up that making a mistake can involve severe punishment. In a punitive family, a belief that "mistakes are fatal" would steer a young person away from sloppiness or other behaviors that could provoke cruelty. Unburdening allows the client to re-evaluate the belief and update or replace it with a more adaptive one, for instance, "It's okay to make mistakes." Unburdening has the following steps:

Witnessing: The therapist invites the client to ask the target Part to share thoughts and feelings related to a moment or situation that was overwhelming for the Part. The client must focus on *listening* to the target Part, allowing previously untold feelings and information to be shared from Part to Self.

Reparenting/Re-Do: The therapist facilitates a corrective emotional experience (Catanzaro et al., 2018), similar to the "mismatch" step in memory reconsolidation (Ecker et al., 2012), which refers to processing new or updated information that contradicts a previously held and constraining belief. For instance, a client with a rageful parent may develop a belief that anger is always dangerous. The therapist guides the client in asking the target Part what needed to be different for the client in the moment accessed in the "witnessing" step and helps the client visualize reparative behaviors or events. Ecker maintains that the original emotions must be activated for the brain to rewire. In this example, the Part may benefit from picturing her rageful parents expressing anger calmly (Ecker et al., 2012).

Retrieval: The therapist guides the client in inviting the target Part to "join them in the present," encouraging creative visualization to reference a place in their current real-life environment where the Part ostensibly will make its new home. This parallels trauma interventions that help a client orient themselves to the safety of the here and now.

Release/Unload: The therapist helps the client identify the limiting belief, or burden, they took on in the original trauma and to consider relinquishing the belief. The belief is often considered essential to self-protection, so a client will give up a belief only if new and trusted information is introduced. For instance, a client who grew up in a family that avoided conflict may carry the "burden" that disagreeing with someone could lead to disconnection. The therapist will then invite the client to imagine a place where their younger self would like to release the burden and visualize the surrender of the outdated belief.

Invitation: The therapist invites the client to identify a more adaptive, resonant belief to replace the burden that was released. For the person who grew up with the burden that conflict is dangerous, the replacement belief might be, "Conflict is part of connection." The new belief must be grounded in realistic, adaptive terms to support buy-in by all the client's Parts.

Integration: The therapist invites the client to reflect on the unburdening process and to discuss how they might anchor the session progress in the following week. The therapist and the client may agree on notes to take about the process and try to predict areas of the client's life where they might look for new experiences related to the unburdening.

CONSIDERATIONS AND NEXT STEPS

It is essential, especially with more complex trauma, to diligently track and follow up on all Parts that come up in each session to make sure unburdenings are completed. It's also important that the therapist checks in with the client protector Parts regularly to prevent backlash.

UTILIZATION OF IFS FOR THE TREATMENT OF TRAUMA

IFS views trauma on a continuum from acute to complex, with no change in the flow of treatment or interventions. However, writers on IFS present several cautions based on the severity and complexity of the trauma presented. Anderson (2021) identifies issues IFS therapists must consider when working with greater levels of trauma:

Therapeutic alliance: Complex trauma usually involves developmental attachment wounds; such clients have Parts that do not trust relationships at all, much less the relationship with a therapist. Therapists must check for Parts that have concerns about therapy or the therapist, and they must maintain their presumption of positive function on even destructive Part behaviors.

Reaction to extremes: Suicidality, reports of extreme horror, and sitting with devastation all activate therapists' Parts. Anderson recommends that therapists conduct self-debriefing after trauma sessions to process their reactions to session content.

Boundary issues: Because of the extremes of trauma, therapists must be on guard for their own Parts that may consider interventions outside of normal boundaries, or distance themselves from the work.

Comorbidity: Clients with trauma may also have conditions such as obsessive-compulsive disorder, or medical issues that add to a client's symptomatology; accurate assessment is essential to account for Parts related to comorbidities.

While IFS is taught as a single, trauma-informed model, Joanne Twombly (2022) distinguishes between "Standard IFS" and "Trauma-Informed IFS." For the latter, Twombly employs "hypnotic language skills," that is, using language that is invitational and allows for feedback from the client; and Safe Space Imagery, which helps clients access self-states associated with safety. Twombly also teaches the "Window of Tolerance," created by Dr. Dan Siegel (1999), to help clinicians monitor for hypo- and hyperarousal that can hinder a client's ability to process emotions. Twombly highlights the importance of therapists' sophistication on the issues of race, gender, and culture to create optimum safety for the client.

An additional component of IFS is the exploration and use of somatic experience. Trauma can begin in utero, before language, thus there are situations where clients cannot verbalize their experience. Many Exile parts manifest somatically, such as through restricted breathing, numbness, demeanor, posture, or turning away. Susan McConnell (2020) has developed a model of IFS that encourages more extensive awareness of the somatic experience of therapist and client. McConnell asserts that both injuries to the body-mind system, *and* individual capacity for healing, can often be accessed only through somatic practices.

ASSESSMENT OF RESEARCH EVIDENCE REGARDING EFFECTIVENESS OF IFS IN TREATING TRAUMA

Research on trauma treatment with IFS is in its early stages. A notable study focused on PTSD symptoms in survivors of childhood trauma. Conducted in a diverse metropolitan area in the Northeastern United States with 17 subjects, the study showed that 92% no longer met PTSD criteria at a one-month follow-up (Hodgdon et al., 2022).

A randomized clinical trial by Zev Schuman-Olivier, MD, at the Cambridge Health Alliance, explored IFS as a PTSD treatment online during the COVID pandemic. Findings suggest IFS can be practiced online effectively; publication is pending. A 2016 study on IFS for depression in female college students demonstrated results comparable to CBT and IPT, showing a substantial reduction in Beck Depression Inventory scores (Haddock et al., 2016).

A 2013 proof-of-concept study on IFS for rheumatoid arthritis supported its recognition as evidence based by NREPP. Results showed sustained improvements in pain and physical function but not in anxiety, self-efficacy, or disease activity (Shadick et al., 2013).

The Foundation for Self Leadership's database includes over 100 IFS–related publications, contributing to evidence supporting IFS efficacy. More diverse research across practice areas and social identities is crucial for IFS to become a standard mental health modality.

CASE EXAMPLE: USING IFS FOR THE TREATMENT OF TRAUMA OF NONCONSENSUAL SEX

The following example is fictionalized from multiple clinical experiences with a wide variety of client identities, and no similarity to an actual person should be construed.

CLIENT BACKGROUND

Peter, a 32-year-old gay man, sought treatment to address an inability to be intimate with men he dated. Peter reported that when he was 20, he had been volunteering at an LGBT advocacy organization, and a staff person had persuaded him to have sex despite Peter's lack of consent. In the first few sessions, the therapist allowed Peter to express his experience in his own words, as the therapist introduced IFS language and helped Peter identify various parts that emerged. These Parts included those concerned with the risks of being vulnerable in treatment, Parts that had different positions regarding his presenting problem, and Parts with concerns the therapist logged as secondary themes for later treatment. Additionally, they identified the Part that was involved in Peter's sexual function, which Peter identified as "antisex." In the session below, Peter expressed interest in doing deeper work with this Part.

BEGINNING WITH PROTECTORS, USING THE SIX FS

THERAPIST (TH):	(*Beginning **Find** step*) Good afternoon, Peter. I'm curious what Parts you are aware of today?
PATIENT (P):	I think I'm ready to work on healing the "antisex" Part of me today.
TH:	Okay, what is it like to say that? *Checking for permission from the system and Parts that might have concerns about working on the "antisex" Part.*
P:	Well, Part of me is nervous.
TH:	I respect that. Does it make sense that you would have a Part of you that would be nervous? *Validating the nervous Part.*
P:	[Laughing nervously] Yes. But it also says it trusts you.
TH:	I'm so glad. Please tell this nervous Part that I am grateful for its trust.
P:	[Laughs] It says "You're welcome." [Pause] So how do we do this?
TH:	Well, tell me about this "antisex" Part (*Using the client's words*). What are you aware of about this Part?
P:	Well, basically there is this wall that stops me from having sex. I don't even feel horny anymore. *The therapist interprets this to mean the Part has a significant "pull" on the Self of the client and may need help "unblending" as explained in the upcoming "Focus" step.*
TH:	And where do you feel that wall in your body?
P:	It's in my chest.
TH:	(*Begins **Focus** step.*) Okay, so maybe, if it feels all right to you, you could close your eyes (*invitational language*), and turn your attention to this Part. Maybe you can even put a hand on your chest to make contact with this Part. What do you notice?
P:	This part is like a "knight in shining armor," but not shining, but you know, that armor they wear. It's encasing my whole torso.
TH:	Let's try something, I wonder if you maybe close your eyes, and ask this Part if it would be willing to give you a little space, so that you could be you, and this Part can be this Part. *The therapist helps Peter "unblend" from the antisex Part.*
P:	Okay … [closes eyes] … okay, the Part is sort of standing in front of me now.
TH:	Okay, and what is it like to have this Part interacting with you like this now?
C:	I actually feel a little relieved. It felt good to get a little space. *Now that a Part has been identified for work, the "Feelings toward" step allows the therapist to assess whether the client has enough compassion or other Self-Energy qualities to allow a useful dialogue with the target Part.*
TH:	Okay let's check in … what feelings do you have toward this "armor" Part?
P:	Well, like I said, Part of me is mad at it – it is fucking up my sex life!
TH:	And does it make sense that you would have a Part that could be angry or frustrated at how this Part protects you? *The therapist is validating the angry Part.*

P: Yes!

TH: Okay, could you let that Part know you understand its frustration, and
           see if it could also step back?

           *The therapist repeats this process with each of the Parts holding the shame, sad-
           ness, and weariness that Peter has toward the "armor" Part. The therapist then
           double-checks with the client about Self-Energy.*

TH: So, Peter, you have done great work getting these different parts of you to
           step back. So maybe just check, how are you feeling toward this Part now?

P: I'm actually feeling more relaxed, like, I'm curious what this part is
           really about. *The therapist interprets this as a sign that the client can interact
           with the antisex Part without activating protector Parts.*

TH: (**Fleshing out** step) That's great, so maybe you can start noticing a little
           more about this part. How does it act?

P: It's sort of dark ... and silent. It's sort of like "standing guard." It's just
           doing its job.

TH: Do you have a sense of what emotional age this part has?

P: Hmm, that is an interesting question. I think it's like a young adult part
           of me. I remember I was much more shy and rigid in my 20s.

TH: And how does this part appear to you right in this moment, as you
           become aware of its emotional age, like it's in its 20s?

P: He's like a part of me, that is like, irritated, and stuck.

TH: (**beFriending** step) Okay, very good, you are getting to see a much
           clearer image of this Part of you. I want to invite you now to let this
           Part know, you are here to listen to anything it wants to tell you, and
           maybe just take some time, and just listen.

P: Okay. [Closes eyes again, reflecting internally] It's saying "Sex isn't
           worth it."

TH: And what do you notice happens when you hear it say that?

P: That frustrated Part of me is screaming.

TH: Okay, that makes sense. See if you can validate that frustrated Part and
           have it step back.

P: Okay. [Takes a moment to communicate with the frustrated Part].
           I think it's okay now.

TH: Do you get why this Part says "Sex isn't worth it"?

P: I guess I do. I think this Part just doesn't want a repeat of what
           happened.

TH: Could you let this Part know that you get that it's trying to prevent
           something bad from happening?

P: The Part is saying, "Of course I am protecting you, it's my job."

TH: (*Identifying **Fear***) Could you ask this Part what it thinks would happen
           if it didn't do its job?

P: Yes, it thinks all men are like that guy, that ... you know [Referring to
           the incident of nonconsensual sex].

TH: Peter, I wonder if you could ask this Part to show you an image about
           what it's most concerned about?

P:	Okay, it's showing me Alan's face when I told him what he did to me was not okay. He just laughed. [Shudders].
TH:	And so, this Part is afraid that …?
P:	It doesn't want me ever to be that humiliated again.

WORKING WITH AN EXILE – THE UNBURDENING PROCESS

The Therapist sees that the Exile Part here is the humiliated feelings Peter experienced when he tried to advocate for himself. He is now going to help Peter complete an Unburdening.

TH:	(Begins **Witnessing** step) Okay, and how are you doing right now? How is it to see that image? *Checking for Parts that might have concerns about this level of vulnerability.*
P:	It's okay.
TH:	Can you see yourself in that scene? The young man you were when this happened, your "20-year-old self?"
P:	Yes.
TH:	Can you see the look on his face? *The therapist is helping to make the image more vivid.*
P:	Yes, he looks so lost and hurt and confused.
TH:	Can you go to him and just be with him?
P:	It's so weird but he is just holding me and crying.
TH:	Does that make sense? *Supporting witnessing and validation.*
P:	Yes, it does make sense. I see he has been blaming himself but looking back on it I see how he had nothing to do with this – Alan was the asshole.
TH:	Let him know that you see that.
P:	[Tearful]. I am. He is also saying how angry he is.
TH:	Let him know you hear him and that you get it.
TH:	(**Reparenting** step) Maybe you can ask him what about this situation needs to change. *Picking up on the boundary-setting theme and beginning a "do-over."*
P:	He says that he wants to erase Alan from our life. He doesn't want to kill him. He kinda knows that Alan is like a broken person – like, he shouldn't die but just go the hell away.
TH:	Okay, take a minute and let him erase Alan in whatever way your mind sees fit.
P:	Yeah, it feels good. Like I was too stunned the first time around and too *nice* and it's like, begone, you bastard! It's like the old me gets it now, he believes he didn't cause this.
TH:	Great, notice how this feels.
P:	It's like, it's sad, but it's good. I feel like that feeling when you know you're in the right. *The therapist moves into the **Retrieval** step, bringing the Exile into the present, away from the original threat.*

TH: That's great, Peter. See if he would like to join you here in the present.

P: Yes, he would!

TH: Okay, can you think of a place in your life, maybe in your apartment, where 20-year-old Peter could come and stay?

P: Yes, I picture him in this chair in my bedroom.

TH: Great, notice how he is doing there.

TH: (*Begins* **Release/Unburdening** *step*) Peter, if you could put into words the belief you had that had you stuck with this situation, what would it be?

P: I think it's something like, "Gay means anything goes." Like, if I were to push back on someone who wants to have sex with me, it's homophobic. I can see that's ridiculous when I say it out loud but I think that's what was happening for me.

TH: Okay, so let me invite you to ask this Part of you if it is ready to release this burden, this idea that "gay means anything goes." *This is a step where some final protectors may express concern about what it will mean to give up a long-held belief.*

P: It says it is scared to give up this belief. It seems to think that being free to be gay is always going to mean people trying to do whatever they want to me.

TH: And does it make sense that this part has this fear? It has wanted to protect you from nonconsensual sex.

P: It does make sense. [Patient reflects for a moment]. I'm letting this part know that we can learn how to say no to people, and still be free to be gay.

TH: That's beautifully put! I wonder if you can see if this Part is able to take that in.

P: It is listening. It likes the idea of me learning to say no and set limits with people.

TH: So, it sounds like you're saying this Part was able to see that the real vulnerability you had was not because of being gay but because of not being comfortable saying no, which it sounds like you and your Parts feel like you could work on.

P: Yes, that's right.

TH: So, I'll make a note of that as a trailhead, and, maybe now, could you ask this Part, where or how would it like to release this burden, "gay means anything goes"?

P: He is showing me an image of the bonfire at this gay men's retreat I went to once. We wrote things on pieces of paper that we wanted to get rid of in our lives and we threw them into the fire.

TH: That's a powerful image, Peter! See if you can be there again with this Part. Maybe you want to picture writing this burden on a piece of paper and putting it in the fire. *The therapist lets Peter's imagery lead and supports making the image as vivid as possible.*

P: Yes, he is doing that.

TH:	Take your time with this. Notice how it feels to 20-year-old Peter.
P:	He feels great! And he feels good knowing that there are other gay men around him who aren't "using" him. They're just friends.
TH:	(*Invitation step*) That's great. Peter, let's come up with a more positive belief you can replace this burden with. How would you put it? *The therapist makes sure to replace the negative cognition with a positive one.*
P:	Huh. I mean I want "gay" to mean "freedom."
TH:	Okay, and what would be the difference this time?
P:	I think it would be, "I get to be me. I'm my own person."
TH:	That sounds good. Take a minute and check with your system, does it resonate?
P:	I think so. Let me check. I think it's more like, "I'm the boss of me. I matter."
TH:	"I'm the boss of me, I matter." How does that feel?
P:	You know what, I think the statement is actually "I matter." Yes.
TH:	Okay, good work, I am glad you took the time to find what fits you. Let's invite that message in, "I matter."

The therapist helps Peter **integrate** his experience of this unburdening with him, listening for any Parts with questions, concerns, or observations, and validating Peter's experience. They also discuss how Peter might remain mindful of how the new positive cognition might show itself in the coming week and what new behaviors might become available.

GOING FORWARD

While this unburdening took place in a single session, more complex trauma can take many weeks and months to work through all the related protectors in order to allow safe access to an Exile. Along the way, the therapist carefully tracks the unburdening, marks progress, and notes areas for later work.

STRENGTHS AND LIMITATIONS OF IFS IN THE TREATMENT OF TRAUMA

STRENGTHS

Non-Pathologizing Stance: IFS has at its core a belief in a powerful, innate, and intact Self that is present in both the client and the therapist. Having Parts normalized reduces the shame and stigma that can often impede the development of a working alliance, allowing deeper and longer-lasting change to occur. This non-pathologizing stance extends to the therapist's Parts as well. Therapists are not expected to be free of Parts but rather to be aware of them and seek support to maintain leadership over their Parts.

Flexibility: There is virtually no client symptom that cannot be framed as the behavior of Parts working with good intentions but sometimes in dysfunctional ways.

Simplicity: IFS is elegantly simple. When navigating the not-always-clear path from symptom to its remission, especially when complex feelings are activated, therapists and clients alike benefit from a way of understanding their work that places minimal demand on cognitive processing during the flow of the session. Because resistance is reframed as expected and valid behaviors from protector Parts, the work has less of a sense of struggle.

Framework for Addressing Countertransference: Due to some of the extreme situations that come along with trauma treatment, it is expected that the therapist will experience considerable countertransference. Because countertransference is understood as the activation of the therapist's Parts, there is a clear method for attending to what arises in the therapist as he encounters his client's Parts.

Framework for Addressing Oppression: Oppressive forces such as racism, sexism, patriarchy, materialism, and many more are accounted for as *legacy burdens*, and there is a process for liberating clients from these harmful beliefs. Therapists are expected to gain awareness of and leadership over their own legacy burdens as well.

LIMITATIONS

There are very few limitations to IFS efficacy in trauma treatment when the aforementioned cautions are taken into consideration. IFS therapists are taught to assess levels of client Self-Energy continually and to respect any present protector Parts that have concern for the client. This approach "focuses on enhancing the ability to attend to difficult and distressing internal experiences with mindfulness" (Hodgdon et al., 2022).

One limitation of note is the possibility that a client is uncomfortable framing their experience in terms of Parts and other IFS language. In such cases, the IFS therapist can revert to "IFS-informed psychotherapy," working in the client's language model, while internally maintaining a compassionate view of defenses, resolving inner conflict, and challenging constraining beliefs. Another limitation is the absence of attachment theory in the model. While IFS sees the Self of the Client as the primary agent of healing, the authors feel there is room for the model to account for the healing aspects of the therapist–client dyad, as well as the well-documented lifelong need for connection with others.

RESOURCES FOR LEARNING

Main IFS Website https://www.ifs-institute.com
IFS Learning Hub https://learn.ifs-institute.com/
IFS Foundation https://www.foundationifs.org/
IFS Publications Database https://grantuoso.org/ifssearch

BOOKS

Anderson, F.G. (2017). *Transcending trauma: healing complex PTSD with internal family systems*. Eau Claire, WI: PESI Publishing.

Schwartz, R.C. & Sweezy, M. (2021). *Internal family systems therapy* (2nd ed.). New York NY: The Guilford Press.

McConnell, S. (2020). *Somatic internal family systems therapy: Awareness, breath, resonance, movement and touch in practice.* Berkeley, CA: North Atlantic Books.

REFERENCES

Anderson, F.G. (2017). *Transcending trauma: Healing complex PTSD with internal family systems.* Eau Claire, WI: PESI Publishing.

Anderson, F.G. (2021). *Transcending trauma: Healing complex PTSD with internal family systems.* Claire, WI: PESI Publishing.

Catanzaro, J., Doyne, E., & Thompson, K. (2018). IFS (Internal family systems) and eating disorders: The healing power of self-energy. In A. Seubert, & P. Virdi (Eds.), *Trauma-informed approaches to eating disorders.* New York, NY: Springer Publishing Company.

Ecker, B., Tcici, R., & Hulley, L. (2012). *Unlocking the emotional brain.* 1st Edition. Routledge/Taylor & Francis Group.

Gutierrez, N. (2022). *The pain we carry: Healing from complex PTSD for people of color.* Oakland, CA: New Harbinger Publications.

Haddock, S.A., Weiler, L.M., Trump, L.J., & Henry, K.L. (2016). The efficacy of internal family systems therapy in the treatment of depression among female college students: A pilot study. *The Journal of Marital and Family Therapy, 43*(1), 131–144.

Hodgdon, H. Anderson, F.G., Southwell, E., Hrubec, W., & Schwartz, R. (2022). Internal family systems (IFS) therapy for post-traumatic stress disorder (PTSD) among survivors of multiple childhood trauma: A pilot effectiveness study, *Journal of Aggression, Maltreatment & Trauma, 31*(1), 22–43, DOI: 10.1080/10926771.2021.2013375

McConnell, S. (2020). *Somatic internal family systems therapy: Awareness, breath, resonance, movement, and touch in practice.* Berkeley, CA: North Atlantic Books.

Pastor, M., & Gauvain, J. (2021). *Internal family systems level I training manual.* Oak Park, Ill: Trailhead Publications.

Schwartz, R.C. (1995). *Internal family systems therapy (Guilford Family Therapy Series).* New York NY: The Guilford Press.

Schwartz, R.C. (2020) *No bad parts.* Louisville, CO: Sounds True.

Schwartz, R.C., & Sweezy, M. (2021). *Internal family systems therapy* (2nd ed.). New York NY: The Guilford Press.

Shadick, N.A., Sowell, N.F., Frits, M.L., Hoffman, S.M., Hartz, S.A., Booth, F.D., Sweezy, M., Rogers, P.R., Dubin, R.L., Atkinson, J.C., Friedman, A.L., Augusto, F., Iannaccone, C.K., Fossel, A.H., Quinn, G., Cui, J., Losina, E., & Schwartz, R.C. (2013) A randomized controlled trial of an internal family systems-based psychotherapeutic intervention on outcomes in rheumatoid arthritis: A proof-of-concept study. *The Journal of Rheumatology, 40* (11) 1831–1841; DOI: 10.3899/jrheum.121465

Siegel, D. (1999). *The developing mind.* New York, NY: The Guilford Press.

Twombly, J. (2022). *Trauma and dissociation informed internal family systems: How to successfully treat C-PTSD, and dissociative disorders.* Self-Published.

13

CHAPTER 13
COHERENCE THERAPY FOR TRAUMATIC MEMORY AND POST-TRAUMATIC SYMPTOMS

Bruce Ecker and Sara K. Bridges

INTRODUCTION

The standard of effectiveness in coherence therapy is transformational change, the complete and lasting disappearance of major symptoms and their associated distressed or dysphoric state of mind. This outcome is not reliably achieved through emotional regulation techniques that counteractively reduce symptoms partially by cultivating a preferred state of mind or behavior. Rather, profound unlearning through the brain's mechanism of memory reconsolidation (MR) is required. Coherence therapy creates the same set of experiences that has been shown to eliminate an acquired emotional reaction through profound unlearning in laboratory neuroscience studies of MR. Many publications since 1996 have documented the effectiveness of this experiential methodology for ending a wide range of symptoms and problems, including post-traumatic symptoms, which are the special focus of this chapter. The non-pathologizing conceptual framework of coherence therapy lays bare the phenomenology of how implicit emotional learnings drive symptom production and how their unlearning occurs for symptom cessation. This chapter identifies the specific elements of emotional learning that make a mental model or schema have the distinctive, potent qualities that are designated as *traumatic* memory, and a case example shows how the experiential process of unlearning is guided to target those elements for transformational change.

BRIEF HISTORY

Coherence therapy was initially developed from 1986 to 1993 by Bruce Ecker and Laurel Hulley (Ecker & Hulley, 1996) and until 2005 was known as depth-oriented brief therapy or DOBT. Its methodology emerged as a result of several years of closely studying, in their own practices, outlier therapy sessions that had somehow suddenly produced transformational change – the lasting disappearance of a major symptom and its associated distressed or dysphoric state of mind. The aim was to identify the essential steps of the process that these initially rare but remarkably effective sessions shared, across a wide range of symptoms and clients: What is it that therapists would have to know and do, or not do, in order to generate that kind of effectiveness regularly in their sessions?

Ecker and Hulley had come to this project strongly influenced by various non-pathologizing frameworks, including constructivist psychotherapies (especially the

DOI: 10.4324/9781003455851-13

concepts of first-order versus second-order change developed by Gregory Bateson and the Mental Research Institute group in the 1960s and 70s, and the foundational principles articulated by George Kelly in the 1950s and 60s), the experiential in-depth therapies of the Human Potential Movement in the 1960s and 70s (Gestalt therapy and Eugene Gendlin's focusing in particular), and the experiential interaction between the conscious personality and the psyche's depths, as well as the mind's thorough functional coherence, in the extensive writings of Carl Jung.

The search arrived at a well-defined process that was reliably producing transformational change:

> We found consistently that the interactions that produced therapeutic breakthrough did not inherently require preparatory months or years of sessions. The crucial exchanges would in most cases have been equally effective if carried out in the very first sessions, if only the therapist had somehow known what they were. Depth-Oriented Brief Therapy developed as we identified how to bring the client and therapist to those pivotal moments very rapidly, without reducing the therapist's role to one of technician or manipulator....
>
> (Ecker & Hulley, 1996, p. 2)

A decade later, Ecker, studying new research on memory reconsolidation (MR) by neuroscientists, recognized that the markers of transformational change that he and Hulley had used for reverse-engineering the causal therapeutic process were identical to the changes that researchers were now interpreting as confirmation that the MR mechanism had "erased" a subcortical, acquired emotional reaction (Ecker, 2006). Subsequent MR studies with both animal and human subjects specifically identified an experiential process required by the brain for such profound unlearning and change to occur (reviewed by, e.g., Clem & Schiller, 2016), and the steps of that empirically identified process were in one-to-one match with the process that Ecker and Hulley had culled from their clinical observations (Ecker, 2021; Ecker & Bridges, 2020; Ecker & Vaz, 2022). That fortunate convergence of clinical observations and memory research makes coherence therapy a very natural and happy marriage of the art and the science of transformational change.

FUNDAMENTAL CONCEPTS

Each specific, unwanted behavior, state of mind, or somatic distress that a person in therapy identifies is termed a *symptom*. Coherence therapy provides verifiable, atheoretical conceptualizations of both symptom production (elucidating the very basis of a symptom's existence as adaptive emotional learning) and symptom cessation (through an evidence-based process of profound unlearning via *memory reconsolidation*).

Coherence therapy's conceptualization of symptom production is that as a rule, any given symptom exists because the person harbors at least one *coherent, adaptive emotional learning* that is *implicit* (outside of awareness) and that urgently requires the symptom, even with the suffering or hardship that it entails, in order to avoid some even worse suffering.

That is coherence therapy's central principle of *symptom coherence*. For example, consider the symptoms presented by "Gary," a man in his mid-40s who wanted relief from what he termed "social anxiety": An inability to think or speak in most social situations, while feeling so tense and tight throughout his body that he is "almost rigid like a statue." Those symptoms are the freeze response, which occurs when perceiving extreme current endangerment. For that to happen in a normal social situation indicates traumatic memory reactivation. Through an experiential process, described in the following case example section, during his first session of coherence therapy, Gary for the first time mindfully recognized his visceral expectation, learned in childhood in his family, that if he says "anything wrong" in front of others, he will be subjected to a searing ordeal of angry shaming, denigration, and rejection. Bringing awareness to that emotional learning made sense of his frozen tenseness and the mutism that was urgently needed for protecting himself from having another agonizing interpersonal experience. This phenomenology is described by coherence therapy's concept of *the two sufferings* – the suffering due to having the symptom and the even worse suffering expected due to *not* having the symptom. The production of the symptom successfully avoids the worse suffering.

A symptom's underlying emotional learning consists of coherent knowledge of a particular suffering or vulnerability that is urgent to avoid (the *problem*) and knowledge of a particular tactic that is urgently necessary for avoiding it (the *solution*). Gary initially regarded his involuntary mutism as the problem – proof of his defectiveness – but he then came to recognize, experientially, that actually it was his solution to the problem of the shaming, denigration, and rejection that he "knows" will assault him if he were to say anything wrong. Even without yet dispelling that emotional learning or the symptoms it was producing, Gary had already experienced a significant shift, a *pivot into agency*: Symptoms that had seemed to be senseless afflictions that happened *to* him with a mysterious life of their own now fully made sense as his own self-protective perception of danger and his own evasive action. This pivot into agency is not a merely cognitive reframing or restructuring, rather it is the natural effect of the client gaining direct, lucid, affective awareness of the symptom's underlying emotional learning, also termed *the emotional truth of the symptom* or the client's *pro-symptom position*. In coherence therapy, the client's presenting symptom is consistently found, experientially, to be either a solution for preventing the true problem or the emotional and somatic effects of feeling vulnerable to the true problem.

Coherence therapy conceptualizes each symptom-generating emotional learning as a *schema* or *mental model* consisting of *knowings* of various kinds, whether they are termed core beliefs, expectations, attributed meanings, or constructs. The knowings in the schema were formed and learned in the presence of strong emotion, which is why the schema is called an emotional learning. It is well established by memory researchers that the encoding of emotional learnings involves the subcortical brain, including the limbic system, and that learning accompanied by strong emotion makes the learnings extremely fast-responding, tenacious, and unfading over time (e.g., McGaugh & Roozendaal, 2002).

Of course, not all presented symptoms or difficulties originate in the contents of memory. Examples of conditions not based in memory, and therefore not dispellable by coherence therapy, include hard-wired neurological situations (such as those causing difficulties with learning or sensory experience) and biological conditions (such as hypothyroidism that causes a mood of depression).

Coherence therapy emphasizes that a symptom-generating schema is closely coupled to, but distinct from, the emotions and body states generated by it. The target of change in coherence therapy is the symptom's underlying schema or mental model, not the emotion or other symptoms produced by it. The aim is a fundamental depotentiation and annulment of the symptom-generating schema, so that the schema no longer feels at all real anymore, and then it no longer produces any symptoms, including emotion. Such transformational change does not relapse. The therapist does not use emotional regulation techniques or any other *counteractive* methods designed to reduce symptoms or build up a preferred, symptom-free state (such as relaxation techniques to reduce anxiety or positive thinking to reduce depression), because such methods as a rule produce partial, incremental change that is susceptible to relapse.

Since the schema is a particular emotional learning, its annulment is brought about by a process of decisive *unlearning*. The brain's process of unlearning has been identified in neuroscience research on MR since 2004. Unlearning occurs through a well-defined, experiential process that has been shown in many laboratory neuroscience studies to eliminate all responsiveness of a target emotional learning (as reviewed by Clem & Schiller, 2016; Ecker, 2021). In this process, the neural encoding of the consolidated (stable, long-term) target learning is *deconsolidated*, described by researchers as a *destabilization* on the cellular and molecular level, which allows the encoding to then be rewritten according to new learning that nullifies and in effect erases the original learning. The revised neural encoding then automatically *reconsolidates* after about five hours, into stable, long-term memory. Operationally, the process is carried out by creating certain *subjective experiences*, using any suitable external procedures or techniques to do so: First, a violation of the expectations of the reactivated target learning triggers its deconsolidation, followed by experiencing a full contradiction of those expectations several times. For example, if the target learning is the visceral (subcortical) expectation of receiving a wrist shock two seconds after a yellow square appears on a computer screen, a single presentation of the square with no shock occurring (or occurring at 10 seconds) is a violation of expectation, or *prediction error* experience, that induces deconsolidation of that memory's neural encoding (e.g., Díaz-Mataix et al., 2013).

As the following case example shows, that process is replicated in coherence therapy sessions, with the same result of total annulment of the target schema (Ecker, 2018; Ecker & Bridges, 2020; Ecker & Vaz, 2022). The lasting, complete disappearance of schema reactivation and all symptoms generated by the schema is termed *transformational change*, which is not susceptible to relapse because the schema or mental model that was the very basis of the symptom no longer exists in memory. There is no loss of autobiographical or *episodic* memory of life experiences because the schema contains not autobiographical memory, but rather *semantic* memory of a pattern that was construed from personal experiences. The schema is not memory of particular experiences of suffering, but rather is *what was learned from what was suffered*. So, the profound unlearning of a symptom-generating schema is the deep and complete resolution of a specific theme of distress in the client's life. Transformational change persists effortlessly once it occurs, without any ongoing counteractive measures or practices, in contrast to the partial, incremental, relapse-prone change typically produced by counteractive methods. A very wide range of symptoms has been ended in coherence therapy by the unlearning and nullification of their underlying schemas. (For a list of ended symptoms, see Ecker & Bridges, 2020).

DESCRIPTION OF THE THERAPY PROCESS

The overall methodology of coherence therapy can be defined in one sentence: *Find the emotional learnings generating the client's symptoms, then guide the thorough unlearning of those learnings.* How to carry out those two activities efficiently and effectively, starting in the first session, is the substance of all coherence therapy writings, presentations, trainings, and videos.

With a new client, the therapist first works to identify what to regard as the symptom(s) – the specific behaviors, states of mind, and/or somatic sensations that the client wants to be free of. That initial step of *symptom identification* is critical, as having a clear definition of the symptom(s) is essential in order to then effectively carry out the *discovery* phase of coherence therapy. Discovery is an experiential process of bringing an implicit, symptom-requiring emotional learning, or schema, into direct, explicit awareness as a personal emotional truth, as mentioned earlier regarding Gary and described in more detail ahead. Crucially, the therapist *learns from the client* what the content of the schema is – how having the symptom is emotionally necessary. In that way, the truth and accuracy of this internally revealed and recognized coherence is immediately self-evident to the client. The therapist does not do any interpreting. The empathy expressed by the therapist for the emotional learning that requires *having* the symptom greatly facilitates the discovery work and is a distinctive element of coherence therapy, so it has the special name of *coherence empathy*.

Next is the *integration* phase of establishing ongoing awareness of the newly conscious emotional truth in daily life. Integration is developed through repeated, mindful experiences of the discovered schema, during and between sessions, as will be further described later. The therapist structures and assigns these integration experiences, and each time, the client feels, recognizes and "owns" the emotional truth of how and why the symptom is necessary – how it exists on the basis of a potent emotional learning. Many schemas have several components and layers, and in such cases, retrieving the entire schema into awareness requires several alternating steps of discovery and integration. A well-integrated schema is a ripe target for unlearning and nullification through the memory reconsolidation process in the next phase, the *transformation* phase.

In the transformation phase, the therapist will *guide the thorough unlearning of those learnings* by subjecting each discovered schema to the unlearning process of memory reconsolidation. That process fulfills the specific, critical condition required by the brain for unlearning and nullifying a target emotional learning through memory reconsolidation. The critical condition consists of inducing two mutually contradictory experiences concurrently: The reactivation of the target learning in awareness as a subjectively felt knowing and expectation, and a personal experience or knowing that decisively contradicts and disconfirms the knowing and expectation of the target learning. That *juxtaposition experience*, as it is referred to in coherence therapy, after being repeated a few times in the course of a session, is observed to result in transformational change: The target learning's knowing and expectation, which for decades had seemed to be a grim or frightening truth of the world, no longer seems at all real and can no longer be cued and reactivated. How that unfolded for Gary is described ahead. Coherence therapy equips the therapist with a large array of techniques for finding or creating contradictory knowledge, guided by schema content (Ecker & Hulley, 2019).

Successful unlearning is then verified by the client reporting long-term nonoccurrence of the symptom(s) and non-reactivation of the schema in all situations where they had been occurring. In summary, these are the steps of coherence therapy's methodology:

- Symptom identification
- Discovery phase utilizing symptom coherence
- Integration phase
- Transformation phase utilizing the unlearning process of memory reconsolidation
- Verification phase confirming transformational change

Coherence therapy is defined by that methodology carried out experientially, not by any particular techniques that may be used to do so. Some form of "resistance" – meaning conscious or nonconscious non-cooperation with the therapist's current step of therapeutic process – can develop during symptom identification, discovery, integration, or transformation. The therapist responds to resistance by applying the usual coherence therapy methodology to it: Temporarily the therapist regards the resistance as the "symptom" and works to discover the emotional truth of the resistance – how and why, for the client, the resistance is necessary to have at this moment. Working with resistance in coherence therapy is mapped out by Ecker and Hulley (2019) and Ecker et al. (2024).

APPLYING COHERENCE THERAPY FOR POST-TRAUMATIC SYMPTOMS

Therapists encounter widely different types of traumatic memory and post-traumatic symptoms, ranging from those created by acute, single-incident, "shock" trauma to those due to multiple chronic, co-occurring forms of traumatization by abusive parents in daily life throughout childhood – the condition usually termed complex attachment trauma or developmental trauma. Between those two categories are *intermediate* cases of traumatization, such as that of Raoul, who was 36 and married, and who sought coherence therapy for his hair-trigger, excessive anger that flared unpredictably at others in a wide range of situations. The therapist and Raoul revisited a number of these instances and discovered that in each case, his anger had flared when he perceived the other person as deviating from what had been agreed upon, even if only in a minor way. This recognition in turn immediately evoked a surge of images, thoughts and feelings from a devastating experience five years earlier, when Raoul discovered that his business partner had taken actions that blatantly violated key agreements between them and had thereby stolen Raoul's sizable investment in the business. This forced the dissolution of the business, which had embodied Raoul's professional aspirations. The intense betrayal, loss, helplessness, humiliation, and impotent rage were overwhelming and traumatizing. Raoul's subsequent explosive anger in response to any degree or form of perceived broken agreement was a post-traumatic symptom. (For a full account of how transformational change resulted for this case, see chapter 5 in Ecker et al. (2024).)

Across that entire range of trauma conditions, coherence therapy has produced transformational change, as is documented in numerous published cases studies, an online index of which is available (Coherence Psychology Institute, 2023). Practitioners understand that whether the trauma was acute, complex, or intermediate, post-traumatic symptoms may be generated in two main ways, by two different forms of coherence:

- *Symptoms generated by the urgent necessity of keeping the unbearable episodic memory of the traumatic experience(s) suppressed out of awareness.* Such symptoms include dissociation, emotional flatness, distraction behaviors, avoidance behaviors, depersonalization, gaps in autobiographical memory, lack of coherent narrative, and dismissive downplaying and normalizing of childhood suffering.
- *Symptoms generated by semantic (schema) memory of what was learned from what was suffered.* Such symptoms consist of (a) the emotional and somatic distress (such as a chronic mood of anxiety or depression) due to feeling ever vulnerable to more traumatic suffering of the type experienced previously, and/or (b) the tactics nonconsciously relied upon to prevent more traumatic suffering of the type experienced previously (such as Gary's mutism and Raoul's rage).

Both of those types of post-traumatic symptoms are understood in coherence therapy as being generated by coherent implicit knowledge acquired through emotional learning.

Suppression of traumatic episodic memory, and the symptoms entailed by that suppression, are coherently necessary according to the nonconscious expectation (the implicit knowledge) that allowing the memory of the traumatic experience into awareness would be an experience of being helplessly engulfed in agony without escape. That expectation of the psychological lethality of the memory is itself a mental model or schema of the nature of the self in relation to the memory: One's self or mind is expected to be overpowered, overwhelmed, and helpless under the memory's destructive and agonizing intensity. This schema is disconfirmed and ceases to exist as soon as the client has been guided skillfully to de-suppress and allow awareness of the memory of the traumatic incident(s), and finds that the expected agonizing, overwhelming feelings have not happened, showing that the self is bigger and stronger than the memory. The de-suppression process must be facilitated in what coherence therapy terms *small enough steps* that feel tolerable and workable to the client at every point, avoiding an excessive degree of subjective immersion that would be retraumatizing and destabilizing. This is what the trauma therapy field recognizes as the necessity of keeping the therapeutic process inside the client's *window of tolerance* so that the client's state allows fruitful participation in the therapeutic process.

Symptoms entailed by semantic (schema) memory of what was learned from what was suffered are coherently necessary according to the particular schema or mental model that was formed, as illustrated by Gary's mutism and Raoul's rage – protective tactics for preventing any more of the same kind of suffering. Any schema learned in trauma includes knowledge of the signs that the particular danger is present, and the schema reactivates in response to any such signs and launches the protective tactic that is also among the knowings in the schema.

Thus, the underlying ingredient that is common to all types of post-traumatic symptoms is the learned expectation of being *helpless* in the face of a particular, learned danger of overwhelming, unbearable suffering. *That knowledge of vulnerability to being rendered helpless in extreme suffering or endangerment is what makes the episodic or semantic memory traumatic,* and hypercharges the schema with extreme urgency to implement self-protective measures such as hypervigilance, avoidance behaviors, and specific situational tactics. Therefore, the understanding within coherence therapy is that *disconfirming and unlearning the expected vulnerability to helplessness is the highest priority for depotentiating traumatic memory and ending post-traumatic symptoms.* How that is done for the helplessness expected from allowing the traumatic incident memory into awareness is described just above. How that is done for the helplessness expected from the danger that was learned in the traumatic incident(s) depends on the client's mental model of that danger.

In complex attachment trauma, also illustrated by the following case example, the client suffered various types of severe mistreatment in childhood regularly in the course of daily life, and across many or all developmental stages, within the child's primary attachment relationships. As conceptualized in coherence therapy, a child's adaptive emotional learning creates a separate schema for each distinct form of suffering repeatedly experienced as part of family life. Each schema consists of the child's knowledge of how that suffering occurs and feels (the problem) and the urgently necessary tactics for preventing or avoiding it (the solution). For example, a schema is formed in response to being again and again unexpectedly blasted with rage and shaming from Dad for making a simple mistake (as Gary experienced), and a different schema is formed from being disallowed dinner and confined to one's bedroom by Mom with frightening coldness and withdrawal of love due to coming home with soiled pants, or a torn shirt, or a missing glove. As chaotic as the client's array of symptoms may seem initially, every symptom proves to be the coherent expression of at least one underlying schema. Therefore, coherence therapy can alleviate complex attachment trauma through persistent implementation of its usual methodology: The client's manifested symptoms are the points of departure for accessing and revealing each of the underlying schemas, which are then subjected to the memory reconsolidation process of unlearning and nullification. The example of Gary, which is continued later, represents complex trauma. Many other coherence therapy case examples of complex trauma have been published (e.g., Ecker (2018), Ecker et al. (2024), and Vaz and Ecker (2020); and session videos are available at coherencetherapy.org).

RESEARCH EVIDENCE SUPPORTING COHERENCE THERAPY

The methodology of coherence therapy is well defined, but it does not consist of a series of specific behavioral actions or techniques that can be predefined. Rather, the therapist facilitates a particular sequence of experiential events using any suitable techniques. For that reason, coherence therapy is not manualizable in the manner that readily allows for conducting randomized controlled trials or other standard types of controlled study. Specialized study design is necessary and has been suggested (Ecker and Vaz, 2022), but has not yet been conducted.

Despite the absence of supporting research, two other factors have enabled coherence therapy to garner widespread interest and respect in the clinical field: First, its methodology consists of creating the same sequence of experiences identified in laboratory studies of memory reconsolidation nullifying an acquired emotional response. Second, numerous published cases of coherence therapy show the moment-to-moment process producing transformational change across a wide range of symptoms and clients. However, these supporting research aspects are not direct, controlled studies, so studies at that level of rigor are needed.

CASE EXAMPLE

TRANSFORMATIONAL CHANGE IN TRAUMATIC MEMORY ENDING POST-TRAUMATIC SYMPTOMS

The case of Gary is presented in this section to illustrate first the experiential process of bringing into direct awareness the implicit, traumatic emotional learning generating his freeze response in social situations and, second, how the transformation phase of coherence therapy carries out the unlearning process of memory reconsolidation. In order to fully protect client confidentiality, this case example weaves together some elements from the work with other clients.

The underlying emotional learning or schema is most accessible in a scene where the symptom happened strongly, so coherence therapy's discovery phase begins by asking the client to bring to mind a recent good example of that, and to be back in that scene in imagination. Gary chose to revisit a dinner party recently given by a co-worker.

TH:	So, there you are. Just notice the tense tightness of your body. *[pause]* Is this a feeling of unsafety? Like something really bad could happen?
CL:	Yeah, it is! *[Said with a note of surprise, indicating new awareness.]*
TH:	OK. Are you ready to find out what's not safe in this scene?
CL:	Mm-hm. Yeah.
TH:	I'm going to say half of a sentence, and then you immediately say it and just let your mind finish it according to the unsafety you're feeling, without any pre-thinking, ok? Here it is: I better *not* talk freely to any people here, because if I did –
CL:	I better *not* talk freely to any people here, because if I did – *[pause]* What comes isn't words, it's this image of my father exploding with rage.

Gary then described a childhood in which unexpected blasts of rage and denigration from his father were frequent. His father would suddenly bellow right next to him, "How can you be so *stupid*!" over even the smallest of little Gary's mistakes, such as an arithmetic error or spilling some milk. Each time, Gary was stunned into a dissociated, frozen state by the scorching intensity of the blast and the terrifying hatred and disgust that he felt in it. This often happened in front of visiting family members or friends, which was searingly shaming, and no one ever came to his defense or objected to his Dad ripping into him like that.

TH: What did that *mean* to you, that no one ever came to your defense?
CL: *[after gazing at the floor for a few seconds]* Well, it meant Dad was right about me and everybody knew it – but I never thought about that before.
TH: Let's keep putting into words what it meant to you and what you learned from that ordeal happening again and again.

By the end of Gary's first session, with the therapist's assistance he had put into words the underlying, discovered emotional truth of his post-traumatic, social anxiety symptoms of frozen mutism:

Dad is right to be that mad at me and scream at me, and everyone sees and agrees that I'm too stupid to be accepted or loved, so I'll always be shamed and rejected by people for saying or doing anything wrong. Saying *anything* around people is so dangerous! I've *got* to make sure I say *nothing* to stay safe!

The therapist wrote those sentences on an index card and gave it to Gary to read daily, "simply to stay in touch with feeling the emotional truth of it, like you are right now." These daily repeated experiences would be progress with the integration phase.

The schema written on the card did not exist in words or linguistic concepts until now, but it consisted of highly specific knowings nevertheless. The therapist had deliberately elicited Gary's learned expectation that *everyone* would respond to him for any mistake in the same way his Dad did, because that generalization construct is the very source of the terrifying danger that Gary feels when among others – the danger of again being helpless under a barrage of angry denigration and shaming – making his mutism urgently necessary. Therefore that generalization construct is the most effective target for being disconfirmed and unlearned. When the target learning is a generalization, finding past contradictory experiences is usually easy, because life is enormously diverse and does not conform to any such monolithic generalization. With that construct of generalization unlearned and nullified, there would be no (subcortical) perception of danger and therefore no need for silencing himself.

In the next session, the therapist first checked with Gary to confirm that he had repeatedly read the card and was now steadily in touch with the emotional truths written on it. Then the therapist began the transformation phase, which subjects the target schema to the memory reconsolidation process of unlearning. This begins with finding contradictory knowledge, which will then become part of the crucial juxtaposition experience of disconfirmation and unlearning. The specific target for disconfirmation was his construct of generalization – the expectation that all people would react like his father – so the therapist directed the search for contradictory knowledge accordingly:

TH: Tell me something: Have you ever visibly said or done something wrong, and the other person *didn't* react in an angry, rejecting way like Dad always did? *[This is the past opposite experiences technique for finding contradictory knowledge.]*

CL: [Gazes into the middle distance for 10 seconds.] Actually, yes, that has happened. [Gary then describes such an incident, and then others come to mind, and the therapist writes them down. Thus, it emerges that Gary is already in possession of contradictory knowledge that can disconfirm the emotional learning that has been tormenting him, but it has been held in a different memory network than the target schema, and the two have never been mindfully experienced in juxtaposition. This is found to be so in a large majority of cases.]

TH: OK. Let's go over some things we know about your life experience of making mistakes, and it would be good if you could let yourself *feel* these things as we review them, to whatever degree you can. On one side is all those many times when Dad became so angry and rejecting over something you said or did wrong, in front of other family members, and that was so stunning, and scary, and shaming for you. And because of all that, you've really expected that most *everyone* would also reject you harshly for any mistake, like Dad did, and would see that you're too stupid to be accepted or loved. You were feeling that expectation at your co-worker's dinner party. Can you feel it again right now, on a gut level? *[That is the first half of a juxtaposition experience that the therapist is creating. Cueing the memory of the dinner party made sure that Gary was freshly feeling the expectation in the present moment.]*

CL: *[nods yes]*

TH: OK. And on the other side, what you have actually *experienced* is all sorts of people who remain *friendly and relaxed* when they see that you've made a mistake. The *store clerk* was friendly and relaxed when you returned the book because you'd bought the wrong one. Your *co-worker* was friendly and relaxed just last week about your mistake of sending him the May figures when he had asked for the March figures. Your *twelfth-grade teacher* was friendly and relaxed about the mistake you made about the structure of the final paper. Your *college advisor* was friendly and relaxed about your mistake over the materials he needed from you. All these people have been so *different* from Dad. Can you feel *that*? *[That creates the juxtaposition experience. Gary had never before held those experiences alongside his experience of his father, in the same field of awareness, in juxtaposition.]*

CL: *[Nods yes, then remains silent as his eyes are now darting around.]*

TH: What are you experiencing now, from being in touch with both sides like that?

CL: I'm feeling sort of surprised, and sort of relieved. *[This indicates that he has allowed the juxtaposition experience to register subjectively, as needed.]*

TH: All your life, you've had that deep old expectation that most everyone will react harshly, like Dad, to any mistake, and yet here are all of your own observations, again and again, that most people *don't* react like Dad to a mistake you've made, and instead they stay friendly and relaxed. And with recognizing that, you have a feeling of *surprise*, and a feeling of *relief*. *[That empathetic review is a deliberate repetition of the juxtaposition experience. A few repetitions complete the unlearning of the generalization via MR.]*

CL: Yeah. Yeah, that's right.

TH: Would you like to get back in touch with this each day for a few seconds – this knowing that so many people *aren't* the same as Dad, even though you expected that they *would* be? *[That is another deliberate repetition.]*

CL: Sure!

TH: OK, then let's create another index card for that. *[Doing so is another repetition.]*

Gary left the session carrying an index card that read:

> All my life, I've been expecting that if I say or do anything wrong, people will react to me like Dad, furious and disgusted with how stupid I am, and somehow I never noticed that actually people have always stayed friendly and relaxed and helpful when they see I've made a mistake – so different from Dad! Noticing that now is a surprise and a relief.

Reading that card daily would repeat the juxtaposition experience each time. In his next session, Gary described a definite easing of his shutting down in various social situations, but he also said, "It wasn't exactly a walk in the park because, well, if everybody *isn't* like Dad – if most people *aren't* like that – now Dad looks really *mean*. Now I feel like I have this cruel father, and I've been pretty agitated about that."

Gary had encountered a distressing consequence of allowing his mental model of people to be disconfirmed: If everyone reacts like Dad, then Dad is a normal parent, but if most people *don't* react like Dad, that means Dad was an *abusive* parent, and that is sharply distressing to recognize. If the distress that would come from schema nullification is strong enough, schema nullification is fully blocked unconsciously, and the schema remains in force, even if the juxtaposition experience was well crafted. That is the phenomenology of resistance to schema disconfirmation. The fact that schema disconfirmation was in progress meant that Gary's distress was tolerable for him, though it needed therapeutic attention. When full resistance occurs, the client is not aware of the distress that is being avoided. That resistance gets cleared away by guiding the client to envision how it will be when the schema no longer feels true, revealing the expected, resulting distress, which then is addressed until it has become either nonexistent or at least tolerable and workable for the client. At that point, the same juxtaposition experience now successfully dissolves the schema.

Gary's shifted perception of his father required several sessions devoted to processing feelings of anger, a need for accountability from his father, and grieving. At that point, with his generalization of his father unlearned and no longer in force, he looked at the therapist, shook his head sadly, and said, "It wasn't *me*. I'm *not* stupid. It was *him*. He *needed* to see me as stupid, so he could feel ok about *himself*." After that, when amongst people he was no longer freezing into mutism. This complex trauma work required a total of eight sessions. Gary may well have had other symptoms maintained by other complex trauma schemas, but he felt no need to continue therapy beyond this point.

STRENGTHS AND LIMITATIONS OF COHERENCE THERAPY FOR POST-TRAUMATIC SYMPTOMS

Strengths include

- Applicable to all types of traumatic memory.
- Therapist is free to use any experiential techniques suitable for discovery, integration, and transformation, including techniques used in other trauma therapies.
- Outcome of transformational change is liberating and life changing for the client and deeply satisfying and sustaining for the therapist.

Limitations include

- The methodology is well defined but there is no fixed protocol of techniques for carrying it out; rather, the therapist chooses from familiar experiential techniques to fit the client's styles and material. Therefore, safety and success with traumatic memory require the therapist to be experienced, comfortable, and skillful in working with intensely distressing emotion, or else to have close supervision by an experienced coherence therapy practitioner.
- Like some other trauma therapies, coherence therapy involves de-suppression of traumatic memory, which requires skillful facilitation of attention process, memory process, and emotional process so that the pace of de-suppression is well controlled, and the emerging episodic memory material stays within the client's range of tolerance and is never retraumatizing.

There is a modification of usual coherence therapy methodology that is often needed when working with severe trauma: Normally, the therapist assigns a between-session task that at least maintains, but may also advance, the current session's new progress in discovery, integration, or transformation. However, when a session has brought new awareness of de-suppressed traumatic memory, the therapist asks the client near the end of the session, "Let's think about how it would be for you to be in touch with this on your own between sessions, without having me accompanying you in it. Does that seem okay, or is it somewhat uneasy?" If the client indicates *any* uneasiness or unsureness about that, the therapist stabilizes the situation by saying, "I understand, and what I suggest is for you to forget all about these things between sessions, and only when we are together *during* sessions will we revisit them. Okay?" Such permission to re-suppress what was retrieved in the session usually results in the client being able to do so.

RESOURCES FOR LEARNING

See the following References section for each of the books, chapters, and articles listed here.

- Book: *Coherence Therapy Practice Manual and Training Guide.*
- Book: Unlocking the Emotional Brain: Memory Reconsolidation and the Psychotherapy of Transformational Change (2nd Edition) has many case examples addressing a wide range of post-traumatic symptoms.
- Book chapter: "Coherence therapy: The roots of problems and the transformation of old solutions."
- Journal article: "Clinical Translation of Memory Reconsolidation Research" has two detailed case examples of coherence therapy for post-traumatic symptoms.
- Journal article: "Memory Reconsolidation in Psychotherapy for Severe Perfectionism Within Borderline Personality" shows complex trauma symptoms ended mainly using coherence therapy.
- On-demand webinar, 75 minutes: "Trauma Creates Emotional Learnings That Are Unlearned and Depotentiated by Memory Reconsolidation" presented by Bruce Ecker, on coherencetherapy.org.
- On-demand webinar, 6 hours: **"Coherence Therapy: Facilitating Transformational Change Through Memory Reconsolidation"** presented by Bruce Ecker, shows several session videos of trauma work, on coherencetherapy.org.

REFERENCES

Clem, R.L., & Schiller, D. (2016). New learning and unlearning: Strangers or accomplices in threat memory attenuation? *Trends in Neuroscience, 39*(5), 340–351. doi:10.1016/j.tins.2016.03.003

Coherence Psychology Institute (2023). Published case studies, indexed by symptom, demonstrating the therapeutic reconsolidation process as facilitated in Coherence Therapy, promptly producing transformational change. https://bit.ly/2tKXdyX

Díaz-Mataix, L., Ruiz Martinez, R.C., Schafe, G.E., LeDoux, J.E., & Doyère, V. (2013). Detection of a temporal error triggers reconsolidation of amygdala-dependent memories. *Current Biology, 23*, 1–6. doi:10.1016/j.cub.2013.01.053

Ecker, B. (2006, July). The effectiveness of psychotherapy. Keynote address, *12th Biennial Conference of the Constructivist Psychology Network*, University of California, San Marcos. Published as: Ecker, B. (2015). Psychotherapy's mysterious efficacy ceiling: Is memory reconsolidation the breakthrough? The Neuropsychotherapist *16*, 6–24. doi:10.12744/tnpt(16)006-024

Ecker, B. (2018). Clinical translation of memory reconsolidation research: Therapeutic methodology for transformational change by erasing implicit emotional learnings driving symptom production. *International Journal of Neuropsychotherapy, 6*(1), 1–92. doi:10.12744/ijnpt.2018.0001-0092

Ecker, B. (2021, November 19). Reconsolidation behavioral updating of human emotional memory: A comprehensive review and unified analysis of successes, replication failures, and clinical translation. PsyArXiv. doi:10.31234/osf.io/atz3m

Ecker, B., & Bridges, S.K. (2020). How the science of memory reconsolidation advances the effectiveness and unification of psychotherapy. *Clinical Social Work Journal, 48*(3), 287–300. doi:10.1007/s10615-020-00754-z

Ecker, B., & Hulley, L. (1996). *Depth oriented brief therapy: How to be brief when you were trained to be deep, and vice versa.* San Francisco, CA: Wiley/Jossey-Bass.

Ecker, B., & Hulley, L. (2019). *Coherence therapy practice manual and training guide.* Albany, CA: Coherence Psychology Institute. Online: www.coherencetherapy.org/resources/manual.htm

Ecker, B., Ticic, R., & Hulley, L. (2024). *Unlocking the emotional brain: Memory reconsolidation and the psychotherapy of transformational change* (2ndEdition). New York, NY and Abingdon, UK: Routledge.

Ecker, B., & Vaz, A. (2022). Memory reconsolidation and the crisis of mechanism in psychotherapy. *New Ideas in Psychology, 66,* 100945, 1–11. doi:10.1016/j.newideapsych.2022.100945

McGaugh, J.L., & Roozendaal, B. (2002). Role of adrenal stress hormones in forming lasting memories in the brain. *Current Opinions in Neurobiology, 12,* 205–210. doi:10.1016/s0959-4388(02)00306-9

Vaz, A., & Ecker, B. (2020). Memory reconsolidation in psychotherapy for severe perfectionism within borderline personality. *Journal of Clinical Psychology, 76*(11), 2067–2078. doi:10.1002/jclp.23058

14

CHAPTER 14
ACCELERATED EXPERIENTIAL DYNAMIC PSYCHOTHERAPY (AEDP)

A Model of Change and Transformation

Ben Medley

INTRODUCTION

Accelerated experiential dynamic psychotherapy (AEDP) seeks to alleviate the negative effects of trauma by harnessing clients' innate healing capacities and facilitating corrective emotional and relational experiences that lead to positive change and transformation. This empirically validated model integrates emotion theory, attachment theory, affective neuroscience, body-based approaches, interpersonal neurobiology, and transformational studies into a comprehensive and coherent framework. Through the lens of AEDP, trauma is defined as unbearable aloneness in the face of overwhelming negative emotions and experiences. The AEDP therapist, therefore, seeks to undo aloneness by helping clients access, regulate, and viscerally process these emotions in the context of a safe, attachment-based relationship. To help guide the therapist in this process, AEDP delineates a four-state phenomenological map of the transformational process. As suffering gives way to relief, AEDP therapists work diligently with experiences of change and transformation to promote feelings of vitality, well-being, and flourishing and to recover the client's sense of their core selves. Over time, these healing emotional and relational experiences with the therapist can be internalized, so that the client has greater access and ability to regulate their emotional life in relationship to others and the burden of trauma is lifted.

BRIEF HISTORY

AEDP officially entered the field of psychotherapy as a new approach and model in the year 2000 with the publication of Fosha's (2000) book *The Transforming Power of Affect: A Model for Accelerated Change*. Developed by Fosha, AEDP has its origins in developmentally oriented relational psychoanalysis, short-term dynamic psychotherapy (STDP), and intensive short-term dynamic psychotherapy (ISTDP) (Fosha, 2021a; Iwakabe et al., 2022; Prenn & Fosha, 2017). Although STDP, ISTDP, and AEDP share similarities both in title and in an emphasis on emotional processing, AEDP differs fundamentally in orientation. Rather than focusing on pathology and challenging defenses, AEDP takes a healing-oriented approach of "radical empathy and emotional engagement through attunement, resonance, affect sharing, affirmation and self-disclosure" (Fosha, 2000, p. 3).

DOI: 10.4324/9781003455851-14

AEDP is a model of transformation and is also itself an ever-transforming model. In the two decades following the publication of *The Transforming Power of Affect*, AEDP has grown considerably in theory, practice, and scope. What started as a three-state model of affective change in 2000 has grown to the current four-state model and the core concepts of AEDP have been expanded and elaborated over time. In fact, AEDP continues to incorporate findings from research in the fields of positive affect, change processes and psychotherapy outcome, as well as from clinical observation and empirical investigation of transformational phenomena contained within video recorded sessions of AEDP clinical work (Iwakabe & Conceiçao, 2016).

In 2005, Fosha founded the AEDP Institute (Prenn & Fosha, 2017) and thousands of clinicians around the world have attended AEDP training courses and seminars. In addition, the AEDP Institute boasts a robust and continuously expanding global community consisting of faculty, certified supervisors, certified clinicians, satellite local communities, an online community, and the AEDP Practice Research Network (Fosha, 2021a).

FUNDAMENTAL CLINICAL CONCEPTS

First and foremost, AEDP is a model of psychotherapy that is healing-oriented in both theory and practice. Rather than focusing on understanding the complexity of one's psychopathology and how to reverse and counteract it, that is, *what's going wrong*, AEDP assumes a healthy core in all individuals, choosing to centralize healing, that is, *what's going right*. As such, AEDP conceptualizes trauma and the development of psychopathology as resulting from one's unwilled and unwanted aloneness in the face of overwhelming, intense, painful, and frightening affective experiences (Fosha, 2021a). Likewise, symptoms of distress and suffering represent one's best efforts to adapt, cope, and stay connected to others at the time in which the trauma occurred. The primary goal of AEDP, therefore, is to utilize a client's natural healing capacities and to undo aloneness by helping the client have a new, *corrective emotional and relational* experience. This is accomplished by assisting the client in fully embodying their affective experience and processing it to completion in the safety of a secure, attachment-based relationship with the therapist. The positive experiences and emotions associated with these new experiences are then dedicated as much attention and focus as the ones associated with trauma and suffering. Thus, through the moment-to-moment visceral processing of emotional and relational experiences, clients are aided in recovering a sense of their core selves and experiencing an increased sense of resilience and renewed vitality (Fosha, Thoma & Yeung, 2019).

This section will focus on seven fundamental concepts in AEDP: 1) Healing from the get-go; 2) Undoing aloneness and the AEDP stance; 3) Relational processing; 4) The processing of emotion to completion; 5) Dyadic regulation of affect; 6) Metaprocessing; and 7) The transformational process: The four-state model of AEDP.

HEALING FROM THE GET-GO

AEDP holds the strong belief that all people have a wired-in, adaptive neurobiological drive toward healing, growth, self-righting, and flourishing. Referred to in AEDP as *transformance* (Fosha, 2004, 2021b), this drive represents the human potential for positive neuroplasticity that is wired deep in the brain, ready to be activated and awakened in the right environment (Doidge, 2007; Hanson, 2017). AEDP maintains that this drive is present in all people, at all times, no matter how severe the pathology (Fosha, 2021b). Like a blade of grass sprouting from a crack in the concrete, if one is looking for it, amidst suffering, distress, anxiety, and defenses, the transformance drive can be found (Fosha, Thoma & Yeung, 2019). Therefore, from the very first moments of therapy, aka "from the get-go," AEDP therapists become *transformance detectives* actively looking for the slightest glimmers of this drive (Iwakabe et al., 2022). These strivings are distinguished by somatic and affective markers of vitality and energy (Fosha, 2021b), referred to in AEDP as *vitality affects.* Once spotted, these glimmers of transformance can be brought front and center in the therapy so that they can be worked with experientially (Fosha, Thoma & Yeung, 2019).

UNDOING ALONENESS AND THE AEDP STANCE

AEDP recognizes the importance of co-creating safety with the client in order to venture into deep therapeutic work. To aid in building safety, the AEDP therapist approaches clients with a therapeutic stance informed by attachment theory and developmental research into caregiver-infant interactions. The AEDP therapist is encouraging and emotionally engaged, shows compassion toward the client's suffering, is deliberately positive, and shows empathy for their experience (Fosha, 2009b; Lipton & Fosha, 2011). The stance is active, and therapists are encouraged to explicitly affirm and delight in the "quintessential qualities" of the client (Fosha, 2009a, p. 181). The AEDP therapist also explicitly communicates a desire to have an authentic relationship with the client and welcomes all their feelings and experiences into the therapeutic relationship. Likewise, AEDP stresses therapists' openness and authenticity with a willingness to self-disclose information about themselves or their experience. Gone is the psychoanalytic notion of the blank screen. Instead, the AEDP therapist allows themselves to explicitly be part of the therapy with the assurance that intentional and judicious self-disclosure aids in encouraging client vulnerability and in fostering secure attachment (Fosha, 2000). Self disclosure can certainly include sharing facts about oneself, but also disclosing one's affective experience with and for the client, always with a goal of undoing aloneness and/or deepening the affective experience. For instance, when a client shares that they feel sad, the therapist may include that they too feel sad to help deepen the emotion and convey that the client is not alone.

RELATIONAL PROCESSING

A distinguishing feature of AEDP is an emphasis on processing the relational experience between the therapist and client. If the AEDP stance is attachment based, then the AEDP therapist aims to be an active attachment figure, consistently tracking the moment-to-moment experiences of attachment the client is having with the therapist (Hanakawa, 2021). Many trauma therapies focus on the impact trauma can have on the individual, while ignoring the impact trauma can have on relationships with others. Thus, AEDP seeks to help restore the client's trust in relational processes. A common question throughout AEDP therapy is "how are we doing?" and "what's it like to do this *with me*?" Like the "good enough" caregiver, the AEDP therapist also seeks to be attuned to the client with a readiness to repair and return to attunement should and when a rupture occurs in the relationship. From a progressively more and more secure base; fear, anxiety, guilt, and shame can be alleviated, and previously overwhelming feelings and experiences can be explored more and more (Fosha, 2000, 2021b).

In addition, the AEDP therapist tracks the client's *receptive affective experience*. AEDP holds that it is insufficient for the therapist to care for a client; in order to be effective and have any impact relationally, this care must be received by the client (Fosha, 2021b). Therefore, the AEDP therapist encourages clients to take in and integrate the care of the therapist to help undo aloneness and expand relational possibilities. For example, a therapist may ask, "What's it like to hear me say that?" after expressing compassion for the client. Likewise, when the therapist is moved by the client in a session and self-discloses this, they may ask, "What's it like to know/see that I am moved by you?" Not only can the therapist help expand the client's receptive affective capacity by matching words with visible affect, but the therapist is also helping to deepen relational experiences and build secure attachment by promoting a felt sense of "existing in the heart and mind of the other" (Fosha, 2000).

PROCESSING EMOTION TO COMPLETION

AEDP places an emphasis on emotional processing, recognizing that emotions bring with them a sense of aliveness and that they provide information about how to respond to the situation evoking the feeling (Fosha, 2009a). Essentially, the categorical emotions – anger, sadness, fear, disgust, surprise, and joy – contain within them *adaptive action tendencies*. These adaptive action tendencies empower people to be aware of their needs and to take action to fulfill them (Fosha, 2004, 2009a). As such, emotions can be viewed as "the experiential arc between the problem and the solution" (Fosha, 2009a, p. 32). When there is danger, fear can lead to escape; when there is a loss, grief can lead to acceptance; and when there is an injustice, anger can lead to assertion on behalf of the self or others.

However, many people enter therapy with difficulty accessing the fullness of their emotional experience and are operating with limited resources. The emotions associated with traumatic events can exceed a person's capacities and be too overwhelming to feel and process. Without anyone to help, survival dictates the use of defenses to manage these feelings and the affected person then loses access to the adaptive action tendencies and all that they bestow (Yeung, 2021). The AEDP therapist, therefore, seeks to help access emotions that have been disavowed, defended against, or excluded from experience out of necessity (Lipton & Fosha, 2011), so that they can be processed to completion. In this sense, "processing emotion to completion" simply refers to the AEDP therapist and the client working together with an emotion until there is a shift from one's experience feeling bad in some way to feeling better in some way. As Fosha (2004) recognizes, processing painful experiences in the context of the therapeutic relationship often feels good. It can bring a sense of relief and relaxation of tension and a felt sense of the experience feeling "right" (Fosha, 2004).

DYADIC REGULATION OF AFFECT

Dyadic regulation of affect experientially links the undoing of aloneness with the processing of emotions (Fosha, 2021b). Not only is the AEDP therapist assuming a stance welcoming of all their client's affective experiences, but the AEDP therapist also helps dyadically regulate these emotional experiences when they are, and historically have been, too overwhelming to process alone (Fosha, 2021b). Often, when the negative affects associated with trauma and suffering come to the fore, they can be intense and exceed the client's window of tolerance (Siegel, 1999). The AEDP therapist, therefore, actively works to assist the client in staying within this window by co-regulating affective experience as needed. What could not be processed alone can then be processed together with an empathetic, attuned, and responsive therapist (Fosha, 2009b, 2011).

METATHERAPEUTIC PROCESSING

One of the major contributions Fosha and AEDP have made to the experiential therapies is the concept of *metatherapeutic processing* (Grotstein, 2002). Fosha (2009b) asserts that although the aim in therapy is to have a new corrective emotional and relational experience, that alone is not sufficient. For these new experiences to truly be effective, the client needs to be aware, both cognitively and somatically, that something new has occurred. Metatherapeutic processing, also referred to as *metaprocessing*, allows for the experience of transformation itself to be explored and integrated as it unfolds in the moment through alternating waves of experiencing and reflecting on the experience. In practice, metaprocessing requires the question, "What is it like to do this piece of work with me?" (Fosha, 2000; Iwakabe & Conceiçao, 2016).

THE TRANSFORMATIONAL PROCESS: THE FOUR-STATE MODEL OF AEDP

AEDP outlines an elaborate four-state map of the transformational process (Fosha, 2009a; 2009c; 2021b). This map acts as a guide for clinicians by delineating the phenomenology corresponding to each state. With this map in mind, the AEDP clinician is then able to not only track the process of change in the moment-to-moment unfolding of the session, but also recognize and systematically work with the experiential markers along the way. Where the client is on the map informs how one intervenes at any given moment, and then what happens next informs the following intervention, and so on. The arc of transformation moves from suffering to flourishing, from negative to positive, from stuck to unstuck, from bad to good, and from experiences of the *self-at-worst* to the *self-at-best* (Fosha, 2000).

DESCRIPTION OF THE THERAPY PROCESS: FACILITATING THE FOUR-STATE TRANSFORMATIONAL PROCESS

In practice, the AEDP therapist is relentlessly experiential. As a general guideline, AEDP therapists make the implicit, explicit; the explicit, experiential; and the experiential, relational (Prenn & Fosha, 2017). Sessions are dually focused on the client's internal affective experience as it occurs in the body and on the here-and-now relational experience in the therapeutic dyad (Fosha, 2021b). As opposed to top-down interventions using cognition and understanding to affect change, AEDP privileges bottom-up processing of bodily based experiences, actively shifting the client away from in-the-head cognitions to in-the-body, present-moment sensing and feeling. As such, the AEDP therapist invites the client to slow down, notice, and stay with their affective experiences. In this section, each of the four states in the AEDP transformational map are defined in the following, with illustrations demonstrating how to utilize AEDP in clinical work.

STATE ONE: STRESS, DISTRESS, SYMPTOMS, AND TRANSFORMANCE

State One (Stress, Distress, Symptoms, and Transformance) is where AEDP therapy often begins as clients present with experiences of stress, distress, and suffering. This state is marked by the presence of defenses and inhibitory affects such as anxiety, shame, guilt, and demoralization. Defenses and inhibitory affects are recognized in AEDP as a client's best attempts to manage trauma and to protect a client against painful emotional and relational experiences. However, right alongside the negative consequences of trauma, lies transformance. The goal then for the AEDP therapist is to help the client relinquish their defenses, reduce the impact of inhibitory affects, and drop down into their core affective experience. This is accomplished in AEDP through the co-creation of safety with the AEDP stance and noticing and focusing on glimmers of transformance (Fosha, 2021b). Defenses can be bypassed with permission, asking, "would it be okay if we stayed with this sadness for a moment?" or "do you mind if we go back to what just happened?" Defenses can also be appreciated and "melted" by empathetically acknowledging their original context and function, saying, for example, "of course you needed to push your feelings aside given what was happening at that time." Likewise, if the client is experiencing high levels of anxiety, blocking the path to emotional experience, the AEDP therapist can help reduce anxiety with dyadic regulation. Several methods may be employed: Slowing down, prosody of voice, eye gazing, synchronized breathing, head nodding, or even paraverbal sounds and holding, with a simple "mmm-hmmm."

During this phase of work, the AEDP therapist uses moment-to-moment tracking to be on the lookout for glimmers of emotional experience (Prenn, 2009). These glimmers manifest in the form of the transitional affects: *Heralding affects* and *green signal affects*. The heralding affects are defined as glimmers of core affective experiences and may manifest as the client's eyes beginning to tear, a clenched fist, or a sigh. In addition to somatic markers, a heralding affect could also be an emotion-rich word, such as "sad" or "heartbroken" that the therapist explicitly notices to explore the accompanying internal emotional experience (Prenn & Fosha, 2017). For example, a therapist might simply say, "I see so much feeling in your eyes" or "Tell me more about feeling heartbroken" then inviting the client, "Can we stay with that for a moment?" Green signal affects then announce the client's openness to or curiosity about their emotional experience, indicating that the client feels safe, or safe enough, to move forward (Fosha, 2000; Russell, 2015). This may manifest as curiosity or hope, a lowering of anxiety or even a verbal agreement to stay with the experience such as the client stating, "Yes, we can stay with this."

STATE TWO: ADAPTIVE CORE AFFECTIVE EXPERIENCE

In State Two (Adaptive Core Affective Experience), the client "drops down" into the core affective experiences that had been defended against and blocked in State One. As such, processing core affects to completion and the dyadic regulation of affect become the primary focus of the therapeutic work. *Core affects* in AEDP are the deeply wired-in, somatically based, adaptive affective experiences which include the categorical emotions of sadness, joy, anger, surprise, and disgust, as well as relational experiences (feeling connected and/or seen and understood), recognition processes (feelings of familiarity when something resonates), receptive affective experiences (feeling seen, understood, and known), authentic self-expression (the undefended truth of one's experience) and others (Fosha 2000, 2021b). This section will focus on State Two processing of emotion as a means for transformation and healing.

Having co-created enough relational safety in State One, the AEDP therapist aids the client in accessing the negative emotions associated with trauma and suffering. Core emotions move like a wave: They rise, they peak, and then begin to disperse. Often, however, the emotions associated with trauma can be scary, overwhelming, and painful. Keeping this in mind, the AEDP therapist utilizes moment-to-moment tracking to carefully monitor clients' emotional experience. As the wave of emotion begins to swell, clients may exit a window of tolerance and require active assistance from the therapist to help regulate arousal back within a window of tolerance (Fosha, 2000). Employing dyadic regulation, emotions may be down-regulated when they become dysregulated or overwhelming (hyperarousal), or they may be up-regulated when the client begins to shut down emotional expression (hypoarousal) (Medley, 2021). For instance, if a client is overwhelmed with feelings of sadness, the therapist may move closer to the client (while asking permission and tracking to make sure this doesn't add to their being overwhelmed), speak slowly in a low, calming tone of voice, place their hand over their own heart, take a big deep breath while making eye contact and say, "So much feeling .... Just stay with it ... I'm right here with you .... You're doing great." Likewise, if a client requires up-regulation when, for example, accessing anger, a therapist may sit upright in their chair, speak more loudly and quicken their speech, bringing attention to somatic activation in the client's body saying, "Really let yourself have this feeling .... Yes! What does your fist want to say or do?" The therapist is affirming and encouraging with each step the client takes in feeling and expressing emotional experience. As the wave begins to fall and dissipate, a positive shift occurs marked by the emergence of the *post-breakthrough affects*, which include a sense of relief or hope and/or feeling lighter, stronger, or more assertive. The post-breakthrough experiences transition the therapeutic work into State Three.

STATE THREE: TRANSFORMATIONAL EXPERIENCES

In State Three (Transformational Experiences), corrective emotional and relational experiences are made explicit and the client's experience of the successful completion of a piece of therapeutic work is explored (Fosha, 2007; Iwakabe & Conceiçao, 2016). This is accomplished with metaprocessing. For example, if after processing a wave of emotion the postbreakthrough affects surface as the client visibly settles into their chair and takes a big breath, the therapist might comment, "That was a big breath" and then ask the client, "What's it like to ride this wave of feeling with me?" Iwakabe and Conceiçao (2016) noted in their study of metaprocessing that focusing on the positive experiences following a wave of emotion led to the emergence of another positive emotion and so on. Thus, metaprocessing can initiate a round of transformational affects, one leading to another, referred to in AEDP as *the transformational spiral*. In this spiral, one may encounter any or all of the six transformational affects: 1) the mastery affects (pride and joy), 2) the mourning-the-self affects (grief and sadness for the self), 3) the healing affects associated with recognition and affirmation (gratitude, tenderness, and/or feeling moved), 4) the tremulous affects associated with the experience of quantum change, 5) the realization affects (the "yes" and "wow" affects and/or the click of recognition) associated with new understanding, and 6) the enlivening affects (experiences of increased energy and excitement) (Fosha, 2000, 2021b; Yeung, 2021).

Once the transformational spiral is set in motion, the AEDP therapist helps the client stay with, explore, and expand the transformational affects so that they too can be processed to completion and then metaprocessed. This is positive neuroplasticity in motion. With each round of metaprocessing, right brain affective experiences become understood and organized in the left brain (Lipton & Fosha, 2011). As this occurs, a new coherent and cohesive narrative begins to emerge, indicating the formation of secure attachment and resilience (Lipton & Fosha, 2011).

STATE FOUR: CORE STATE AND THE TRUTH SENSE

In State Four (core state and the truth sense), the negative consequences of trauma are gone, replaced by a sense of one or more of the following: Openness, increased empathy with others and with the self, clarity, confidence, creativity, relaxation, wisdom, generosity, a sense of sacredness, and/or connection to self and others (Fosha, 2021b). Clients often report a sense of ease, presence, and deep calm. In this state of being, *the truth sense* begins to emerge, a deeply pleasurable affective experience of rightness and the subjective truth of one's experience (Fosha, 2000, 2004, 2009a). The truth sense is not about things *being right*, but rather, things *feeling right*. As such, neural integration comes to the fore and the benefits of the preceding therapeutic work become integrated into the self. New coherent and cohesive auto-biographical narratives coalesce, reflective of the new, positive experiences in therapy. For instance, a client may experience greater clarity and compassion about the trauma they experienced and how they managed it, as well as how they have changed and transformed. In core state, the client also encounters their *core self*. This experience is often accompanied by a profound sense of revelation and recognition at feeling deeply one's self, without the need for defenses or inhibitory affects. When this occurs, a client may remark simply, "This is me."

The therapeutic task in State Four is to be with and explore core state experiences. More than anything, the therapist seeks to offer their own presence and allow for the spaciousness of the client's experience, encouraging the client to savor each moment with phrases like, "Really let yourself be with this calm feeling" and "Soak this in." In this state, metaprocessing the experience deepens the truth sense, feelings of calm and peacefulness, and the connection to the felt core self. The therapist may simply ask, "What's it like to know this about your experience?" or "What's it like to be so you?" The relational experience can also be made explicit and metaprocessed as well, asking the client "What's it like to experience this *with me?*"

UTILIZATION OF MODEL FOR THE TREATMENT OF TRAUMA

AEDP was originally conceptualized as helping clients with attachment trauma, experiences of omission or commission with caregivers and significant attachment figures in childhood that resulted in an unbearable sense of aloneness for the infant/child. Trauma is not defined by an event itself, as it has been established that people can have varied responses to difficult situations and overwhelming events. Rather, trauma occurs as a result of the absence of a soothing, regulating other to effectively process these negative experiences and events. For this reason, AEDP therapists seek to be there for the client in the ways that others were not, for whatever reason, in order to process these difficult experiences with the client. Over time, this model has also expanded to address other forms of trauma, recognizing that this can occur in other situations beyond childhood, and that AEDP can be useful in addressing symptoms of trauma like PTSD, depression, anxiety, and low self-compassion (Iwakabe et al., 2020, 2022).

In recent years, AEDP has also begun to specifically address the trauma of oppression, recognizing the negative impact systems of power, privilege, and oppression can have on an individual. The trauma of oppression includes the institutional and inter-relational expression of stereotypes, prejudice, and discrimination based on race, sexual orientation, gender, religious affiliation, nationality, ethnicity, age, class, size, and/or ability (David & Derthick, 2017). Recognizing that people form attachments to groups as well as individuals (Smith, Murphy & Coats, 1999), Medley (2024) developed the Triangle of Social Experience, a representational schema of internal working models and affective experience. This tool aids the AEDP therapist in conceptualizing and being mindful of how models of social groups, both social groups of the self and social groups of others, have been internalized by clients. What has been internalized through experiences of oppression institutionally and inter-relationally can have a negative impact on how one views the self, what can be expected of others, and what can be expected of particular social groups. In turn, the trauma of oppression can also affect the amount of access one has to emotional and relational experiences. In psychotherapy, therefore, therapists explicitly recognize and explore how social dynamics and the social experience of the client may contribute to their negative symptoms. AEDP can then be utilized to help clients move through the four states and liberate the core self from internalized oppression.

ASSESSMENT OF RESEARCH EVIDENCE REGARDING EFFECTIVENESS IN TREATING TRAUMA

The AEDP Research Network conducts research on the effectiveness of AEDP based on 16 sessions with follow-up research at the six-month and one-year markers. Research published by Iwakabe et al. (2020, 2022) supports the empirical validity of AEDP, showing that AEDP is effective in alleviating a wide variety of psychological symptoms associated with trauma, including depression, a subjective sense of distress, negative thoughts, emotional dysregulation, interpersonal problems, and experiential avoidance. It has also demonstrated effectiveness in improving positive psychological functioning such as self-compassion and a sense of well-being (Iwakabe et al., 2020, 2022). These improvements were found to be long-lasting at six months, 12 months and beyond (Iwakabe et al., 2022).

LIMITATIONS AND CONSIDERATIONS

AEDP, like most models of therapy, is not well-suited or recommended for all clients. Research into AEDP conducted by Iwakabe et al. (2020, 2022) excluded individuals reporting certain symptoms and diagnosis including active suicidality, addiction, and substance misuse; psychosis and severe impulse disorders, bipolar disorder, moderate to severe autism spectrum diagnosis; and a crisis situation that required immediate crisis intervention, such as intimate partner violence (Iwakabe et al., 2020, 2022). Clients experiencing any of these situations may better be treated by a physician or psychiatrist and/or another form of therapy that specifically addresses the client's needs and immediate concerns. More research is needed into the application of AEDP with clients experiencing these conditions.

CASE EXAMPLE

The following case example will illustrate how AEDP can be utilized in clinical practice. This section will outline a single session using AEDP in all four states in the transformational process, though this is not meant to imply that every AEDP session will, or should, include work in all four states. This example of an early session in AEDP will focus on work with Matteo, an Italian American, gay, cisgender male in his mid-30s. Matteo entered AEDP therapy to address symptoms of anxiety and feeling overwhelmed. In the prior session, the therapist and client uncovered that, at a very early age, Matteo experienced multiple attachment ruptures with peers and family members based in heterosexism that were never repaired. Any self-expression deemed "feminine" or "gay" was met with hostility and rejection. As a result, he began to hide his true self, defensively exclude emotions, and protect himself relationally from the potential pain of attachment ruptures with others. As this was an early session, the therapist was focused on co-creating enough relational safety with the client to begin accessing and processing his emotional experience. Snippets of dialogue have been included to help give the reader an in-the-moment experience of the client and of the therapist's interventions.

WORKING IN STATE ONE

When the client entered the session, he reported that he had not slept well due to anxiety. He expressed frustration about experiencing these symptoms and reported negative self-talk, including blaming himself for his struggles. Alongside these State One symptoms, however, were also glimmers of the client's transformance strivings. The client reported that he had been "stressed and anxious" and that he wanted to "move forward" and "get out of the cycle" that he was in. Assuming the AEDP stance, the therapist focused on and affirmed the client's transformance drive to move forward. After doing so, the client took a risk to be vulnerable and stated that he needed help. The therapist then affirmed this risk and asked what it was like to be vulnerable in this way with him, focusing on the in-the-moment relational experience. The client recognized that his defenses were lowering "like a wall going down." The therapist affirmed the client again and appreciated that the walls must have been there for a very good reason.

CLIENT:	*Yeah. It's kind of a self-preservation thing. If I ask for help, I'm afraid I'm going to be seen as a weak person. So right now, I imagine a wall going down.*
THERAPIST:	*Ok …. Wow. It's like a wall going down right now?* [Affirming client; focusing on transformation and in the moment experience]
C:	*Yeah. And right now, I'm fine but then I start thinking about how I'm going to be able to put that wall down without feeling unsafe in other aspects of my life.*
TH:	*Right, yeah. Good question. Would it be okay if we hold onto that question?* [Asking permission to bypass client's intellectual defense, to return to in-the-moment experiencing]
C:	(Nodding) *Ok.* [Green signal that client is willing to move ahead]
TH:	*Great. So, we'll hold onto it, just to give us space to be with this experience of letting that wall down and to acknowledge together that there's a part of you that wants and needs help … because that's such an important thing to acknowledge.* [Affirming client, focusing on transformance strivings] *And as you're saying, it's a little scary because there's a fear that I might see you as weak* (C nods), *is that right?* [Asking for confirmation to be collaborative and so that we can work directly with the relational experience]
C:	*Yeah, but it's more me thinking about that … because otherwise I wouldn't be here.*
TH:	*Right, sure. So, if I'm understanding you correctly, you're seeing that maybe I don't think that about you? Is that right?* [Focusing on relational experience to help relinquish need for defense and build relational safety]
C:	*Yeah, that's right.* [Green signal]
TH:	*Yeah, great. I'm so glad you can see that because it's true. I don't see you as weak. Not at all. In fact, I'm appreciating that you're being vulnerable with me and that it feels safe enough to do that. That feels good to me.* [Self-disclosing to build relational safety]

WORKING IN STATE TWO

With the relinquishing of defenses and the co-creation of more relational safety, the client then began to drop into State Two affective experience as tears appeared in his eyes.

TH: *What's coming up inside?* [Noticing and focusing on emotional experience, speaking slowly and waiting]

C: *It's just been so hard.* [Recognizing the truth of his experience and deepening affective experience.]

TH: (Speaking slowly in deep tones) *Yeah. It has. I see that. I feel that. Let's just stay with it and make lots of space together.* [Inviting client to stay with emotion and explicitly communicating therapist's openness to feeling]. (After a moment) *What would you name this feeling?*

C: (Beginning to cry) *Sadness. I feel sad.*

TH: *Yeah … just welcome it … yeah … (as client begins to cry more) I'm right here.* [Affirming client, welcoming emotion, encouraging him, dyadically regulating to relationally undo aloneness]

Matteo continued to cry while the therapist used moment-to-moment tracking to look for signs that the client was keeping within a window of tolerance. At one point, the client was no longer looking at the therapist and appeared to be struggling to manage affect. The therapist moved his chair closer to the client to help dyadically regulate his experience, checking with the client to make sure that moving closer felt okay to him. When he replied that it was okay, the therapist stated, "Good I just want you to know that I'm here with you as you feel this" and inquired about his receptive affective experience, adding, "Can you feel me here with you?" Matteo responded that he could, and another wave of emotion arose as he continued to cry. After a moment, the crying lessened, and he visibly settled. Matteo reached for a tissue, took a deep breath, and looked up at the therapist as he wiped his eyes. The State Two wave of emotion seemed to be completed, and the client began to experience the post-breakthrough affects as indicated by a visible relaxation in the body. Matteo took another big breath and the therapist leaned back in his chair and joined him, stating, "That was a big wave of feeling." Matteo nodded and responded, "Yes, it certainly was."

WORKING IN STATE THREE

The therapist then began to metaprocess this piece of therapeutic work, asking "What's that like to ride that wave of feeling together?" The client replied that it felt "good" and when asked to "say more," he stated that he felt "safe, comfortable, and more relaxed." The therapist affirmed the client with a simple "Wow" and continued to metaprocess, asking "What's that like to feel safe, relaxed, and comfortable?"

C: *It's weird.*

TH: *It's weird. Yeah, sometimes weird means new … is that right?* [Making the implicit explicit]

C: *Yeah. It's new.* [Green signal]

TH: *Great. And if I'm getting this right, you seem to be saying that this is a new experience to let that wall down and feel all your emotions with me … with someone else?* [Making the new experience explicit, while also making sure this feels right to the client]

C: (Nodding) *Yeah ….*

TH: *Yeah, wow … what a great new thing ….* [Affirming client's experience]

C: *It is great … and I feel like there's nothing wrong with being emotional in this way.* [Realization affect]

TH: *Me neither. I'm starting to tear up too. It's moving to hear you say, "I feel safe" and "I can be me with all of my feelings." Especially given all that we talked about in the last session.* [Self-disclosing, letting client know that he has an impact on the therapist to deepen experience] *What's that like to see and hear?* [Checking receptive affective capacity]

C: *It feels good. I'm feeling that too.* [Healing affect] *I feel connected.* (He motions from self to therapist) *It's like we are here together. It's you and it's me.*

As the dyad continued to metaprocess, the client experienced a deeper sense of relief and the therapist inquired, "How is relief showing up in your body?" Focusing on the bodily sensations helped expand the positive experience and Matteo noticed a sense of openness in his chest and a contrast between the before, a sense of tension, and the after, an in-the-moment experience of relaxation and openness. He smiled and the therapist asked, "You're smiling, what's that like to notice?" Matteo responded, "It feels like a weight is lifting."

WORKING IN STATE FOUR

As the therapist and Matteo continued to metaprocess, Matteo began to move into State Four.

C: *I just feel like … it's like … this is what I wanted.*

TH: *"This is what I wanted." What's 'this?'"* [Asking for client specificity to make the implicit explicit]

C: *To feel connected.*

TH: *Good. Yes. I'm so glad you feel connected. And what's that like, to feel connected? If we pay attention to how that feels inside?* [Affirming the client's new experience, metaprocessing]

C: *Calm. I feel calm inside.* [State Four]

TH: *Nice. Make lots of room inside for that feeling of calm.* [Expanding positive affect]

         The client took a deep breath and, after a moment, looked up.

TH:	*Where do you feel that inside?* [Focusing on somatic experience, expanding positive affect]
C:	*Here* (motioning to his belly). *I feel it here. Like* … (he makes a downward motion with his hands)
TH:	*What are your hands saying?* [Moment-to-moment tracking to bring attention to somatic experience]
C:	*It's settling. Yeah, it's settling. It feels like me. Like I am here.*
TH:	*Wow. You are here. I'm so glad … really make space inside for this. (He takes a few breaths) Good. Great. What's it like to be here, to be so you?* [Affirming client, metaprocessing.]
C:	*It's good … I feel hopeful … like it is possible to change.*

The therapist affirmed the client and continued to metaprocess these transformational experiences with him. A common practice in AEDP at the end of the session is to save time to metaprocess the entire session together, that is, to explore and reflect on what it is like to have done everything that occurred. When the therapist asked this question, Matteo responded with tears in his eyes, "It's a lot. It feels really big and really important."

CONCLUSION

AEDP is an empirically validated model for working with trauma to help clients lessen emotional suffering and distress. This chapter outlined seven of the core tenets of AEDP and how to maximize a client's innate biological healing processes to undo aloneness and help facilitate a transformational process with AEDP's four-state map. By taking an attachment-based AEDP stance, focusing on the client's transformance drive, and then accessing and processing to completion the warded-off and defensively excluded emotions intertwined with trauma, clients release the emotion's adaptive action tendencies and experience the post-breakthrough affects. This process launches another phase of healing as the therapist begins to work with the client to reflect on the corrective emotional and relational experiences that have occurred. With round after round of metaprocessing in an expanding transformational spiral, clients then begin to form new, coherent narratives and experience a sense of calm, cohesion, well-being, and/or flourishing. As exemplified in the case study, clients regain a sense of their core selves, unfettered by the negative impact of trauma. After repeated rounds of therapeutic work, clients have greater access to their affective experience, connection to self, and connection to others.

RESOURCES FOR LEARNING

Several books and countless articles have been written about AEDP. Two of the mainstays of AEDP training are *The Transforming Power of Affect: A Model for Accelerated Change* (Fosha, 2000) and *AEDP 2.0: Undoing Aloneness & the Transformation of Suffering into*

Flourishing (Fosha Ed., 2021). AEDP also has a series of training videos offered with the American Psychological Association, and the AEDP Institute offers numerous live and on-demand training courses and workshops. For more information, please visit the AEDP Institute website: www.aedpinsitute.org.

REFERENCES

David, E.J.R. & Derthick, A.O. (2017). *The psychology of oppression.* Springer Publishing Company.

Doidge, N. (2007). *The brain that changes itself: Stories of personal triumph from the frontiers of brain science.* Penguin Books.

Fosha, D. (2000). *The transforming power of affect: A model of accelerated change.* Basic Books.

Fosha, D. (2004). "Nothing that feels bad is ever the last step:" The role of positive emotions in experiential work with difficult emotional experiences. *Clinical Psychology and Psychotherapy, 11,* 30–43. http://doi.org/10.1002/cpp.390

Fosha, D. (2007). AEDP: Transformance in action. Connections & Reflections. Retrieved from https://www.aedpinstitute.org/publications/articles/

Fosha D. (2009a). Emotion and recognition at work: Energy, vitality, pleasure, truth, desire & the emergent phenomenology of transformational experience. In D. Fosha, J. Siegel & M.F. Solomon (Eds.), *The healing power of emotion: Affective neuroscience, development, clinical practice* (pp. 172–203). Norton.

Fosha, D. (2009b). Healing attachment trauma with attachment (and then some!). In M. Kerman (Ed.) *Clinical pearls of wisdom: 21 leading therapists offer their key insights.* Norton.

Fosha, D. (2021a). Introduction: AEDP after 20 years. In Fosha, D. (Ed.) *Undoing Aloneness & the Transforming of Suffering into Flourishing: AEDP 2.0.* (pp. 3–23). American Psychological Association. https://doi.org/10.1037/0000232-000

Fosha, D. (2021b). How AEDP works. In Fosha, D. (Ed.) *Undoing aloneness & the transforming of suffering into flourishing: AEDP 2.0.* (pp. 27–52). American Psychological Association. https://doi.org/10.1037/0000232-000

Fosha, D., Thoma, N., & Yeung, D. (2019). Transforming emotional suffering into flourishing: Metatherapeutic processing of positive affect as a trans-theoretical vehicle for change. *Counseling Psychology Quarterly.* http://doi.org/10.1080/09515070.2019.1642852

Grotstein, J. (Fall 2002). *The transforming power of affect: A model for accelerated change (Book Review).* American Psychological Association Division 39. http://www.apadivisions.org/division-39/publications/reviews/transforming.aspx

Hanakawa, Y. (2021). What just happened? and what is happening now?: The art and science of moment-to-moment tracking in AEDP. In Fosha, D. (Ed.) *Undoing aloneness & the transforming of suffering into flourishing: AEDP 2.0* (pp. 107–131). American Psychological Association. https://doi.org/10.1037/0000232-000

Hanson, R. (2017). Positive neuroplasticity: The neuroscience of mindfulness. In J. Loizzo, M. Neale, & E. Wolfe (Eds.), *Advances in contemplative psychotherapy: Accelerating Transformation (pp. 48–60).* Norton. https://doi.org/10.4324/9781315630045-5

Iwakabe, S., & Conceiçao, N. (2016). Metatherapeutic processing as a change-based therapeutic immediacy task: Building an initial process model using a task-analytic research strategy. *Journal of Psychotherapy Integration, 26* (3): 230–247. https://doi.org/10.1037/int0000016

Iwakabe, S., Edlin, E., Fosha, D., Gretton, H., Joseph, A.J., Nunnink, S., Nakamura, K. & Thoma, N., (2020). The effectiveness of accelerated experiential dynamic psychotherapy (AEDP) in private practice settings: A transdiagnostic study conducted within the context of a practice research network. *Psychotherapy, 57* (4), 548–561. https://doi.org/10.1037/pst0000344

Iwakabe, S., Edlin, J., Fosha, D., Gretton, H., Thoma, N., Joseph, A.J., Nunnink, S., & Nakamura, K. (2022). Maintenance of change following Accelerated Experiential Dynamic Psychotherapy: 6- and 12-month follow-ups. *Psychotherapy, 59* (3), p. 431–446. ISSN: 0033-3204 https://doi.org/10.1037/pst0000441

Lipton, B., & Fosha, D. (2011). Attachment as a transformative process in AEDP: Operationalizing the intersection of attachment theory and affective neuroscience. *Journal of Psychotherapy Integration, 21*(3), 253–279. http://doi.org/10.1037/a0025421

Medley, B. (2021). Portrayals in work with emotion in AEDP: Processing core affective experience and bringing it to completion. In Fosha, D. (Ed.) *Undoing Aloneness & the Transforming of Suffering into Flourishing: AEDP 2.0* (pp. 217–240). American Psychological Association. https://doi.org/10.1037/0000232-000

Medley, B. (2024). The triangle of social experience: A new AEDP representational schema for working with the trauma of oppression and the experience of internal liberation. Manuscript in preparation.

Prenn, C.N., & Fosha, D. (2017). *Supervision essentials for Accelerated Experiential Dynamic Psychotherapy*. American Psychological Association.

Prenn, N. (2009). I second that emotion! On self-disclosure and its metaprocessing. In Bloomgarden, A. & Mennuti, R.B. (Eds.), *Psychotherapist revealed: Therapists speak about self-disclosure in psychotherapy* (pp. 85–99). New York: Routledge.

Russell (2015). *Restoring resilience: Discovering your clients' capacity for healing*. Norton.

Siegel, D. (1999). *The developing mind*. Guilford.

Smith, E.R., Murphy, J., & Coats, S. (1999). Attachment to groups: Theory and measurement. *Journal of Personality and Social Psychology, 77*(1), 94–110. https://doi.org/10.1037/0022-3514.77.1.94

Yeung, D. (2021). What went right?: What happened in the brain during AEDP's metatherapeutic processing. In Fosha, D. (Ed.) *Undoing Aloneness & the Transforming of Suffering into Flourishing: AEDP 2.0* (pp. 349–376). American Psychological Association. https://doi.org/10.1037/0000232-000

15

CHAPTER 15
COMPASSION FOCUSED THERAPY FOR THE TREATMENT OF TRAUMA

Dennis Tirch and Talya Vogel

INTRODUCTION

Founded by Paul Gilbert, compassion focused therapy (CFT; Gilbert, 2010) is an experiential therapy modality that leverages human compassion to enhance emotion regulation, overcome shame-based difficulties, and transform psychological suffering. As this chapter will demonstrate, the foundations of CFT are distinctively well suited to help people wo have experienced trauma and PTSD. CFT was designed to be modular and adaptable, allowing coherent integration of compassion-focused experiential practices with existing modes of psychotherapy. Standard triphasic protocols for trauma treatment, such as the one proposed by Judith Herman (1992), are particularly compatible with CFT, and the approach in this chapter involves just such an integration. CFT draws on many psychological disciplines, including affective neuroscience, evolutionary psychology, Buddhism, attachment theory, CBT, and Jungian psychotherapy. Guided imagery and mindfulness techniques are prominent experiential methods used in CFT. Nevertheless, CFT is more than a skills-based therapy, as nuanced work within the psychotherapy relationship is central to this modality. Individuals with a history of trauma are particularly vulnerable to high levels of shame and self-criticism, which can make treatment challenging. However, cultivating compassion can be helpful in addressing shame. CFT methods can facilitate working with shame and contribute to therapeutic growth, when integrated with a comprehensive, trauma-informed approach.

BRIEF HISTORY OF CFT

CFT came into being as a distinct therapy modality around 2006. The first years of the 21st century witnessed a remarkable change in evidence-based psychotherapy, as experiential practices found in Eastern contemplative traditions were adopted by cognitive behavioral therapy (CBT) and other modalities (Hayes et al. 2011; Tirch et al., 2014). In this context, CFT founder Paul Gilbert realized that his shame-prone patients responded better to the presence of compassion and a warm inner monologue than they did to rationality and cognitive restructuring. Many of the techniques and concepts found in CFT relate to various disciplines which include Buddhism, affective neuroscience, evolutionary psychology, attachment theory, and Jungian psychotherapy.

DOI: 10.4324/9781003455851-15

CFT was first developed for people who have high levels of shame and self-criticism. These are elements of clients' experiences that are present trans-diagnostically and are known to be vulnerability factors in a variety of psychopathologies (Gilbert & Irons, 2005; Zuroff et al., 2004). Both shame and self-criticism can seriously interfere with therapeutic progress, regardless of the initial reason for seeking treatment (Rector, et al., 2000). Feelings of shame and self-criticism often involve a person's fixation on condemning thoughts and emotions like anger, anxiety, or disgust (Gilbert & Irons, 2005). Across various diagnoses, higher levels of shame and self-criticism (Kannan & Levitt, 2013) and lower levels of self-compassion (Neff, 2011) have been linked to symptoms of anxiety and depression. This preoccupation with negative thoughts and emotions can lead to narrowed attentional focus and a constricted range of behaviors, as a person becomes preoccupied by their social worth relative to others, as well as reduced empathy (Fredrickson, 2001; Wachtel, 1967).

Clients who have experienced trauma in their lives often manifest considerable shame and self-criticism. However, developing compassion and positive emotions can be helpful in addressing these painful emotions, making meaningful therapeutic change more likely for persons living with trauma. Several CFT professionals and colleagues have applied compassion work to trauma. Deborah Lee (2022) developed a CFT approach to living with trauma and established many of the conceptual bridges between CFT and trauma-informed psychotherapy (Lee & James, 2013). To date the effectiveness of CFT has been demonstrated in helping individuals with a variety of complex and long-term mental health challenges, including those with personality disorders (Lucre & Corten, 2012), psychosis (Braehler et al., 2013; Mayhew & Gilbert, 2008), eating disorders (Gale et al., 2014), and co-occurring diagnoses (Judge et al., 2012). Meta-analyses and literature reviews of CFT continue to demonstrate significant effects of this therapy for an increasing range of problems (Wilson et al., 2019).

THE CFT DEFINITION OF COMPASSION IN THEORY AND PRACTICE

CFT uses a simple definition of compassion, but one that has powerful implications for the use of compassion cultivation in psychotherapy. In CFT, compassion is defined as *a sensitivity to the presence of suffering and its causes, in oneself and others, combined with a motivation to take action to alleviate or prevent such suffering.* In the context of CFT, compassion is seen as a complex process that has emerged from humans' evolved care-giving and care-receiving motives. These motives are biological imperatives that guide basic human functioning according to the way that we have evolved to interact with the world (Gilbert, 1992). As such, dimensions of the compassion motive are clearly present in human parental care and childrearing. Situating our understanding of compassion in evolved, species-preservative algorithms means that CFT views compassion as encompassing a range of emotional, cognitive, and motivational components.

Importantly, the CFT definition of compassion involves two primary components, which practitioners sometimes call "The Two Psychologies of Compassion." The first dimension, known as "The Psychology of Engagement," involves deploying mindful awareness and flexible attention to actively engage with suffering (Gilbert, 2010). This aspect of compassion can be understood as openness and willingness to notice and work through suffering. The second component, known as "The Psychology of Alleviation/Prevention" involves taking action to alleviate or prevent suffering by developing the skills needed to translate a compassion motive into action.

These two main dimensions, in turn, are composed of various elements, known as the "competencies of compassion." These competencies represent different emergent qualities of the compassionate mind that can be strengthened through CFT practices. CFT techniques seek to stimulate and cultivate the compassion motive and to develop and enact the competencies of compassion. These competencies include six processes related to mindful engagement with suffering, including a motivation to care, present moment-focused sensitivity to suffering, sympathy, empathy, distress tolerance, and non-judgment. We also find six skills that are related to alleviation and prevention of suffering: Compassionate attention, compassionate reasoning, compassionate behavior, experiential work with the five senses, compassion imagery, and compassionate mindfulness of emotions.

One primary pathway to developing compassion and personal transformation in CFT is found in how we work with, and better understand, our emotions. CFT centers on the development and enhancement of deep, evolved emotional and motivational systems, specifically those related to regulating affect. This approach aligns with the premise that emotions are driven by evolutionary emergent motives. Emotions can also play a role in augmenting and reinforcing these motives through facilitating patterns of action. As proposed by Gilbert (1989, 2010), these important behavioral trajectories include forming social connections, seeking status, cultivating relationships, finding sexual partners, creating attachments, and caring for offspring. All of these actions serve evolved motives such as the motive to cooperate, to compete, to mate, or to care. Emotions can draw our attention to certain motives and can give us feedback about how well we are actualizing evolutionary imperatives embedded in biosocial motives. Ultimately, our emotions provide a signal of how successful we are in fulfilling these species-level evolutionary needs, as well as how successful we are in realizing individual aims.

Emotions have evolved to guide our behaviors in the present moment, and it is often the anticipation of these emotions that influences our actions. Based on research in evolutionary analysis and affective neuroscience (DePue & Morrone-Strupinsky, 2005), Gilbert's CFT model (2010) posits that three emotional systems play a role in guiding human actions. These three systems involve: (1) Threat Focused Emotions – emotions that help us survive against harm or loss, including anger, anxiety, and disgust (Ledoux, 1998). (2) Seeking/Acquiring Focused Emotions – emotions that drive us to acquire resources for survival and reproductive success, also known as "drive systems" that involve "seeking" behaviors (Panksepp, 1994). These emotions include joy, pleasure, and excitement and are associated with winning, succeeding, and acquiring. (3) Calming/Soothing Focused Emotions – emotions that have evolved to promote a sense of safeness and peace, often referred to as the "rest and digest" state. Once animals are no longer under threat or seeking resources, they can rest and relax. For many animals, simply removing a threat can induce this state. However, for mammals, additional mechanisms have developed to promote calming and soothing behaviors. As mammals evolved, their attachment systems also underwent changes to allow for affiliative signals to trigger a state of calmness and safety (Porges, 2007). This is evident in the way that infants become calmed by the presence and physical contact of their parents during times of distress. As mammals began giving birth to immature offspring, the attachment system became integral in regulating emotions between the infant and the parent (Cozolinio, 2006; Mikulincer & Shaver, 2007). The parasympathetic and sympathetic nervous systems have undergone significant changes to enable the parasympathetic nervous system to produce a calming response in response to caring and safe relationships (Porges, 2007). Specialized brain systems have also evolved to detect and respond to affiliative signals, such as oxytocin (Carter, 1998), which is involved in trust and affiliative relationships. Oxytocin has also been shown to directly impact threat processing in the amygdala (Kirsch et al., 2005). This evidence supports the idea that affiliative behavior plays a key role in regulating emotions, especially those related to threats (Uvnäs Moberg & Prime, 2013). Attachment theorists propose that healthy attachment bonds provide a secure base from which individuals can explore their world and face challenges (Bowlby, 1969; Mikulincer & Shaver, 2007). CFT builds upon attachment theory, acknowledging that internal beliefs about others as stable sources of support may be problematic. Many individuals have experienced abuse, trauma, or neglect from caregivers or within caregiving relationships. These traumatic experiences can lead to a distorted association between seeking comfort and feeling threatened due to classical conditioning. This can result in a fear of receiving compassion and difficulty activating self-soothing mechanisms (Gilbert, 2009). As a result, CFT focuses on gradually stimulating the affiliative system as an internal point of reference and organizing process. Patients learn to cultivate an inner compassionate self and visualize a compassionate figure that can serve as a nurturing, parental presence within themselves.

USING CFT IN THE TREATMENT OF TRAUMA

CFT is an integrative therapy and is often utilized alongside other evidence-based forms of treating trauma including CBT, EMDR, and other forms of exposure-based therapy. While CFT is used to effectively treat a number of clinical presentations including depression, anxiety, addictive behaviors, and personality disorders (Leaviss & Uttley 2015), CFT's emphasis on working with shame and self-criticism is especially relevant in working with trauma (Irons & Lad, 2017). Research shows that shame can strongly contribute to the development and maintenance of PTSD, and not addressing this core aspect of PTSD can be an obstacle to recovery (Rushford et al., 2022). As noted, CFT was designed to work more effectively with shame and self-criticism that may not often respond effectively to traditional talk therapy. Many clients may note that they *logically know* they had no role in their traumatic experiences, but *feel* an embodied sense of self-blame and shame. This is where CFT can be highly effective in working with both top-down and bottom-up processes in an experiential way to help clients bridge the gap between knowing and understanding.

It has been widely recommended that the gold-standard way of working with trauma, especially complex trauma, is through a phased approach (Cloitre et al., 2011; Herman, 1992) where phases included (1) safety and stabilization, (2) trauma processing, and (3) integration. Depending on the client, type of trauma, and symptomatology, these phases will span different numbers of sessions and will include different interventions. As CFT is easily integrated into a wide range of modalities, a compassion-focused perspective and integration of compassion-focused interventions can be utilized throughout the phased approach.

Generally, Phase I focuses grounding, stabilization, and preparing clients for processing traumatic memories. This phase is designed to provide psychoeducation and to build coping resources and tools. The clinician will help the client frame their symptoms through an evolutionary and neurophysiological lens to help provide compassionate understanding of their symptoms. Often, individuals who experience trauma present with shame around symptomology. Helping clients understand the three emotion systems (drive, threat, and soothing) along with the basics of how the nervous system is designed to respond to threat can be hugely impactful to clients in early stages of treatment. Deborah Lee (2022) calls this first phase "Compassionate Insights" and includes discussion of: Evolution, human suffering, tricky brain, affect regulation, threat/shame/self compassion, attachment, and compassion.

The first phase can also include specific psychoeducation on the nervous system such as soothing rhythm breathing, developing mindful attention, and guided imagery. This is also a phase of treatment where the tone of the psychotherapy relationship and a CFT therapeutic stance is established. The primary goal of this phase is to help clients learn how to shift from threat-based processing, with dominance of the sympathetic nervous system into their soothing based processing, with a more dominant parasympathetic nervous system. Clients learn the CFT "Reality Check," an exercise in evolutionary functional analysis, in Phase I. During the reality check, the therapist takes a radically de-shaming and accepting stance, enacting the "wisdom of no blame" (Tirch et al., 2014). Clients reflect that they did not choose to be born, nor did they choose their genetic inheritance or the environment that they were raised in. So many of the causes and conditions that bring forth our behaviors and that drive our suffering were not of our choosing, and, from a certain point of view, were not our fault. In this way, Phase I involves cultivation of awareness and insight, as well as a practical understanding of nervous system grounding, somatic techniques, and distress tolerance.

Once clients can begin to effectively utilize distress tolerance and ground themselves in the presence of difficult emotions, clinicians can shift to Phase II which focuses on processing past traumatic experiences. Whether the clinician utilizes TF-CBT, EMDR, CPT, PE, or other more manualized forms of trauma-focused psychotherapy, CFT can be effectively integrated. The benefit of integrating a compassion-focused perspective in processing is to help clients embody their evolved compassion motive, which can transform a person's relationship to traumatic experiences and re-experiencing of emotional memories that are rooted in trauma. During Phase II, clients begin viewing these memories from a lens of self-compassion and centeredness, rather than from habitual shame-based and self-critical lenses. In Phase II, clients can become more familiar with competencies of compassion, such as building their ability to get unhooked from judgmental thinking, developing their ability to accept and tolerate challenging emotional states, and cultivating flexible perspective taking through enhancing empathy. Phase II fully immerses clients in the embodied experience of compassion and a compassionate perspective toward one's own suffering and traumatic experiences. Experiential practices can include guided imagery and multiple chair work, among other techniques. Once clients can contact trauma memories without significant impairment or overwhelming distress, and once clients begin noticing significant improvement in dealing with hypervigilance, hyperarousal, and other trauma-related symptoms, clinicians move clients to Phase III.

Phase III focuses on reconnecting clients to themselves, others, and the world. Often, when clients describe a decrease in posttraumatic symptoms and improvement in daily functioning, this phase may be cut short or skipped altogether. However, spending time on this phase helps clients begin to answer the question, "now what?" Depending on trauma type, severity, and duration, clients may be unsure of how to view themselves outside the context of their "trauma self." Therefore, CFT helps clients explore ways to reclaim their narrative from a compassionate and values-based perspective. Clients can also begin to explore values, goals, and meaning/purpose, using methods imported from acceptance and commitment therapy (ACT) (Tirch et al., 2014). EMDR "future templates," which are similar to the guided imagery used in CFT, can be utilized in this phase of work to help clients imagine formerly avoided situations and how their current self would effectively navigate through them. Exercises may include values authorship, loving-kindness meditation, and compassionate behavioral actions. In this phase, clients explore how to embody and access their compassionate self in daily living and how to connect their behaviors to their values.

CASE EXAMPLE AND DESCRIPTION OF THE THERAPY PROCESS

Jane was a 32-year-old Caucasian female who sought treatment to address symptoms of intense emotional fluctuations, dissociation, angry outbursts, and shame. Jane was married and wanted to have children, but feared that her difficulty managing her intense emotions would keep her from being a good mother. Jane recognized the historical patterns of traumatic parenting in her family and told the therapist that she wanted to break this cycle. She experienced intense daily fluctuations in mood and used marijuana as a way to numb her emotions. Jane and her husband had frequent arguments in which she yelled and then felt an intense amount of shame. She worked at a high paying job that she stated she "should" feel good about, but constantly felt anxious about not being good enough and worried constantly about being fired. Jane noted a lack of warm, compassionate, comforting attachment figures growing up.

CASE CONCEPTUALIZATION

A compassion-focused formulation includes four essential elements: (1) The client's biological and environmental contexts, both past and present, viewed through a functional analytic lens to understand antecedents, behaviors, and consequences that have shaped the client's patterns of coping; (2) What the client fears most and is least willing to experience, such as fears around themes of abandonment, rejection, shame, abuse, or harm; (3)

The client's internally and externally focused "protective" safety strategies and behaviors; and (4) The intended and unintended consequences of those safety strategies (both public and private) for the client, such as shame-based self-criticism, beliefs about coping, or views on the nature of the client's own suffering, including depression and anxiety (Tirch et al., 2014). Each of these dimensions was explored with Jane.

1. The Client's Biological and Environmental Contexts, Both Past and Present:
   Jane's childhood was characterized by an emotionally dysregulated mother who would frequently and unexpectedly yell or hit her. Throughout Jane's life, her mother's care and compassion was paired to trauma and distress, compromising Jane's ability to regulate her emotions through activation of her soothing system and contributing to anxiety and emotional dysregulation.
2. Internal and External Experiences the Client Fears Most and Is Least Willing to Experience:
   Jane noted that when she had thoughts about her childhood or intrusive images about her abuse, she felt emotionally numb and would frequently dissociate. At other times, Jane felt intensely anxious and reported frequent panic attacks at work. She told her therapist that she felt guilty when she experienced sadness because she knew "other people have it worse." Jane described frequently beating herself up for not being good enough and that this manifested itself at work, at home, and around friends.
3. The Client's Internal and Externally Focused "Protective" Safety Strategies and Behaviors:
   Jane described the need to smoke marijuana in the evenings as a way to manage her anxiety. She noted that it was "the only thing that helps my emotions." Jane also described people-pleasing tendencies and the desire to do things perfectly so that people will not become angry at her. Jane avoided thinking about the future because she felt overwhelmed and hopeless about things not getting better. She told the therapist that she worried that if she were to let go of her inner critic, she would be complacent and not be motivated to try hard.
4. The Consequences (Both Intended and Unintended) of Jane's Safety Strategies:
   Jane's dependence on marijuana stopped her from exploring other coping strategies and developing a sense of mastery or control over her internal world. She also stated that her marriage constantly felt rocky because of frequent arguing. Jane recognized that her inability to think about the future without panicking stopped her from being able to set meaningful goals.
   Being able to understand Jane through a compassion-focused lens indicated repetitive themes of avoidance, control, and unhelpful ways of coping in response to her years of childhood trauma. From the outside looking in, Jane's colleagues saw a highly functioning individual, married, with a high paying job, but Jane's constant inner criticism, fluctuations in mood, intrusive memories of trauma, and nearly daily arguments with her husband kept her from connecting to meaningful goals. Her history of abuse and lack of a caring, nurturing attachment figure made it difficult to self-soothe in the presence of close relationships, as her nervous system had fused closeness with fear/threat. A compassion-focused case formulation demonstrated a painful history and the development of an inner critic that continued to reflect Jane's mother's constant early criticism of her. From a CFT perspective, the clinician could see fears of compassion, avoidance of the present moment, and difficulty connecting to sources of meaning.

PHASE I: CONNECTING SAFELY TO THE PRESENT THROUGH PSYCHOEDUCATION AND NERVOUS SYSTEM GROUNDING

Aligned with the first phase in trauma therapy, the clinician worked with Jane on developing distress tolerance tools to navigate moments of overwhelming panic and anxiety. Initial sessions focused on building rapport and embodying a compassionate stance toward Jane's present and past experiences. Additionally, the clinician worked on framing Jane's current symptoms through a trauma-focused, compassion-oriented, and nervous system-informed perspective. Jane learned to identify the physical and emotional aspects of sympathetic nervous system activation and how these symptoms were designed evolutionarily to protect her from danger. She also learned about her parasympathetic nervous system response to threat (i.e., dissociation and emotional numbing) as her body's attempt to protect her from pain in situations where she was unable to escape danger. The clinician discussed how we do not choose the bodies we are born with, nor do we choose the families we are born into. Yet, these experiences that we do not choose strongly shape how our nervous system responds to both external and internal sources of threat. Embodying this CFT perspective of "no-blame" and explaining symptoms through an evolutionary lens, helped Jane tap into more validating responses to her own suffering.

Initial sessions worked to give Jane alternative and healthy ways to respond to distress. The clinician provided Jane with a list of coping strategies, informed by DBT TIPP skills, for her to practice in moments in which she felt high levels of anxiety and panic. These strategies included using ice, sour candy, salt, grounding objects, and scents. The clinician helped Jane understand how grounding through the body and the senses would start to shift her into her soothing parasympathetic nervous system. Additionally, these strategies could help Jane begin the important trauma goal of differentiating between past and present. Jane began to practice contacting the present moment through CFT interventions including soothing rhythm breathing, safe/calm place, and other methods.

PHASE II: PROCESSING THE PAST

Once Jane was able to develop a "coping toolkit" to navigate overwhelming emotions, sessions pivoted toward revisiting her traumatic experiences and addressing the unhelpful trauma narratives. Jane and her therapists worked on Jane's development of self-empathy and her ability to validate her own emotional experiences. Phase II involved a transition from simpler experiential grounding techniques such as soothing rhythmic breathing and a visualization of a safe calm place. More advanced imagery and compassion cultivation methods were used in Phase II, such as Jane's visualization of a compassionate version of herself, or the construction and imagining of a "perfect nurturer" (Lee, 2022). This imagery allowed Jane the opportunity to gradually stimulate and embody her compassionate self. Enacting and embodying this care-giving and receiving motive allowed Jane to transform her relationship to difficult emotions and helped her to cultivate resilience. Recordings of many compassionate mind-training practices can be found at https://www.mindfulcompassion.com.

Phase II also includes forms of exposure to traumatic memories, as well as troubling thoughts and emotions. Jane used her compassion-focused imagery to help cultivate nervous system grounding, acceptance, and willingness, before she engaged in direct exposure to difficult and avoided internal experiences in session. The form of exposure Jane's therapist used is known as the compassionate exposure and response sequence (CERES). This sequence involves the client: (1) Engaging in a brief mindful compassion practice to ground and prepare for the exposure session; (2) Imagining a compassionate other, perfect nurturer, or compassionate version of themselves; (3) A brief internal dialogue with this compassionate guide where the compassionate figure encourages and supports the client's engagement with feared or avoided material; (4) Imaginal exposure to the challenging material, with an emphasis on full willingness to encounter and deeply feel the sensations and emotions that arise during exposure; (5) A period of grounding and compassionate imagery, where the client takes a few minutes to imagine a dialogue between their supportive, compassionate guide, and their everyday self. The compassionate guide emphasizes the courage and strength that the client is developing in this process; (6) The client sets an ongoing intention to continue in the process of compassion-focused exposure and recovery from trauma.

EMDR methods can also be integrated into this CERES process. By doing this, the client is not only engaged in mere imaginal exposure, but also in a relational EMDR process with bilateral stimulation occurring throughout the exposure segment of CERES. Other somatic trauma therapy methods can also be integrated as Phase II encourages the client to shift their perspective on their chronically challenging cognitions and private experiences, building flexible responding and transforming the stimulus functions of trauma memories. Jane engaged in exposure that used EMDR techniques, and this combination allowed her to build up a "toolbox" of both coping methods and ways to turn toward her feared experiences in a way that was theoretically consistent and easy to follow and practice. Jane reported that having specific coping strategies and techniques blended with a specific way to face her fears allowed her to "keep going" and to eventually reclaim much of her life from avoidance, distress, and functional impairment.

PHASE III: CONNECTING TO A MEANINGFUL FUTURE

Through the exercises in Phase II, Jane became able to revisit elements of her traumatic experience with less distress and noted improved ability to regulate, validate, and communicate her emotions. Therefore, the clinician shifted to Phase III, which focuses on reconnecting with self, others, and the world. Jane had long associated her view of self as "broken" and "traumatized," so once these narratives were less potent, sessions explored meaningful aspects of self. Sessions focused on connecting to values and on building goals around these values. For example, Jane noted that community was an important value, but she had avoided opportunities to connect to others due to her anxiety that she would be judged or would let people down. Once Jane identified ways that her compassionate self would approach these social situations, she engaged in behavioral experimentation to try bringing her compassionate coping tools into opportunities to connect with others. During this phase, Jane also focused on healing her relationship with her husband, now that she was able to be more regulated and present at home. The clinician helped Jane explore other aspects of self that she did not have the opportunity to cultivate in childhood such as playfulness, curiosity, and fun. Jane noted that her ability to contact compassionate self, self-regulate, and find meaning in the present moment made her more confident in her future self's ability to have a child.

ASSESSMENT OF RESEARCH EVIDENCE

As a relatively young psychotherapeutic approach, the research evidence of the effectiveness of CFT in treating trauma is in its nascent stages. The most recent review and meta-analysis examining the effectiveness of CFT for clinical populations only included two studies focusing on PTSD/trauma-related symptomatology (Millard et al., 2023). In these studies, CFT was not found to have had a significant intervention effect on a posttraumatic questionnaire (Rycroft, 2016) or on prolonged grief disorder (Johannsen et al., 2022). However, there were significant limitations in these studies that are important to note. The Rycroft study only examined self-administered CFT rather than clinician-administered CFT, had high rates of attrition, and a low number of participants (N = 6). The Johannsen et al. study noted that while CFT was not shown to have significant effect on symptoms of prolonged grief disorder, the group-based CFT intervention showed a significant positive effect on reducing posttraumatic stress symptoms. Rushforth and colleagues noted that "much of the research regarding the efficacy of compassion-based interventions in PTSD treatment lacks statistical significance, control groups or causal considerations" (Rushforth et al., 2022, p. 5).

A 2020 systematic review (Winders et al., 2020) examined self-compassion in the context of trauma and PTSD. The review examined nine compassion-focused interventions for PTSD. Five of the nine studies utilized comparison groups, and among these five, one showed greater significant reduction in PTSD symptoms in the compassion-based group relative to the control group (Lang et al., 2020). Among the four remaining studies utilizing comparison groups, one study demonstrated alleviation of PTSD symptoms in both the compassion-based condition (imagery rescripting) and in the comparison clinical intervention condition (traditional imaginal exposure), with a slightly larger improvement in the traditional intervention condition (Hoffart et al., 2015). The remaining three studies (Beaumont, et al., 2012; Beaumont, et al., 2016; Held & Owens, 2015) showed a nonsignificant improvement in the compassion-based conditions. However, a review by Rushforth et al. (2022) noted that due to the small sample sizes, these studies were potentially underpowered, and the nonsignificant results should be interpreted with caution. Within the Winders (2020) review, three of the four studies without control groups found a significant reduction in PTSD symptoms following compassion-based interventions (Au et al., 2017; Kearney et al., 2013; Müller-Engelmann et al., 2019).

Pilot studies and other studies not included in the previously mentioned meta-analyses are more promising when it comes to the research for utilizing CFT for trauma. A 2022 study by McLean, Steindl, and Bambling (2022) examined the effectiveness of a CFT group therapy for adult women who had experienced childhood sexual abuse. This study found significant improvement across all outcome variables (symptoms of posttraumatic stress, shame, self-criticism, fears of compassion, depression, anxiety, and stress) from pre-to post-intervention, which were maintained at follow-up. A 2023 study by Romaniuk et al. (2023) examined the effect of group compassionate mind training (CMT) for ex-service personnel with PTSD and their partners. The study found a significant reduction in fears of compassion, PTSD symptoms, anxiety, stress, external shame, and self-criticism at the three-month follow-up along with a reduction in depression and increase in quality of life and social safeness. Au et al. (2017) used a multiple baseline design to examine a brief compassion-focused therapy derived intervention for trauma-related shame and PTSD symptoms. The study found significant reductions in PTSD symptoms among nine of the ten participants and significant decreases in shame among eight of the ten participants. While more high-quality and large-scale research is needed, the current state of the research highlights CFT as a promising treatment for trauma-related symptoms, particularly among individuals experiencing high levels of shame and self-criticism.

STRENGTHS AND LIMITATIONS OF A CFT APPROACH TO TRAUMA

CFT founder Paul Gilbert intentionally named the approach "compassion *focused* therapy" rather than "compassion therapy." This is meant to emphasize that CFT can serve as a way to focus therapy on cultivating compassion, without needing to jettison all of the hard-earned techniques and clinical skills that therapists acquired over their career as psychotherapists. This flexibility is a particular strength of CFT. Best practices in treatment of specific problems, such as exposure and response prevention for anxiety disorders, behavioral activation for severe depression, or triphasic approaches for trauma, can be blended with CFT elements to help clients overcome shame-based difficulties. Furthermore, the cultivation of compassion in and of itself can provide benefits across levels of functioning. Similarly, mindfulness cultivation in CFT can impart the same benefits found in other forms of mindfulness training. The CFT case formulation model provides a rubric to intelligently integrate these elements of treatment in a user-friendly and accessible way. The CFT model of emotion regulation can guide a clinician's understanding of how trauma and developmental experiences of attachment can shape a client's present day emotion regulation capacity. Many of the elements of triphasic treatment of trauma are also prime areas of emphasis in CFT, such as nervous system grounding, working with challenging shame-based narratives, and building patterns of action that build meaning and purpose.

Like many treatments for trauma, CFT research needs to be expanded and methodologically improved before it could be more widely disseminated as a gold-standard treatment for trauma. The limited outcome research for trauma-specific CFT interventions needs to be addressed but need not foreclose clinicians from adapting CFT methods to their evidence-based practice treatment plans. Indeed, practice-based research is a promising avenue for future CFT development. Training in CFT remains difficult to access for many clinicians, as this is a newer modality, with a small community of dedicated therapists and trainers working to bring the approach to a large group of practitioners. As such, it may not be feasible for many therapists to shift to an exclusively CFT–focused approach to the treatment of trauma. CFT practitioners need to be particularly sensitive to the resistance many clients may have to the concept of compassion. Therapists are advised to take the time to understand the underlying evolutionary model of motives, emotion, and compe-tencies that serves as CFT's foundation, rather than simply adapting a few imagery tech-niques to their typical practice routines. This will allow clinicians to better integrate CFT and compassion cultivation into their trauma work, with sensitivity to the functional anal-ysis of client's fears, blocks, and resistance to compassion cultivation (Tirch et al., 2014).

RESOURCES

The Compassionate Mind Foundation (www.compassionatemind.co.uk) is the interna-tional hub for ongoing training and treatment development for CFT. Their website has many resources, including video, journal articles, and email discussion lists. The Founda-tion maintains an ongoing certificate program for post-graduate education in CFT.

In the United States, The Compassionate Mind Foundation of The United States of America (http://www.compassionfocusedtherapy.com/) and The Center for CFT (www.mindfulcompassion.com) host a range of workshops, trainings, and online meetings for clinicians who are interested in developing their knowledge and skill in practicing CFT. This includes the Trauma, Transformation, & Resiliency (TTR) program, specifically designed for using CFT for working with clients impacted by trauma. The website for The Center for CFT hosts a range of meditations and CFT imagery practices that are free to use or download.

REFERENCES

Au, T.M., Sauer-Zavala, S., King, M.W., Petrocchi, N., Barlow, D.H., & Litz, B.T. (2017). Compassion-based therapy for trauma-related shame and posttraumatic stress: Initial evaluation using a multiple baseline design. *Behavior Therapy*, 48(2), 207–221. https://doi.org/10.1016/j.beth.2016.11.012

Beaumont, E., Durkin, M., McAndrew, S. & Martin, C.R. (2016). Using Compassion Focused Therapy as an adjunct to Trauma-Focused CBT for Fire Service personnel suffering with trauma-related symptoms. *The Cognitive Behaviour Therapist*, 9(34), 1–13. doi: 10.1017/S1754470X16000209

Beaumont, E., Galpin, A. & Jenkins, P. (2012). Being kinder to myself: a prospective com-parative study, exploring post-trauma therapy outcome measures, for two groups of clients, receiving wither cognitive behaviour therapy or cognitive behaviour therapy and compassionate mind training. *Counselling Psychology Review*, 27, 31–43.

Bowlby, J. (1969). *Attachment and loss* (Vol. 1). Basic Books.

Braehler, C., Gumley, A., Harper, J., Wallace, S., Norrie, J., & Gilbert, P., (2013). Exploring change processes in compassion focused therapy in psychosis: Results of a feasibility randomized controlled trial. *Randomized Controlled Trial, British Journal of Clinical Psychology, 52*(2), 199–214. https://doi.org/10.1111/bjc.12009

Carter, C.S. (1998). Neuroendocrine perspectives on social attachment and love. *Psycho-neuroendocrinology, 23*(8), 779–818. https://doi.org/10.1016/s0306-4530(98)00055-9

Cloitre, M., Courtois, C.A., Charuvastra, A., Carapezza, R., Stolbach, B.C., & Green, B.L. (2011). Treatment of complex PTSD: Results of the ISTSS expert clinician survey on best practices. *Journal of Traumatic Stress, 24*(6), 615–627.

Cozolinio, L.J. (2006). *The neuroscience of human relationships: Attachment and the developing social brain.* (Norton Series on Interpersonal Neurobiology). WW. Norton and Company.

Depue, R.A. & Morrone-Strupinsky, J.V. (2005). A neurobehavioral model of affiliative bonding: Implications for conceptualizing a human trait of affiliation. *Behavioral and Brain Sciences, 28*(3), 313–350. https://doi.org/10.1017/S0140525X05000063

Fredrickson, B.L. (2001). The role of positive emotions in positive psychology: The broaden and- build theory of positive emotions. *American Psychologist, 56*(3), 218–226. https://doi.org/10.1037/0003-066X.56.3.218

Gale, C. Gilbert, P., Read, N., & Goss, K. (2014). An evaluation of the impact of introducing compassion focused therapy to a standard treatment programme for people with eating disorders. *Clinical Psychology & Psychotherapy, 21*(1), 1–12. https://doi.org/10.1002/cpp.1806

Gilbert, D.T. (1989). Thinking lightly about others: Automatic components of the social inference process. In J.S. Uleman & J.A. Bargh (Eds.), *Unintended thought* (pp. 189–211). The Guilford Press.

Gilbert, P. (1992). *Human nature and suffering.* Lawrence Erlbaum Associates., Inc.

Hayes, S.C., Strosahl, K.D., & Wilson, K.G. (2011). *Acceptance and commitment therapy: The process and practice of mindful change.* Guilford press.

Gilbert, P. (2009). Introducing compassion-focused therapy. *Advances in Psychiatric Treatment, 15*(3), 199–208. https://doi.org/10.1192/apt.bp.107.005264

Gilbert, P. (2010). *Compassion focused therapy: Distinctive features.* Routledge/Taylor & Francis Group. https://doi.org/10.4324/9780203851197

Gilbert, P. & Irons, C. (2005). Focused therapies and compassionate mind training for shame and self-attacking. In P. Gilbert (Ed.), *Compassion: Conceptualisations, research and use in psychotherapy*, (pp. 263–325) Routledge. https://doi.org/10.4324/9780203003459

Held, P., & Owens, G.P. (2015). Effects of self-compassion workbook training on trauma-related guilt in a sample of homeless veterans: A pilot study. *Journal of Clinical Psychology, 71*(6), 513–526. https://doi.org/10.1002/jclp.22170

Herman, J. (1992). *Trauma and Recovery.* New York, NY: Basic Books.

Hoffart, A., Øktedalen, T., & Langkaas, T.F. (2015). Self-compassion influences PTSD symptoms in the process of change in trauma-focused cognitive-behavioral therapies: a study of within-person processes. *Frontiers in Psychology, 6*, 1273.

Irons, C., & Lad, S. (2017). Using compassion focused therapy to work with shame and self-criticism in complex trauma. *Australian Clinical Psychologist, 3*(1), 1743.

Johannsen, M., Schlander, C., Farver-Vestergaard, I., Lundorff, M., Wellnitz, K.B., Komischke-Konnerup, K.B., & O'Connor, M., 2022. Group-based compassion-focused therapy for prolonged grief symptoms in adults – results from a randomized controlled trial. *Psychiatry Research, 314*, 1–9.

Judge, L., Cleghorn, A., McEwan, K. & Gilbert, P. (2012). An exploration of group-based compassion focused therapy for a heterogenous range of clients presenting to a community mental health team. *International Journal of Cognitive Therapy, 5*(4), 420–429. https://doi.org/10.1521/ijct.2012.5.4.420

Kannan, D. & Levitt, H.M. (2013). A review of client self-criticism in psychotherapy. *Journal of Psychotherapy Integration, 23*(2), 166–178. https://doi.org/10.1037/a0032355

Kearney, D.J., McManus, C., Martinez, M.E., Felleman, B., & Simpson, T.L. (2013). Loving-kindness meditation for posttraumatic stress disorder: A pilot study. *Journal of Traumatic Stress, 26*(4), 426–434. https://doi.org/10.1002/jts.21832

Kirsch, P., Esslinger, C., Chen, Q., Mier, D., Lis, S., Siddhanti, S., Gruppe, H., Mattay, V. S., Gallhofer, B., & Meyer-Lindenberg, A. (2005). Oxytocin modulates neural circuitry for social cognition and fear in humans. *Journal of Neuroscience, 25*(49), 11489–11493. https://doi.org/10.1523/JNEUROSCI.3984-05.2005

Lang, A.J., Casmar, P., Hurst, S., Harrison, T., Golshan, S., Good, R., Essex, M. & Negi, L. (2020). Compassion meditation for veterans with posttraumatic stress disorder (PTSD): A nonrandomized study. *Mindfulness, 11*, 63–74.

Leaviss, J., & Uttley, L. (2015). Psychotherapeutic benefits of compassion-focused therapy: An early systematic review. *Psychological Medicine, 45*(5), 927–945. https://doi.org/10.1017/S0033291714002141

LeDoux, J. (1998). Fear and the brain: Where have we been, and where are we going? *Biological Psychiatry, 44*(12), 1229–1238. https://doi.org/10.1016/s0006-3223(98)00282-0

Lee, D. (2022). Using compassion focused therapy to work with complex PTSD. In P. Gilbert & G. Simos (Eds.), *Compassion focused therapy: Clinical practice and applications (pp. 565–583)*. Routledge.

Lee, D.A., & James, S. (2013). *The compassionate-mind guide to recovering from trauma and PTSD: Using compassion-focused therapy to overcome flashbacks, shame, guilt, and fear*. New Harbinger Publications.

Lucre, K.M., & Corten, N. (2012). An exploration of group compassion-focused therapy for personality disorder. *Psychology and Psychotherapy: Theory, Research, and Practice, 86*(4), 387–400. https://doi.org/10.1111/j.2044-8341.2012.02068.x

Mayhew, S.L. & Gilbert, P. (2008). Compassionate mind training with people who hear malevolent voices: A case series report. *Clinical Psychology & Psychothery, 15*(2), 113–138. https://doi.org/10.1002/cpp.566

McLean, L., Steindl, S.R., & Bambling, M. (2022). Compassion Focused Group Therapy for adult female survivors of childhood sexual abuse: A preliminary investigation. *Mindfulness, 13*(5), 1144–1157.

Mikulincer, M., & Shaver, P.R. (2007). *Attachment in adulthood: Structure, dynamics, and change*. The Guilford Press.

Millard, L.A., Wan, M.W., Smith, D.M., & Wittkowski, A. (2023). The effectiveness of compassion focused therapy with clinical populations: A systematic review and meta-analysis. *Journal of Affective Disorders, 326*, 168–192.

Müller-Engelmann, M., Schreiber, C., Kümmerle, S., Heidenreich, T., Stangier, U., & Steil, R. (2019). A trauma-adapted mindfulness and loving-kindness intervention for patients with PTSD after interpersonal violence: A multiple-baseline study. *Mindfulness*, *10*(6), 1105– 1123.

Neff, K.D. (2011). Self-compassion, self-esteem, and well-being. *Social and Personality Psychology Compass*, *5*(1), 1–12. https://doi.org/10.1111/j.1751-9004.2010.00330.x

Panksepp, J. (1994). The role of brain emotional systems in the construction of social systems. *Politics and the Life Sciences*, *13*(1), 116–119.

Porges, S.W. (2007). The polyvagal perspective *Biologicall Psychology*, *74*(2), 116–143. https://doi.org/10.1016/j.biopsycho.2006.06.009

Rector, N.A., Bagby, R.M., Segal, Z.V., Joffe, R.T., & Levitt, A. (2000). Self-criticism and dependency in depressed patients treated with *cognitive* therapy or pharmacotherapy. *Cognitive Therapy and Research*, 24(5), 571–584. https://doi.org/10.1023/A:1005566112869

Romaniuk, M., Hampton, S., Brown, K., Fisher, G., Steindl, S.R., Kidd, C., & Kirby, J.N. (2023). Compassionate mind training for ex-service personnel with PTSD and their partners. *Clinical Psychology & Psychotherapy*, *30*(3), 643–658.

Rushforth, A., Kotera, Y., & Kaluzeviciute, G. (2022). Theory Paper: Suggesting Compassion-Based Approaches for Treating Complex Post-traumatic Stress Disorder. *International Journal of Mental Health and Addiction*, 1–12. https://doi.org/10.1007/s11469-022-00856-4

Rycroft, C.M., 2016. *The Development and Evaluation of a Brief Self-practice Compassion-Focused Therapy (CFT) Intervention as a Precursor to Treatment as Usual (TAU) for Trauma Patients: A Pilot Randomised Controlled Trial (RCT)*. University of Lincoln.

Tirch, D., Schoendorff, B., & Silberstein, L.R. (2014). *The ACT practitioner's guide to the science of compassion: Tools for fostering psychological flexibility*. New Harbinger Publications.

Uvnäs Moberg, K. & Prime, D.K. (2013). Oxytocin effects in mothers and infants during breastfeeding. *Infant*, *9*(6), 201–206.

Wachtel, P.L. (1967). Conceptions of broad and narrow attention. *Psychological Bulletin*, 68(6), 417–429. https://doi.org/10.1037/h0025186

Wilson, A.C., Mackintosh, K., Power, K., & Chan, S.W.Y. (2019). Effectiveness of self-compassion related therapies: A systematic review and meta-analysis. *Mindfulness*, *10*(6), 979–995. https://doi.org/10.1007/s12671-018-1037-6

Winders, S.J., Murphy, O., Looney, K., & O'Reilly, G. (2020). Self-compassion, trauma, and posttraumatic stress disorder: A systematic review. *Clinical Psychology & Psychotherapy*, *27*(3), 300–329.

Zuroff, D.C., Mongrain, M., & Santor, D.A. (2004). Conceptualizing and measuring personality vulnerability to depression: Comment on Coyne and Whiffen (1995). *Psychological Bulletin*, *130*(3), 489–511. https://doi.org/10.1037/0033-2909.130.3.489

CHAPTER 16
USING CHAIRWORK PSYCHOTHERAPY IN THE TREATMENT OF TRAUMA

The Way of the Four Dialogues

Scott Kellogg and Amanda Garcia Torres

INTRODUCTION

This chapter introduces readers to the practice of chairwork psychotherapy and its application for the treatment of trauma, PTSD, and inner suffering. Chairwork psychotherapy is a dynamic experiential modality that involves: (a) inviting a patient to sit in one chair and have an imaginal encounter with someone from the past, the present, or the future in the chair opposite; (b) creating a storytelling chair in which the patient can express and work through difficult, painful, or secret narratives; and/or (c) using several chairs to create dialogues among different parts of the self. The principal aspects of chairwork psychotherapy will be explained and illustrated in this chapter. This includes the *Four Dialogues*, which are: *Giving Voice, Internal Dialogues, Telling the Story*, and *Relationships and Encounters*. These serve as the foundation and the core components of all chairwork dialogues. Two case examples will then be presented demonstrating the use of chairwork psychotherapy for the treatment of trauma.

A BRIEF HISTORY OF CHAIRWORK PSYCHOTHERAPY

Chairwork psychotherapy is a synthesis and a celebration of over 60 years of chairwork practice and experimentation by a wide range of integrative and experiential therapists. First created by Dr. Jacob Moreno, the originator of psychodrama (Moreno, 2019) in the 1950s, it was later adopted and further developed in the 1960s by Dr. Friedrich "Fritz" Perls, the creator of Gestalt therapy (Perls, 1969). At its most basic, chairwork involves "(a) inviting a patient to sit in one chair and have an imaginal encounter with someone from the past, the present, or the future in the chair opposite" and/or (b) "using several chairs to create dialogues among different parts of the self—with love, desire, fear, and courage often emerging as core themes" (Kellogg & Garcia Torres 2021, p. 171–172). This approach not only draws on the foundations provided by Gestalt therapy (Perls, 1969) and psychodrama (Moreno, 2019), but also on the insights and practices of redecision therapy (Goulding & Goulding, 1997), schema therapy (Young, Klosko, & Weishaar, 2003), emotion focused

DOI: 10.4324/9781003455851-16

therapy (Greenberg, Rice, & Elliott, 1993), cognitive behavioral therapy (Burns, 2006), voice dialogue (Stone & Stone, 1989), and transformational chairwork (Kellogg, 2014).

FUNDAMENTAL CLINICAL CONCEPTS

The core components of chairwork psychotherapy are the *Four Principles* and the *Four Dialogues*. The *Four Principles* affirm that:

1. It is clinically useful to understand people as containing different parts, modes, voices, or selves;
2. It is healing and transformative for people to give voice to these different parts;
3. It is also healing and transformative for people to enact or re-enact scenes from the past, the present, or the future; and
4. The ultimate goal of chairwork, the "True North" of the practice, is the strengthening of what is known as the ego in psychoanalysis (Freud, 1969), the healthy adult mode in schema therapy (Young et al., 2003), or the Inner Leader in the chairwork approach (Kellogg & Garcia Torres, 2021).

In 2001, Kellogg, in the context of his work as a schema therapist (Young et al., 2003), began an intense exploration of the therapeutic possibilities of chairwork. In his efforts to better understand this healing art, he searched through clinical reports and case examples from the previous 40 years to learn how clinicians had used dialogue work in their sessions. He focused on the specific actions that therapists were taking when working with method – *regardless of their theoretical orientation*. Essentially using a "grounded theory" approach (Kellogg, 2023), he looked at the successful cases through the lens of the "chairs," and, out of this, he was able to develop his first framework for using chairwork in psychotherapy (Kellogg, 2004). Building on this initial formulation, the *Transformational Chairwork Psychotherapy Project* (Kellogg, 2014) was created in 2008 as a vehicle for training other therapists in this method of therapy, and, in 2013, Garcia Torres (2020; 2021) joined in the effort. In 2018, inspired by a training in the voice dialogue method (Gaspard, 2020; Stone & Stone, 1989), Kellogg created the *Four Dialogues*, which bears some similarity to the *Integrated Gestalt Practice* model of Sonne and Tønnesvang (2015). This new understanding became the foundation for *Chairwork Psychotherapy*.

The Four Dialogues are: Giving Voice, Internal Dialogues, Telling the Story, and Relationships and Encounters; they serve as the foundation and the core components of all chairwork dialogues. *Giving Voice* involves: (1) isolating and amplifying an emotional state to transform it into a part (e.g., the Sad Part); (2) interviewing a part to understand its role, history, and function in the person's life; and (3) empowering people to claim personal authority and to say "No" to that which imprisons them and "Yes" to life and positive changes; *Internal Dialogues* involves creating encounters between the different parts of the self so that not only is the inner world of the individual more harmonious, but also the functioning of the patient in the outside world is more effective and less conflicted. *Telling the Story* is a way to engage with and work through difficult, troubling, and traumatic memories so that the patient is less haunted by them. Lastly, *Relationships and Encounters* involve dialogues with other people that often involve the expression of feelings of love, anger, fear, and grief; the intention is to help people resolve grief and work though experiences of mistreatment or abuse (Kellogg & Garcia Torres, 2021).

DESCRIPTION OF THE CHAIRWORK PSYCHOTHERAPY PROCESS

Drawing on schema mode therapy, chairwork psychotherapy can be seen as using a trans-diagnostic approach to treatment. With the Four Dialogues as a framework, all patients can be understood as having various combinations of challenges with parts, difficult memories, and relationships. The core therapeutic questions for each session are: "What is the problem and why is it a problem now?" This connects us to the "Here and Now" emphasis of Gestalt therapy (Perls, 1969). While a range of dialogical interventions are used in the work, the overarching goal is to strengthen the Inner Leader as this is a mechanism for working through each of these challenges.

The Inner Leader has its roots in the ego of the Freudian structural model (Freud, 1969), the adult ego state of redecision therapy (Goulding & Goulding, 1997), and the healthy adult mode of schema therapy (Rafaeli, Bernstein, & Young, 2011; Young et al., 2003). It is the executive of the system, and it is challenged to take authority in three areas (Kellogg & Tatarsky, 2012). The first is that of regulating the other parts. While each of these have their specific function, role, and history, in a healthy system they are subordinate to the Inner Leader. In many ways, this is the core challenge of psychotherapy as critical, frightened, angry, self-soothing, or aggressive parts may be too strong – which is why the patient is in therapy (Rafaeli et al., 2011). The parts dialogues (*Giving Voice* and *Internal Dialogues*) will always include work with the Inner Leader.

The second challenge is that of learning how to successfully engage with and form successful relationships with other people. The third is the capacity to "take assertive, meaningful, and effective action in the world" (Kellogg & Tatarsky, 2012, p, 115). This means that the Inner Leader holds and embodies the individual's values and makes decisions and chooses life directions based on them. Given this, the Inner Leader may be understood as having a heroic dimension in the world.

UTILIZATION OF CHAIRWORK PSYCHOTHERAPY FOR THE TREATMENT OF TRAUMA

Trauma can be organized into two categories: (1) acute trauma – which would include experiences such as a criminal attack, a natural or man-made disaster, or an automobile accident; and (2) developmental or complex trauma – which would refer to ongoing abuse, mistreatment, or impingements on the self that occurred during childhood or during a long-term adult relationship. The good news is that there is an array of chairwork dialogues that can be used to bring healing and freedom to patients living with the effects of trauma or mistreatment – whether acute or developmental. One question that is helpful to ask of these patients is: "How is that living in you today?" This captures the idea that patients who come to therapy for trauma treatment are challenged by a past that is living in the present – rather than a painful but historical memory.

TELLING THE STORY

The approach to therapeutic storytelling was initially inspired by an acute stress disorder study by Bryant and colleagues (Bryant 2008). In the original chairwork model, patients who wanted to work through their experiences of abuse or mistreatment would begin by sitting in the Center or the Inner Leader chair. They would then be asked to recall a relevant difficult or problematic memory. Next, they would be invited to move to another chair and tell the story, as best they could, of the troubling or disturbing incident. The chairs were set up in such a way that they were not directly looking at the therapist, which allowed the patient to go into their own private space while still feeling the presence of the therapist. After telling the story, they were encouraged to stand up, move around, shake it off, and then sit down and tell the story again. This process was repeated three to five times (Kellogg, 2018). Not surprisingly, this was often a very emotionally intense experience. What was quite striking about it, however, was that more details emerged with each iteration. This was interpreted as a sign that the trauma narrative was being integrated by the patient – which is a pathway to healing.

In 2019, inspired by the work of Roediger, Stevens, and Brockman (2018), the creators of chairwork psychotherapy moved to a *third-person storytelling model*. In the original model, if a patient named Harper had been in a car accident, they could move to another chair and tell the story in the first-person: "I was in a car accident, and these are some of the things that happened to me." With third-person storytelling, Harper would move from Center to another chair and tell the story of the car accident in the third person: "Harper was in a car accident, and these are some of the things that happened to them." This is a compelling way of working as it is less intense than first-person storytelling, while also providing sufficient emotional activation to facilitate the integration of the traumatic material. This has now become the favored form of trauma storytelling in chairwork psychotherapy.
To be clear, the patients who are engaging in these dialogues are in therapy because they want to work through their traumas or difficult memories; no one is pressured to do any more than they wish to. Sometimes the story can only be told once, and this is completely acceptable. For cases where the patient is unable to complete the storytelling, they also have the option to speak a part of the story, or even just the first sentence: "There was a girl named Charlotte and when she was five something scary happened to her." In such an instance the patient and therapist can revisit the work over the course of many sessions, or until the patient is able to give a full expression of the story.

There is another, perhaps unexpected, benefit here. While the telling of trauma stories can be difficult for the patient, it can also be hard for the therapist to hear them. With repetitive storytelling, the therapist can undergo a process of habituation; a process in which they become less triggered by very disturbing material. As their anxiety declines, they will gain the freedom to engage with the material more actively and may even be able to work with very intimate details. In short, both the patient and the therapist have something to gain from this process.

RELATIONSHIPS AND ENCOUNTERS

While each of these approaches can be used in a stand-alone manner, *Telling the Story* and work in the interpersonal realm often flow together. With interpersonal trauma or mistreatment, the core dialogue work involves the patient – in their Inner Leader mode – speaking, respectively, with the perpetrator or the abuser, the people who might have known what was going on and did not intervene to help them, and/or themselves at an earlier developmental stage. To start, the patient sits in Center, or the Inner Leader chair, and imagines the relevant person in the chair opposite. Using the *Cycle of Emotions*, the therapist invites them to express their love, anger, fear, or grief – as appropriate to that person. When working with figures who abused or mistreated the patient, there are some strategies to be considered.

Role reversal is an essential part of psychodrama (Moreno, 2019), and it is core to chairwork psychotherapy as well. In general, role reversal involves inviting a patient to switch chairs and "become" the other person – the person that they are concerned with. The therapist not only interviews this person to better understand them, but also facilitates a dialogue between this person and the patient. This is, fundamentally, an exercise in empathy and it can be profoundly healing. When working with trauma, however, role reversal needs to be used selectively. It is important that patients be able to fully express their anger – as well as other emotions – to the people who hurt or mistreated them (Young et al., 2003). Given that, one should not invite the patient to do a role reversal with an abuser as the increase in empathy with the perpetrator can decrease the patient's ability to fully express their anger – which can interfere with the healing process (see also Kellerman, 2000).

Again, some patients may find it to be quite difficult to speak to someone who mistreated them, as the level of fear may be quite high – even in an imaginal setting. When this occurs, it can be very therapeutic for the therapist to step in and confront the abuser while defending the patient. This can be understood as a form of *reparenting* – which is a fundamental mechanism of healing in schema therapy (Young et al., 2003).

With people who knew about the abuse – especially childhood abuse – the *Cycle of Emotions* can be used as well. Here, the dialogue structure would be the same while the range of emotions may be different with a greater emphasis on anger, grief, and love. With these dialogues, which are often with a mother, father, or some kind of caregiving figure, a role reversal strategy might be considered. The patient may want to know why they were not protected, as this may feel unresolved for them. If they decide to go ahead, they may learn that the caregiver felt responsible for other children and was an economic prisoner, that they were being abused and terrified by the perpetrator, and/or that they were depressed or addicted, and so on. The therapist can ask the caregiver if they had an opportunity to go back in time and do it all over, would they do something different? If they say yes, that can certainly be healing for the patient.

Perhaps of greatest importance in the therapy of experiences of childhood abuse is for the patient to be able to speak with care, compassion, and empathy to their child self – the part of them that experienced the abuse. Strikingly, many patients have difficulty speaking to their child self with any kindness. If this is the case, it is important that the therapist step in and dialogue directly with the child in the chair. Some strategies to consider are: (1) Affirmations of the goodness and the beauty of the child and distress over what they are going through: "You are such a lovely and beautiful child, and I am so angry and so upset about what you are going through." (2) Affirmations that they are seen and that they are not alone:

> "I know what you are going through. Big [Patient's Name] told me what is happening, and I hate them for doing this to you. I want you to know that I see you. I cannot fix this, and I cannot stop this, but you are seen – you are no longer alone."

MIXED EMOTIONS

While the emotions evoked and expressed in the relationship dialogues may sometimes be quite clear and straightforward, other patients may have quite complex and confused feelings toward those who mistreated them or those who did not protect them. These relationships may have included a wide range of experiences – good, bad, and neutral. For example, a parent may have had episodes of being emotionally abusive due to marital, economic, or psychiatric pressures, but was quite loving and warm when things were better. These "mixed emotions" resonate with Perls' (1969) emphasis on ambivalence and the importance of being able to express both appreciations and resentments. Relationships between adults can also be a source of deeply conflicting feelings.

> I was in love with my spouse, and we were making plans to have a child. I was happy about this – I was excited to move into the next stage of our lives together. You cannot even begin to imagine my horror when one day she stopped coming home and started telling her friends that I was a bad partner. I have tried to reach out repeatedly and she won't speak to me. I am beside myself.

Clearly this level of betrayal is extremely difficult to process. The *Rhombic Dialogue* (Chesner, 2019; Kellogg, Trapp & Rizzon, in press; Pugh, 2019), which is a four-chair dialogue structure, is a powerful method for engaging with this kind of pain. With this dialogue structure, the patient begins in Center – in the Inner Leader chair. There is a chair that is in front of them and six or eight feet away; this is for the personification of the person toward whom they have mixed feelings (Pugh, 2019). There are chairs, several feet away, at a 45-degree angle to their right and left, respectively; these chairs will be facing the other person. The patient then chooses one of the side chairs to hold the positive feelings and the other side chair to hold the negative feelings. Sitting in Center, the patient can look at the person in question, check in with themselves to assess their emotional state, and then move to the diagonal chair that embodies the dominant emotions. Going to the *resentments* chair, this patient could begin by saying: "I am horrified and enraged at what you did. How could you do this to me? So many lies! And telling our friends – and not letting me talk to you? It was so wrong" – and continues from there. They then move to the *appreciations* chair and give voice to this part:

> "My heart hurts. I loved you. I loved you. I was hoping we would have a beautiful life together. I would never purposefully hurt you. I am completely confused. You seemed to love me. When I am not enraged, I am filled with grief."

The patient does several rounds of going back and forth between these middle chairs – expressing their feelings to the problematic person. They then go back to Center, the Inner Leader chair, look at the person in the chair opposite, and assess where they are now emotionally and share that with the problematic person. The goal is to develop a more integrated sense of the person so that there is greater emotional stability within.

Another source of complex emotions is when the person has changed over time:

> Growing up with my father was a nightmare. He was a complete alcoholic, and he terrorized all of us. He has been sober for 15 years, and he has worked hard to turn his life around. He is one of my best friends.

This can leave the patient with a sense of the parent as two different people – which can be emotionally confusing. The *Vector Dialogue* structure – which uses three chairs – provides an opportunity to begin to work this through (Kellogg, 2019). The patient will start in the Center, in the Inner Leader chair; two chairs are placed at 45-degree angles to their right and left – facing the patient. These will embody the "good" part and the "bad" part of the problematic figure. They should be further away than in the Rhombic Dialogue – perhaps at a distance of five or six feet. The patient can be asked to set the distance that feels comfortable to them. The patient then decides which chair will embody the good person and the bad person, respectively, and they speak to each of them accordingly. Here, the goal is to conceive and experience them as two different people – one with whom there is a possibility of a positive or affirming relationship and the other who can be released and left in the past. With both the Rhombic and the Vector Dialogues, it may take several sessions of chairwork to sort through these emotional complexities before any kind of resolution is achieved.

ENACTMENTS AND RE-ENACTMENTS

Enactments and re-enactments have deep roots in psychodrama (Hudgins & Kellerman, 2000), and it can be seen as a combination of *Telling the Story* and *Relationships and Encounters*. The goal is to re-work a memory or a story so that the patient is in a place of greater power at the end. As M.M. Goulding and R. Goulding (1997) emphasized in their work, they want to "turn the scene from [a] tragedy to a drama that ends well" (p. 168).

The patient can begin by calling up a troubling memory; the therapist and the patient can organize the chairs to represent the different figures in the story. The therapist and patient begin by standing and looking at the situation laid out before them. They can then move around and confront the abuser, protect the child or the younger self, and engage with other people who may have been involved. Chairs embodying beneficial forces such as the police or angels can be introduced. They can also confront the abuser and protect and affirm the patient. Yelling and the use of invective is invited. The abuser's chair can be knocked over and/or removed from the room after the confrontation is complete. The Child chair can be moved to a safe place and a wall of chairs can be put around them for protection. If it is an adult trauma, a wall of chairs can be set up, and the patient, with the therapist standing nearby, can stand behind the wall and confront and yell at the abuser in the other chair. The patient and therapist can also work to challenge thoughts of self-blame for the mistreatment that might be taking place in the child and/or challenge cognitive distortions that might be taking place in the adult. Again, the goal is to challenge victimhood and move the client to an empowered state (Goulding & Goulding, 1997).

INTERNAL DIALOGUES

The trauma therapy literature refers to trauma-related schemas or modes. In chairwork psychotherapy, trauma-related beliefs and strategies are seen as being embodied in different parts and behaviors. These often take the form of parts that are either perceiving high levels of danger, or fomenting critical attacks on the self; they may also take the form of behaviors connected to avoidance and self-soothing. These are understood, engaged with, and healed using *Internal Dialogues*.

As noted earlier, while some patients come into therapy because of histories of childhood abuse and mistreatment, others are wrestling with extreme experiences that have occurred when they were adults. Resick (2001), in her cognitive processing therapy, laid a central emphasis on the role of schemas in PTSD. Over time, people develop schemas about themselves and the way the world functions. These schemas serve to guide behavior and help make the world seem more predictable or manageable. When a traumatic event does occur, it may so deeply challenge the worldview of the current schema or schemas that a new schema is created. This new schema is typically very fear driven and rigid. The world is now seen as dangerous or more dangerous than it was before, while the individual is felt to be lacking in power. Resick believes that this new schema is not connected to the older, pretrauma schema and it is this disconnection that is a driver for PTSD.

Hudgins (2002) tells the story of Andrea, a young woman who was gang-raped just as she began college. Andrea described her situation this way:

> I used to be this lively, happy girl, ready to take on the world. I was so excited about starting college .... I knew good things were ahead of me. ... But now ... I'm a scared, lonely, and ugly girl inside and out. ... I have no ambition .... All I care about is being left alone so I can be safe.
>
> (p. 13)

Building on Resick's conceptualization, chairwork could be used to create an encounter between the old schema and the new, threat-driven schema. On the one hand, the old schema was not capable of integrating the traumatic experience; on the other, the trauma-driven schema is full of cognitive distortions and does not allow for healthy functioning in the world.

Building on work by de Oliveira (2016), the two schemas could be envisioned as two people making different arguments (Pugh, 2019; Roediger et al., 2018). Before seeking to challenge the trauma-centered part, it is important to check in with the Inner Leader to see if they, in fact, want to change or give up this trauma-driven schema. This is an important motivational piece that can be easily overlooked. Using a Rhombic Dialogue and Burns' (2006) cost-benefit analysis structure, the patient could start in Center – or the Inner Leader chair – with the trauma-based perspective personified in the chair opposite ("I believe we should hide from the world"). At 45 degrees to the left and the right could be two "attorneys" – one that would argue for the benefits of keeping the trauma-centered belief ("it will keep me safe") and one arguing that the costs are too high ("I am completely losing my life"). With the therapist's guidance, the patient can move among all four chairs, speaking from the different perspectives and reacting to them in the Inner Leader chair. After this, the patient can decide whether they want to go forward.

Having decided to go forward, the patient could begin in Center with two chairs in front – at 45-degree angles – facing each other. One is the personification and the embodiment of the threat-centered schema ("I believe that the world is filled with evil men and I want nothing to do with it"), and the other chair is the embodiment of the pretrauma schema ("While it is true some men are evil and dangerous, I have found many others to be good; there are a number of them that I have loved and who have been good to me"). The patient is invited to decide which chair will embody which part; they can then move back and forth between the two chairs – giving voice to the different perspectives. To increase the emotional intensity, patients are encouraged to stand behind the chairs – which helps them to speak more authoritatively from each perspective. Referring to the preceding example, the "Happy Girl" and the "Traumatized Girl" could engage and dialogue with each other.

After doing this numerous times, the patient returns to Center and reflects on the experience. With sufficient emotional intensity, a third perspective will likely emerge that integrates aspects of the other two. The Inner Leader can then choose to embrace this new perspective, which will allow them to function more effectively in the world (Kellogg & Garcia Torres, 2021).

RELATIONAL SELF DIALOGUES: WHAT WAS I THINKING?

Trauma is complex – which means that some patients may see themselves, rightly or wrongly, as partly or completely responsible for what happened. As they look back with hindsight, they may castigate themselves for the decisions they made. However, the decisions made at an earlier time each have their own logic – using the worldview and the values that they embraced at that time. The decisions they made in the past might have been the correct ones – even if something traumatic occurred.

The *Relational Self Dialogue* model, which is drawn from the *Attachment Timeline* work of Dayton (2023), is a blend of *Relationships and Encounters* and *Internal Dialogues*, and it is appropriate when the younger self is an adolescent or an adult – not a child. The patient starts in Center – in the Inner Leader chair. In the chair opposite, they imagine their younger self – the self that was alive at the time of the trauma. They begin by expressing their thoughts, feelings, and concerns about what happened. They then switch chairs, do a role reversal, and become this younger self. In this chair, with the assistance of the therapist, the younger self describes their current situation and makes the case for their decision in as vigorous a manner as possible. The goal is for them to defend their life. The patient then moves back to the Inner Leader/Center chair, pauses for a moment or two to take in what the younger self said, and then responds. This cycle is repeated several times. The goal is for the Inner Leader to not only understand, but also to feel what the younger self was going through. The hope is that the self-castigation will stop, and there will be an emergence of self-compassion.

ASSESSMENT OF RESEARCH EVIDENCE REGARDING THE EFFECTIVENESS OF CHAIRWORK PSYCHOTHERAPY

The world of psychotherapy is currently witnessing a chairwork renaissance. More clinicians are using this method, integrating it into their therapeutic approaches, writing about it, training others in it, and doing research on its effectiveness. A recent meta-analysis on "Chairwork in Individual Psychotherapy" by Pascual-Leone and Bahar (2023) is likely the best summation statement on the clinical power of chairwork. There are several essential findings from their study:

1. In single-session studies, the use of chairwork did lead to a decrease in symptoms – but not more than other interventions. In this context, chairwork is equally effective with other therapeutic interventions in a one-session scenario.
2. Including chairwork as a central part of ongoing treatment does lead to somewhat better outcomes than therapies that do not use chairwork.
3. There may be differences in the effectiveness of different therapies that use chairwork. Emotion focused therapy did better than therapies that did not use chairwork and the impact of chairwork increased over time – even after therapy was completed.

These findings should give hope and encouragement to clinicians who are considering using chairwork in the treatment of their patients – whether they are suffering from trauma or some other form of inner anguish.

CASE EXAMPLES OF USING CHAIRWORK PSYCHOTHERAPY IN TRAUMA TREATMENT

JAMES: A SURVIVOR OF CARJACKING AND A CAR CRASH

A man named James has experienced a carjacking and a major accident. He is in therapy to address depression and PTSD symptoms. Using the *third-person storytelling* dialogue structure, his therapist might say, "I want you to move to this chair and tell the story of what happened, but I want you to tell the story as if someone else were talking about you." Before beginning, the therapist might ask him to "take some breaths" to mindfully shift into the storytelling work. The patient may start with, "There was a man named James and one night when he was leaving work to drive home, someone threatened him with a weapon and forced himself into his car." With encouragement from the clinician, the patient would continue: "James was terrified. He thought he would be killed." If James begins to struggle with continuing the story, the therapist might gently ask questions like, "And then what happened?" "What was James feeling/thinking?" or "How has this impacted James?" The patient can expand with, "James froze and could not get out of the car," "After driving for a while, James pushed the gas. He thought he might escape if he crashed the car," and "He has nightmares and cannot get himself to drive. He feels ashamed that he was not able to protect himself."

After the patient completes the initial round, the therapist would instruct James to stand up, move around, and sit back down to complete another retelling of the story. "I'd like you to do that again. When you are ready, please begin." This storytelling process would be repeated a total of three to five times, depending on the emotional tolerance of the patient. More details may emerge with each subsequent retelling, and the patient may begin to expand his perspective of what happened to the protagonist of the story: "James was distracted that night because he wanted to get to his wife who needed his help. He was trying to be a good husband," and "James crashed the car because he thought it was the only way to survive. He got hurt, but he lived. It worked!" After the final retelling, the therapist might say, "After being with James's story, what do you feel about what happened to him?" The patient might share and increase his understanding and compassion for the protagonist, and develop a larger perspective on the forces at play in the traumatic story. The therapist and the patient would both move to different chairs to debrief the experience.

In a following session, the therapist can invite the patient to engage in a *Relationships and Encounters* dialogue so that James can confront the perpetrator. The clinician would set up two chairs and invite the patient to imagine the perpetrator in the empty chair across. James would then be invited to stand behind a chair, imagine the perpetrator in the empty chair, and express his feelings and thoughts about what happened, "You scared me so much. Because of you, I feel like I cannot protect myself; especially at night. This fear is crippling me," and "I also drink to forget what happened." As the dialogue progresses, the patient would be asked to express any anger they may have, "You had no right to hurt me. You could have taken my money and let me go. I hate you!" Once this patient has spoken for some time, the clinician would ask him to describe the perpetrator and note if his appearance or energy has changed, "You seem much smaller than I remembered. You wait in the dark to sneak up on people. You pick unfair fights. I pity you."

In a final step, the clinician can ask James to speak from and embody his Inner Leader: "I wonder if you might express your intention of how you want to live your life now?" to which James might tap into his existential empowerment and say, "I refuse to hide away because of you. I am going to get behind the wheel of my new car. You do not control me." After this dialogue is complete, the therapist and patient would both move to new chairs to debrief the dialogue experience.

EMMA: A SURVIVOR OF SEXUAL ASSAULT AT A PARTY

A 30-year-old woman named Emma seeks therapy due to persistent PTSD symptoms and social difficulties which emerged following a sexual assault by a college teammate. While it would be good to complete *Storytelling* work with her, she would likely also benefit from a *Relational Self Dialogue*. Using two chairs, the clinician may facilitate a dialogue between Emma and her younger self that experienced the assault. The patient would begin in Center, tapping into their Inner Leader: "I am Emma, I am the Inner Leader, and this is my life."

Then this patient would be asked, "Can you imagine 19-year-old Emma? I'd like you to speak to her about what she experienced." This can sound like,

> "You are so eager and naive and something so terrible happened to us. While I have been distressed about this for a long time, I want you to tell me your story. I want to know how you made sense of it."

The patient would then be asked to do a role reversal and to speak from the perspective of their young adult self: "I can't believe this happened to me. My freedom and joy were taken. I feel I was so stupid to trust anyone." After expressing her emotional distress, the therapist might then ask Emma to walk through her decision-making around the assault,

> "I am young, but I am not stupid or reckless. I stayed away from the party drugs; I made my own drinks. I did everything right and I still got hurt. That guy was someone I knew and seemed okay; I just wanted to have fun."

Switching chairs and becoming the Inner Leader, Emma would take a few moments to see if she can take it in; if not, she would be invited to switch chairs and become younger Emma and again defend herself by affirming that she made fairly good decisions. This may take a few rounds. The therapist would then invite adult Emma to see if she could speak to her younger self with compassion. The goal would be for her to be able to say something like this:

> "For a long time, I did not understand the decisions you made that night; but now I see you did your best to be cautious. He was an acquaintance, so you thought he was safer than the other guys. I see you and I hear your pain."

After this is complete, the clinician and patient can debrief the experience. Emma may begin to feel less responsible for the assault, and more accepting of her 19-year-old self who was simply doing her best.

Moving into a *Cognitive Restructuring* dialogue, the therapist and patient would complete an exploration of Emma's pre- and posttrauma informed schemas. Setting up two chairs, both facing outward, the therapist would ask Emma to stand behind one chair and speak from that part that is centered in the trauma: "All men are predators. I will keep them far away." Moving to stand behind the second chair, the clinician would ask the patient, "Would you speak from the part that embodies what you believed prior to the assault?" Emma might say, "I love making friends and having new experiences! I never want to miss out on anything or anyone." The patient would be asked to shuttle back and forth between the chairs, speaking from the two perspectives. After doing this for several rounds, a third voice might begin to emerge: "I want safety, but I am so sad and lonely." Moving to Center, the Inner Leader might say,

> "I want safety, and I want to be a part of the world. I am allowed to welcome some people and to keep others out. I can accept the fun of new experiences and I can accept the regret of missing out."

The therapist can check in with the patient and ask her to assess how she is feeling with this new belief: "I am a bit nervous, but I feel good when I say that I can choose who I hang out with and that I can also deal with missing out. I feel that I can live with this." The therapist and patient would then move to different chairs to debrief the dialogue work and to begin discussing how Emma might embody her new schema system in her daily life.

STRENGTHS AND LIMITATIONS OF CHAIRWORK PSYCHOTHERAPY AS A TREATMENT FOR TRAUMA

The "rule of thumb" for us has been that if the patient can do psychotherapy, they can do chairwork. The caveat is that the clinician will want to make adjustments in terms of speed and intensity to meet the specific needs and capabilities of the patient. The way to help ensure safety is to repeatedly assess their level of motivation. Does the patient want to work through the trauma? There is usually a part that wants to go into it and get better and a part that does not. An *Internal Dialogues* chairwork session is a perfect way to sort this out; in fact, it may be necessary and important to return to the motivation dialogue several times during the treatment as the Inner Leader must be in alliance with the therapist for the treatment to proceed.

Another way to approach this is to keep the essential elements of the *Four Dialogues* in mind. The releasing of the burden of the secrets and the confronting of that which is terrifying is often central to the restoration of the self. It can be done in many small steps. Whether done by the patient or the therapist, interacting with the people involved and the traumatized child or self is vital. Challenging problematic or skewed beliefs, schemas, or cognitions is essential for improved functioning. If the therapist stays anchored in these principles, they will likely find ways to do chairwork that are healing and transformative.

RESOURCES FOR LEARNING

BOOKS

Kellogg, S. (2014). *Transformational Chairwork: Using psychotherapeutic dialogues in clinical practice.* Lanham, MD: Rowman & Littlefield.

Pugh, M. (2019). *Cognitive behavioural chairwork: Distinctive features*. Abingdon, Oxon: Routledge.

van der Wijngaart, R. (2023). *Chairwork: Theory and practice*. Shoreham by Sea, West Sussex, UK: Pavilion Publishing.

ARTICLE

Kellogg, S., & Garcia Torres, A. (2021). Toward a Chairwork Psychotherapy: Using the Four Dialogues for Healing and Transformation. *Practice Innovations, 6*(3), 171–180. http://dx.doi.org/10.1037/pri0000149

WEBSITES

Chairwork Psychotherapy Initiative (https://www.chairworkpsychotherapy.com/)
Chairwork (https://chairwork.co.uk/about-us/)

REFERENCES

Bryant, R. et al. (2008). A randomized controlled trial of exposure therapy and cognitive restructuring for posttraumatic stress disorder. *Journal of Consulting and Clinical Psychology, 76*, 695–703. doi:10.1037/a0012616

Burns, D.D. (2006). *When panic attacks: The new drug-free anxiety therapy that can change your life*. Harmony Books

Chesner, A. (2019). Working with addictions: The addictions compass and intergenerational action genogram. In A. Chesner (Ed.), *One-to-one psychodrama psychotherapy: Applications and technique*. Abingdon, Oxon: Routledge.

Dayton, T. (2023). *Treating adult children of relational trauma: 85 experiential interventions to heal the inner child and create authentic connections to the present*. Eau Claire, WI: PESI Publishing.

de Oliveira. I.R. (2016). *Trial-based cognitive therapy: Distinctive features*. London: Routledge.

Freud, S. (1969). *An outline of psycho-analysis*. New York: W. W. Norton.

Garcia Torres, A. (January 9, 2020). Using psychotherapeutic dialogues for healing and liberation: Chairwork y La Raza. *Public Seminar*. https://publicseminar.org/essays/using-psychotherapeutic-dialogues-for-healing-and-liberation/

Garcia Torres, A. (March, 2021). Using Chairwork Psychotherapy to combat the psychological impact of oppression. *Schema Therapy Bulletin, 21*.4–11. https://transformationalchairwork.com/wp-content/uploads/2021/09/Garcia-Torres-ISST-Social-Justice-Chairwork-Psychotherapy.pdf

Gaspard, B.D. (2020). *The final 8th: Enlist your inner selves to accomplish your goals*. Novato, CA: New World Library.

Goulding, M.M., & Goulding, R. (1997). *Changing lives through decision therapy*. New York: Grove Press.

Greenberg, L.S., Rice, L.N., & Elliott, R. (1993). *Facilitating emotional change: The moment-by-moment process*. New York: Guilford Press.

Hudgins, K. (2002). *Experiential treatment for PTSD: The therapeutic spiral model.* New York: Springer Publishing Company.

Hudgins, M.K. & Kellerman, P.F. (2000). *Introduction.* In P.F. Kellerman & M.K. Hudgins (Eds.), *Psychodrama with trauma survivors: Acting out your pain* (pp. 11–19). London: Jessica Kingsley.

Kellerman, P.F. (2000). The therapeutic aspects of psychodrama with traumatized people. In P.F. Kellerman & M.K. Hudgins (Eds.), *Psychodrama with trauma survivors: Acting out your pain* (pp. 23–38). London: Jessica Kingsley.

Kellogg, S. (2014). *Transformational Chairwork: Using psychotherapeutic dialogues in clinical practice.* Lanham, MD: Rowman & Littlefield.

Kellogg, S. (July, 2018). Transformational Chairwork: The four-dialogue matrix. *Schema Therapy Bulletin.* http://transformationalchairwork.com/wp-content/uploads/2018/07/Kellogg-TCW-Four-Dialogue-Matrix-ISST-Bulletin1.pdf

Kellogg, S. (October, 2019). Transformational Chairwork: Therapeutic change using the four dialogues. *InPsych: The Bulletin of the Australian Psychological Society Limited,* 41, 16–21. https://www.psychology.org.au/formembers/publications/inpsych/2019/october/Transformational-chairwork

Kellogg, S. (Spring, 2023). Chairwork Psychotherapy: Using the Four Dialogues in the Treatment of Trauma. *New York City Cognitive Therapy Association Newsletter.* https://www.chairworkpsychotherapy.com/traumafourdialogues

Kellogg, S., & Garcia Torres, A. (2021). Toward a Chairwork Psychotherapy: Using the Four Dialogues for Healing and Transformation. *Practice Innovations,* 6(3), 171–180. http://dx.doi.org/10.1037/pri0000149

Kellogg, S., Trapp, R., & Rizzon, A. (in press). Bringing it to life: Using Chairwork and the four dialogues in Schema Therapy. In J. Monteiro & B. Cardosa (Eds.). *Como eu faço Terapia do Esquema. Brazil.* https://www.chairworkpsychotherapy.com/chairworkschematherapy

Kellogg, S.H. (2004). Dialogical encounters: Contemporary perspectives on "chairwork" in psychotherapy. *Psychotherapy: Research, Theory, Practice, Training,* 41, 310–320.

Kellogg, S.H., & Tatarsky, A. (2012). Re-Envisioning addiction treatment: A 6-point plan. *Alcoholism Treatment Quarterly,* 30, 1–20. http://www.tandfonline.com/doi/abs/10.1080/07347324.2012.635544

Moreno, J. (2019). *Psychodrama.* Psychodrama Press.

Pascual-Leone, A., & Bahar, T. (2023). Chairwork in individual psychotherapy: Meta-analyses of intervention effects. *Psychotherapy,* 60(3), 370–382. doi:10.1037/pst0000490

Perls, F.S. (1969). *Gestalt Therapy verbatim.* Moab, UT: Real People Press.

Pugh, M. (2019). A little less talk, a little more action: A dialogical approach to cognitive therapy. *The Cognitive Behaviour Therapist,* 12, E47. doi:10.1017/S1754470X19000333

Rafaeli, E., Bernstein, D.P., & Young, J. (2011). *Schema therapy: Distinctive features.* East Sussex, UK: Routledge.

Resick, P.A. (2001). Cognitive therapy for posttraumatic stress disorder. *Journal of Cognitive Therapy: An International Quarterly,* 15, 321–329.

Roediger, E., Stevens, B., & Brockman, R. (2018). *Contextual schema therapy: An integrative approach to personality disorders, emotional dysregulation & interpersonal functioning.* Oakland, CA: Context Press.

Sonne, M., & Tønnesvang, J. (2015). *Integrative Gestalt practice: Transforming our ways of working with people.* London: Karnac Books.

Stone, H., & Stone, S. (1989). *Embracing our selves: The voice dialogue manual.* Novato, CA: New World Library.

Young, J.E., Klosko, J.S., & Weishaar, M.E. (2003). *Schema Therapy: A practitioner's guide.* New York: Guilford.

CHAPTER 17
CONCLUSION

Synthesis and Future Directions

*Evan Senreich, Shulamith Lala Ashenberg
Straussner and Jordan Dann*

INTRODUCTION

From the descriptions of the 15 experiential therapies in this book, it is apparent that they represent a wide diversity of theoretical underpinnings and clinical processes with their own language and techniques. One might wonder how these different treatment modalities fall into a single category called "experiential psychotherapy." For example, there would seem to be little similarity between the psychoanalytic basis of intensive short-term dynamic psychotherapy (ISTDP); the creative metaphoric processes of expressive arts therapy (EXA); the "bottom-up" body sensation foci of somatic experiencing therapy (SE) and sensorimotor psychotherapy (SP); the focus on memory reconsolidation in coherence therapy; the strong influence of attachment theory utilized in accelerated experiential dynamic psychotherapy (AEDP); the emphasis on an individual's "parts" in internal family systems therapy (IFS); and the bilateral brain stimulation of eye movement desensitization and reprocessing (EMDR). When this wide array of therapies is utilized to treat the ramifications of exposure to trauma, their differences may seem more obvious than their similarities.

In reality, in spite of these major theoretical differences, the 15 experiential therapies explicated in this book share major aspects in common that far outweigh their diversity, which in particular informs their conceptualization of how to work with trauma survivors. This chapter begins with a delineation of the similarities of these therapies in working with clients impacted by trauma and concludes with an exploration of some of the issues regarding the future use of experiential therapies for the treatment of trauma.

COMMONALITIES AMONG EXPERIENTIAL THERAPIES FOR TREATING TRAUMA

PHENOMENOLOGICAL PERSPECTIVE

Phenomenology is a philosophical concept that can be defined as "the study of structures of consciousness as experienced from the first-person point of view" (Smith, 2013, p. 1).

DOI: 10.4324/9781003455851-17

Noting that it was primarily developed by the philosopher Edmund Husserl in the early 20th century, Längle and Klaasen (2021) state: "Phenomenology is an attitude of perception that does not focus on facts and 'objective' data but rather on that which appears subjectively to human beings" (p. 746). In all of the therapies described in this book, a phenomenological approach is key, with therapists helping clients focus on what individuals are experiencing in the moment and how they are experiencing it. "The phenomenological work is traditionally done by observation and focusing. The therapist inquires about the patient's actual experience on a rather continuous basis. The prototypical question is 'What are you experiencing now?' or 'What are you aware of now'" (Yontef & Fuhr, 2005. p. 94). No matter what the theoretical basis is of each of the experiential therapies in this book, the therapist is repeatedly drawing clients' attention to what they are experiencing in the room from moment to moment with total acceptance of the clients' subjective reactions.

When working with reactions resulting from trauma, therapists utilizing experiential therapies elicit clients' feelings, thoughts, memories, bodily sensations, and behaviors associated with the traumatic event in the present moment, but always attuned to supporting the client and not overwhelming them with what they cannot handle emotionally at the time. The 15 therapies in this book accomplish this in diverse ways. For example, Sensorimotor Psychotherapy, somatic experiencing therapy, focusing-oriented therapy, and Hakomi therapy may focus more intensely on bodily sensations, whereas emotion focused therapy (EFT) may focus more on the feelings arising from the traumatic situation. Expressive arts therapy focuses more on the client's artistic creative processes in the moment, whereas internal family systems therapy and psychodrama may focus more on what parts of the person are being activated by the trauma. However, in all of the 15 therapies, the client's experience in the room in relation to the ramifications of the trauma is central.

THE PRIMACY OF THE CLIENT-THERAPIST RELATIONSHIP

Another major commonality seen in the experiential therapies in this book is how the relationship between the client and therapist is figural, with the latter maintaining continuous attunement to what is occurring in this dyad. In all of these therapies, there is an emphasis on the therapist working with the client for them to discover a felt experience of safety in the therapeutic relationship and to create opportunities for clients to have an accepting human being in their lives with whom they can share their innermost experiences. When working with survivors of trauma, this becomes an essential feature of the collaborative nature of the client-therapist dyad, as traumatic experiences often have a profound impact on a human being's ability to trust and feel present with others. This is particularly true for individuals who have endured developmental trauma where they could not depend on abusive or neglectful caregivers and therefore currently utilize unfulfilling ways to survive in social environments. In this regard, the 15 experiential therapies in this book in their own ways maintain a major focus on the client's experience of what is happening in the therapeutic relationship in the moment both as a way for clients to gain awareness regarding how they relate to others in order to survive and also as a means for the client-therapist dyad to be used as a reparative experience to restore trust. Therapies that usually utilize a group process such as psychodrama and expressive arts therapy also focus on the relationships between group members in order to accomplish this goal.

ATTENTIVENESS

Very much related to the phenomenological perspective and primacy of the client-therapist relationship is the level of attentiveness to the process in the room exhibited by the 15 experiential therapies described in this book. One might be struck by the intensity of focus that the experiential therapist needs to maintain. Whereas therapists sitting back in their chair while clients recount what occurred in the past week or at different points in their lives can certainly be a part of the process in these modalities, the nature of these therapies all call for a very high degree of observant attunement to what is happening in the moment. This is not to state that other forms of psychotherapy do not call for this quality. However, these experiential therapies all require a particular high degree of awareness of the processes occurring in the moment, with active interventions a continual feature of each session. This level of awareness is not solely relegated to the client's verbal expressions and the observable phenomena in the room during the session, but also to the attentiveness of the therapist to themselves. Experiential modalities require that therapists track not just the client's reactions, but also pay close attention to their own kinesthetic resonance as a source of information to guide interventions, especially as they relate to overall safety, containment, and affect regulation. This is quite different from the procedure of classical psychoanalysis described as follows:

> Freud felt that all that was needed was to simply make no effort to concentrate the attention on anything in particular, and to maintain a regard for all that one hears with the same measure of calm, quiet, and attentiveness of evenly hovering attention.
>
> (Twemlow, 2001, p. 23)

In essence, therapists who choose to be trained in and utilize experiential therapies need to be open to engaging in these active processes both with clients and with themselves during each session.

CREATIVITY

A feature common to experiential modalities is the frequent use of imagery, fantasy exploration, play, and metaphor. Whereas this may seem obvious for creative arts therapy, the case examples of most of the other modalities in this book provide examples of the therapist asking clients to engage with their creativity by imagining different parts of themselves or visualizing people and situations either in their actual lives or in their fantasies. Examples would be the taking on of roles of others in psychodrama; the visualization of a safe, calm place in compassion-focused therapy; the use of chair work in Gestalt therapy and chairwork psychotherapy; the use of imaginal confrontation in emotion focused therapy; or tapping into strong associations of body sensations to memories and imaginary scenes in focusing-oriented therapy and the somatic-oriented therapies.

Neuroscientists Allan Schore (2010) and J. Douglas Bremner (2006) have revealed the negative impact that developmental trauma has on the healthy growth and trajectory of the right-brain capacities that are related to affect regulation, attachment, and creativity. Experiential therapeutic modalities include the use of creative interventions as a means to work with neuroplasticity and target particular regions and neural pathways in the brain to stimulate new functioning. Across the various case examples in this book, therapists direct clients to work with visualization as a means to develop increased feelings of safety when engaging traumatic memories. The somatic experiential therapies invite clients to use imagery in order to describe their kinesthetic experience with an intention of working with a creative process that includes the right hemisphere's embodied and implicit experience.

Creativity also includes the responsiveness, spontaneity, and aliveness of interpersonal functioning, which enhances one's feelings of authenticity in human relationships. The capacity to play is directly tied to one's feelings of safety with others. As a greater sense of interpersonal security is restored, clients can reclaim their creativity and are able to find resilience and agency to transform traumatic experience. Creativity includes our ability to transform suffering into meaning. As the existential therapy theorist, Victor Frankl (1962), wrote: "Suffering ceases to be suffering at the moment it finds a meaning ..." (p. 114).

HOLISM

The vast majority of the experiential therapies described in this book emphasize the integration of mind and body. Cognition, emotion, and behavior are viewed as fused with the biological systems of the body. Whereas this aspect of experiential therapies is obvious among the more somatic bottom-up experiential therapies, such as sensorimotor psychotherapy, somatic experiencing therapy, focusing-oriented therapy, and Hakomi therapy, most of the other experiential therapies emphasize a mind-body connection as well, with the therapist repeatedly directing the client to notice what they are experiencing throughout their body. As it is increasingly recognized in the mental health field, individuals who have experienced trauma are not able to process what occurred to them solely through the use of their cognition (van der Kolk, 2014). Consequently, the at least partly somatic "bottom-up" approaches of many of the experiential therapies have great potential in treating survivors of trauma. This integrative holistic approach does indeed set experiential therapies apart from other schools of psychotherapy such as cognitive-behavioral, psychoanalytic, humanistic, and narrative therapies. However, psychoanalyst Wilhelm Reich's body-oriented character analysis, along with related therapies that were derived from it such as Alexander Lowen's bioenergetics and John Pierrakos' core energetics are forerunners of aspects of many of the experiential therapies in this book (Gilbert, 1999; Wilner, 1999).

SAFETY

An aspect of treatment greatly emphasized by the authors of the chapters in this book is the need for the therapist to be exquisitely attuned to the window of tolerance of their clients in exploring their traumatic histories. The issue of safety is certainly an essential element of all reputable therapy approaches to trauma treatment and is not unique in any way to experiential therapies. However, it is important to emphasize how each of the experiential therapy chapters in this book particularly focuses on titrating the therapeutic work with safety mechanisms in order not to emotionally and physiologically overwhelm the client. As experiential therapies, with their phenomenological "in the moment" approaches, tend to elicit strong emotions and quick body responses, ensuring safety in the therapeutic dyad is of utmost importance. Therapists utilizing experiential approaches must keep the issue of emotional safety in the forefront of their work. It is also important to note that most of the experiential therapies relate these safety mechanisms to the development of a strong client-therapist relationship, which, as previously discussed, is a hallmark of these therapies. A large part of the trusting bond that clients develop for the therapist centers around clients deeply feeling that the latter has complete respect for their pace in re-experiencing the events of the traumatic situation and will be careful in trying not to exceed their emotional limits. For those who have suffered from traumatic experiences, safety can be an alien and unknown experience. Regarding developmental trauma, feeling safe includes an ability to adequately discern whether another person is trustworthy, kind, available to respond to their needs, and has the ability to self-regulate. Therapists must therefore monitor their own ability to regulate themselves, which in turn supports the capacity of the client to self-regulate.

FUTURE DIRECTIONS FOR EXPERIENTIAL THERAPY IN THE TREATMENT OF TRAUMA

In order to explore the future of experiential therapies, this section includes discussions of the need for more evidence-based outcome studies, issues regarding training therapists in these modalities, and the adaptation of these therapies for online virtual practice.

OUTCOME RESEARCH

There are diverse psychotherapy treatment modalities whose effectiveness in treating clients with posttraumatic stress disorder (PTSD) have been supported by research. A literature review by Lancaster et al. (2016) found that prolonged exposure therapy and a number of cognitive-behavioral therapies, as well as the experiential therapy EMDR, which is described in this book, have the strongest evidence base of support for treating PTSD. Furthermore, narrative-based therapies such as STAIR and narrative-exposure therapy have at least some degree of research support for trauma treatment (Wei & Chen, 2021), with dialectical behavioral therapy also demonstrating effectiveness in this regard (Choi-Kain et al., 2021). However, apart from the ubiquity of EMDR in discussions of evidence-based therapy modalities for treating trauma, the other 14 experiential therapies described in this book are usually not mentioned. For example, the 2024 Clinical Practice Guidelines of the American Psychological Association (APA 2024) for the treatment of PTSD "strongly recommends" only cognitive behavioral therapy (CBT), cognitive processing therapy (CPT), cognitive therapy, and prolonged exposuret, and "conditionally recommends" EMDR, narrative exposure therapy (NET), and brief eclectic psychotherapy, the latter which combines elements of CBT with psychodynamic therapy.

There are far fewer literature reviews and comprehensive meta-analyses regarding effective treatments for developmental and complex trauma (C-PTSD), and they tend to support the same treatment modalities as those pertaining to PTSD (Karatzias et al., 2019).

However, Mahoney and Markel (2016) posit that although evidence-based CBT models are beneficial for the symptom alleviation of complex trauma, much more is needed therapeutically. They note that complex trauma in childhood is usually perpetrated by the client's primary attachment figure and state: "While we recognize that symptom alleviation is necessary to recovery [as provided by Trauma-Focused CBT] ... such an approach neglects to address the underlying issues related to the client's sense of self" (p. 5). They recommend an integrative approach utilizing psychoanalytic theories such as self-psychology with CBT trauma models. Most of the experiential therapies described in this book do indeed target the attachment issues that need to be addressed for survivors of developmental and complex trauma. Therefore, well-designed outcome studies are badly needed to validate their effectiveness for complex trauma.

The authors of the vast majority of the chapters in this book call for the need for far more research to evaluate the effectiveness of the experiential treatment modality they describe. This would certainly seem to be a major direction that adherents of the experiential therapies need to take in order to ensure that these treatment methods are effective for treating trauma. If such studies do indicate that the modality is indeed effective, then the results need to be published in respected professional journals in order to enhance the use of these creative therapeutic models for trauma treatment. It is important to note that although there are only a limited number of studies regarding the effectiveness of experiential therapies in treating trauma, there is a far greater body of research that does support the use of many of these experiential modalities for other mental health conditions. In a comprehensive literature review of meta-analyses regarding the effectiveness of person-centered and experiential therapies, Elliot et al. (2013) found that they were at least as effective as CBT in the treatment of most mental health conditions.

A number of the authors in this book note in their chapters that the creative processes involved with the experiential therapies render them difficult to manualize for quantitative randomized controlled trial studies, which at the present time are usually considered to be the gold standard for determining effectiveness of a treatment modality. First, this issue has resulted in an insufficient number of such research projects, as they may be difficult to design. Second, this has resulted in resistance to promoting such studies among some proponents of a number of the experiential therapies. However, Brownell (2016), a Gestalt therapist, strongly counters this perspective, emphasizing the need for methodologically solid research to confirm the value of the experiential modalities so that these therapies do not become locked out of current recommendations for effective practice.

An important need for future research that is not often discussed are studies determining what types of trauma treatment are suitable for each client based on the latter's personality style. For example, it would be helpful to have some way of knowing which client who has survived trauma might ideally benefit from one of the experiential therapies, as opposed to a CBT or exposure therapy modalities. A 2011 issue of the *Journal of Clinical Psychology* was devoted to research articles regarding this question for psychotherapy in general (e.g. Norcross & Wampold, 2011), but not specifically for the issues of trauma treatment. Currently, clients impacted by trauma may begin treatment based on referrals and/or according to what is available to them without their knowing about the different types of therapy that might best suit their needs. As each human being is so different, such matching may be unrealistic. Apart from research, this actually points to a future need for clients seeking trauma treatment to have greater access to descriptions of different suitable therapeutic modalities and where they can utilize them according to their financial and health insurance situation.

TRAINING THE BEHAVIORAL HEALTH WORKFORCE IN EXPERIENTIAL THERAPIES

When reading the descriptions of the experiential therapies in this book, it is quite obvious that each of them is quite complex in regard to both theory and practice. Using them for clients impacted by trauma adds yet another layer of complexity to them particularly in regard to maintaining emotional safety for the client and preventing re-traumatization. Therefore, the editors of this book would like to emphasize that those clinicians who would like to use these therapy modalities undergo the extensive training process that most of them require, many of which may take at least several years to complete. Besides levels of didactic course work, these programs often require that the trainee participate in ongoing supervision, engage in their own therapy with a certified clinician of that modality, attend retreats, and complete case study presentations. Although one could certainly add aspects of the different experiential therapies to one's clinical practice through continuing education courses, one must be careful not to advertise oneself as a particular type of experiential therapist without having completed a sufficient level of training in that modality. All too often, therapists will complete one or more continuing education courses in particular modalities and subsequently create the impression on their websites that they have expertise in them. This is misleading to clients and is a breach of ethics in the mental health profession.

It is important to note that many experiential therapists have received comprehensive training in more than one type of therapy, whether another experiential modality or one from a different category of therapy. This is the case for many of the authors in this book. In doing so, therapists often find that this synergy is highly beneficial to their clients.

EXPERIENTIAL PSYCHOTHERAPY AND TELEHEALTH

Since the COVID-19 pandemic, the use of online therapy sessions has greatly increased, with therapists having to adapt to providing their services in a virtual environment. Although both therapists and clients have identified challenges to online sessions, the easy accessibility and increased convenience of virtual psychotherapy has increased clients' request for this service.

With the increase in usage of this virtual format, the question arises regarding its effectiveness in comparison to traditional in-person therapy. Although recent studies have generally indicated positive outcomes for the effectiveness of virtual therapy, Smith et al. (2022) note that the research into this issue is new, limited in quantity, and not sufficiently specific in regard to who might or might not benefit from online therapy. In particular they note that much of the evidence supporting the effectiveness of online therapy pertains to cognitive-behavioral therapy, and it is not clear that this can be applied to person-centered and humanistic approaches. In a review of the literature regarding the practice of person-centered and experiential therapies online, Rodgers et al. (2024) conclude that "good person-centred and experiential psychotherapy and/or counseling online is possible, but may require increased attentiveness from the therapist" (p. 17).

For the 15 experiential therapies described in this book, increased attention in the future must be paid to training therapists in how to adapt these modalities to virtual sessions in two distinct categories.

First, as experiential therapies emphasize a strong client-therapist bond, the question of how to develop and maintain this on a computer screen is extremely important. On this subject, a literature review of studies of the perceptions of psychologists and their clients of virtual therapy by Cataldo et al. (2021) found that clients reported more satisfaction with the therapeutic alliance developed online than did their therapists. Therefore, the ability to create a strong relationship online is certainly possible, but needs far more attention in training programs and supervision. Certainly, when working with clients impacted by trauma, this issue is of paramount importance in regard to the client's emotional safety.

Second, the question arises as to how to adapt the phenomenological methods of experiential therapies to the virtual space. In-person therapy allows for the use of physical office space to support physical movement, provides accessibility to art supplies and therapy props, and allows for visual observation of both patients' and therapists' entire body. Therefore, when providing experiential therapy via telehealth, the therapist must be intentional and creative about how to effectively modify experiential modalities and interventions. For instance, creative arts therapists might incorporate the use of screen sharing for collaboration with art-making programs and software. While somatic therapists can see a patient's feet and legs during face-to-face therapy, during a telehealth session they might direct a patient to verbally report what they are observing about the lower half of their body. EMDR therapists may consider the incorporation of technology that supports synchronized bilateral stimulation. When providing virtual experiential therapy services, therapists should pursue training and supervision in order to make modifications that respond to the constraints of telehealth. There is already literature available regarding how to make these modifications to experiential therapy methods for virtual sessions (e.g. Biancalani et al., 2021; Banack, 2021; Fisher, 2021; Pugh et al., 2021). However, much more needs to be explored on this subject, and training programs need to give much more consideration to the adaptation of these methods to telehealth.

SUMMATION

The editors hope that this book has provided a meaningful exploration of how 15 diverse contemporary experiential psychotherapies can be utilized to help clients recover from the severe impact of trauma in their lives. This concluding chapter has focused on how experiential therapies can accomplish this through their emphasis on phenomenological methods, the primacy of the client-therapist relationship, the profound attentiveness of the therapist to what is occurring in the moment, the use of creativity, a holistic mind-body perspective, and a continuous focus on the safety of the client in the therapeutic space to avoid re-traumatization. This chapter strongly emphasizes that far more research needs to be performed to validate the efficacy of the experiential therapies for the treatment of trauma. If the findings demonstrate their effectiveness, then it would be of utmost importance if clients impacted by trauma become aware of their value and have access to well-trained mental health professionals who can provide them with these creative, holistic psychotherapy modalities.

REFERENCES

American Psychological Association (2024). *Clinical practice guidelines for the treatment of post-traumatic stress disorders*. Washington, DC: Author.

Banack, K.D. (2021). Adapting emotion-focused therapy for teletherapy. *Person-Centered and Experiential Psychotherapies, 20*(4), 303–311. doi: 10.1080/14779757.2021.1993968

Biancalani, G., Franco, C., Guglielmin, M.S., Moretto, L., Orkibi, H., Keisari, S., & Testoni, I. (2021). Tele-psychodrama therapy during the COVID-19 pandemic: Participants' experiences. *The Arts in Psychotherapy, 75*: 101836. doi: 10.1016/j.aip. 2021.101836

Bremner, J.D. (2006). Traumatic stress: Effects on the brain. *Dialogues in Clinical Neuroscience, 8*(4), 445–461. doi: 10.31887/DCNS.2006.8.4/jbremner

Brownell, P. (2016). Warrant, research, and the practice of Gestalt therapy. In J. Roubal (Ed.), *Towards a research tradition in Gestalt therapy* (pp. 18–34). Newcastle upon Thyne, UK: Cambridge Scholars Publishing.

Cataldo, F., Chang, S., Mendoza, A., & Buchanan, G. (2021). A perspective on client-psychologist relationships in videoconferencing psychotherapy: Literature Review. *JMIR Mental Health, 8*(2), e19004. doi: 10.2196/19004

Choi-Kain, L., Wilks, C.R., Ilagan, G.S., & Iliakas, E.A. (2021). Dialectical behavior therapy for early life trauma. *Current Treatment Options in Psychiatry, 8*(11), 111–124. doi: 10.1007/s40501-021-00242-2

Elliott, R., Greenberg, L.S., Watson, J., Timulak, L., & Friere, E. (2013). Research on humanistic-experiential psychotherapies. In M.J. Lambert (Ed.), *Bergin & Garfield's Handbook of Psychotherapy and Behavior Change* (6th edition) (pp. 495–538). New York: Wiley.

Fisher, N. (2021). Using EMDR therapy to treat clients remotely. *Journal of EMDR Practice and Research, 15*(1), 73–84. doi: 10.1891/EMDR-D-20-00041

Frankl, V.E. (1962). *Man's search for meaning: An introduction to logotherapy*. Boston, MA: Beacon Press.

Gilbert, C. (1999). Breathing: The legacy of Wilhelm Reich. *Journal of Bodywork and Movement Therapies, 3*(2), 97–196. doi: 10.1016/S1360-8592(99)80029-1

Karatzias, T., Murphy, P., Cloitre, M., Bisson, J., Roberts. N., Shevlin, M., Hyland, P., Maercker, A., Ben-Ezra, M., Coventry, P., Mason-Roberts, S., Bradley, A., & Hutton, P. (2019). Psychological interventions for ICD 11 complex PTSD symptoms: Systemic review and meta-analysis. *Psychological Medicine, 49*(11), 1761–1775. doi: 10.1017/S0033291719000436

Lancaster, C.L., Teeters, J.B., Gros, D.F., & Back, S.E. (2016). Posttraumatic stress disorder: Overview of evidence-based assessment and treatment. *Journal of Clinical Medicine, 5*(11), 105. doi: 10.3390/jcm5110105

Längle, A., & Klaasen, D. (2021). Phenomenology and depth in existential psychotherapy. *Journal of Humanistic Psychology, 61*(5), 745–756. doi: 10.1177/0022167818823281

Mahoney, D., & Markel, B. (2016). An integrative approach to conceptualizing and treating complex trauma. *Psychoanalytic Social Work, 23*(1), 1–22. doi:10.1080/15228878.2015.1104640

Norcross, J.C., & Wampold, B.E. (2011). What works for whom: Tailoring psychotherapy to the person. *Journal of Clinical Psychology, 67*(2), 127–132. doi: 10.1002/jclp.20764

Pugh, M., Bell, T., & Dixon, A. (2021). Delivering tele-chairwork: A qualitative survey of expert Therapists. *Psychotherapy Research, 31*(7), 843–858. doi: 10.1080/10503307.2020.1854486

Rodgers, B., Tudor, K., & Sutherland, A. (2024). An integrative review of the person-centred and experiential therapy literature on delivering individual video counselling and psychotherapy. *Counselling and Psychotherapy Research, 24*(1), 16–26. doi: 10.1002/capr.12600

Schore, A.N. (2010). Relational trauma and the developing right brain: The neurobiology of broken attachment bonds. In T. Baradon (Ed.), *Relational trauma in infancy: Psychoanalytic, attachment and neuropsychological contributions to parent–infant psychotherapy* (pp. 19–47). Routledge/Taylor & Francis Group.

Smith, D.W. (2013). Phenomenology. *Stanford Encyclopedia of Philosophy.* Department of Psychology, Stanford University. https://plato.stanford.edu/entries/phenomenology/

Smith, K., Moller, N., Cooper, M., Gabriel, L., Roddy, J., & Sheehy, R. (2022). Video counselling and psychotherapy: A critical commentary on the evidence base. *Counseling & Psychotherapy Research, 22*(1), 92–97. doi: 10.1002/capr.12436

Twemlow, S.W. (2001). Training psychotherapists in attributes of "mind" from Zen and psychoanalytic perspectives, Part II. *American Journal of Psychotherapy. 55*(1), 22–39. doi: 10.1176/appi.psychotherapy.2001.55.1.22

van der Kolk, B.A. (2014). *The body keeps the score.* New York, NY: Penguin.

Wei, Y., & Chen, S. (2021). Narrative exposure therapy for posttraumatic stress disorder: A meta-analysis of randomized controlled trials. *Psychological Trauma: Theory, Research, Practice, and Policy, 13*(8), 877–884. doi: 10.1037/tra0000922

Wilner, K.B. (1999). Core energetics: A therapy of bodily energy and consciousness. In D.J. Weiner (Ed.). *Beyond talk therapy: Using movement and expressive techniques in clinical practice* (pp. 183–203). Washington DC: American Psychological Association. doi:10.1037/10326-000

Yontef, G. & Fuhr, R. (2005). Gestalt therapy theory of change. In A.L. Woldt & S.M. Toman (Eds.), *Gestalt therapy: History, theory, and practice* (pp. 81–100). Thousand Oaks, CA: Sage Publications. doi: 10.4135/9781452225661

INDEX

Pages in *italics* refer to figures.